How to

Doctor Your Feet

Without the Doctor . . .

Myles J. Schneider, D.P.M.

Mark D. Sussman, D.P.M.

CHARLES SCRIBNER'S SONS
New York

Library of Congress Cataloging in Publication Data

Schneider, Myles J.
How to doctor your feet without the doctor . . .

Reprint of the 1980 ed. published by Running Times, Woodbridge, Va.
1. Foot–Care and hygiene. 2. Self-care, Health. I. Sussman, Mark D., joint author. II. Title. III. Title: Doctor your feet.
[DNLM: 1. Podiatry–Popular works. WE890 S359h]
[RD563.S28 1981] 617'.585024 80-24805
ISBN 0-684-16841-3

1 3 5 7 9 11 13 15 17 19 X/P 20 18 16 14 12 10 8 6 4 2

Cover photo: Patrick M. Olmert
Drawings: Melody Sarecky

Printed in the United States of America

Contents

Dedications

For the special people in my life, especially my sons Frankie and Sammy
Myles J. Schneider, D.P.M.

For my wife Meryl, my best friend, and my superstar sons Brian and Scott
Mark D. Sussman, D.P.M.

Acknowledgments

We would like to thank our good friend and editor Ed Ayres, the publisher of *Running Times* magazine, who shared our enthusiasm for producing this book. We also want to thank the following individuals for their great energy and patience: Melody Sarecky, whose instructive drawings appear throughout the book; Monica Reid Spence, who typed the manuscript (over and over) while cheerfully managing our office; and Stephen F. Stern, D.P.M., our friend and associate who provided valuable professional criticism and saw many of our patients while we were away from the office doing our research, despite his busy schedule as president of the Virginia Podiatry Society.

1. Introduction

A Note from the Authors

Dear Friends:

As podiatrists, we have always been interested in helping people who have problems with their feet to take better care of *themselves*, as easily and inexpensively as possible. The purpose of our book is not to provide theories or explanations of how the feet work, but to provide practical techniques for relieving pain and preventing it from recurring. We are delighted to have produced a guide which will not only show folks how to treat the problems they *can* treat safely and effectively, but also explains clearly and forcefully just what kinds of conditions require professional care.

At a first glance, a book on "how to doctor your feet without the doctor" might appear to be against the best interests of the medical profession, as well as of the public. We have anticipated the objections that might be raised: that people who are not trained in medical care may do themselves more harm than good; that even if untrained individuals can safely care for themselves they might need more instruction than can be provided in a book; and—to be completely forthright—that books of this sort may compete with medical professionals for the consumer's health-care dollar!

We feel that all three objections can be addressed satisfactorily by simply pointing out that there are some 55 million Americans who need foot care services but have never visited a podiatrist's office. Since there are only some 8,000 podiatrists in the U.S., it is obvious that each one of us would be inundated with feet if all those who could benefit from our expertise decided to actively seek our help. More to the point, we would be so busy taping blisters and telling patients to replace those worn soles that we would be unable to give proper attention to the kinds of serious injuries or conditions that *must* have professional treatment.

What are the alternatives to a guide like this? With only a limited number of podiatrists available to treat millions of troubled feet, many of the people who walk (or hobble) on those feet will (1) turn to another kind of doctor who may not have the expertise and perspective necessary to provide proper treatment, (2) they will do nothing at all, simply letting their problems accumulate, or (3) they will attempt some sort of self-treatment. For those who would otherwise have no treatment at all, we think the value of a book which provides step-by-step guidance is quite obvious.

For those who might otherwise turn to professionals who are not specialists in foot care, there is more of a trade-off. On one hand, the patient may find a doctor who can provide better treatment than would be possible at home. On the other hand, he might walk into the office of a practitioner who would be more likely to rely on surgery or drugs than we would like to see.

But there is more than a question of "home-made" versus "professional" involved here. There is the broader question of how much each person in our society should assume responsibility for his own health. The traditional view is that such matters should always be left "up to the doctor," and that it is a mistake for any non-professional to meddle in matters that he would "not understand." But that view is changing rapidly. Our society's growing awareness of the value and all-pervasive nature of preventive medicine changes the picture completely around.

It is now apparent that *everyone* participates in his own health-care services *whether or not he or she intends to do so.* Every adult makes his own decisions regarding such vital questions as what nutrients will be taken into his body, what exercises his muscles will get from day to day, how much of that exercise will be aerobic, and so on. Relatively few people have any formal physiological or medical training on which to base such decisions, and few have the time or money to consult their doctors about such matters. Yet most survive, and it is partly because of the growing availability of basic health-care information (such as simple rules of good nutrition) that they do.

This book is not the product of any judgement on our part that medical information should be dispensed to the public. Rather, it is an outgrowth of our observation that people everywhere are *already in the business of taking care of themselves.* In the coming years, millions of Americans suffering from athlete's foot or achilles tendonitis will "take their feet into their own hands" whether we podiatrists encourage them or not. Our job is not to encourage or to discourage them, but to help those who wish to do so by providing whatever specific information they may find useful. At the same time, we can help those who are enthusiastic about self-care to make careful distinctions between the kinds of problems they can cope with on their own, and those for which they need the services of a doctor. In each chapter, we have clearly indicated the conditions under which a doctor should be called.

As podiatrists with special interests in sports, we have seen a tremendous growth of interest in preventive medicine and self-care during the past few years. The thousands of runners and other athletes we have met have often showed an ability to become quite expert at taking care of themselves. In fact, we owe many of the techniques and tips described in this book to them as much as to our own medical educations. We are highly confident of our readers' ability to take the information we have compiled here, and use it well. In doing so, we think they will not only save themselves the costs of medical bills they don't need (while freeing us to do the work we have to do); they will also have far more appreciation of the wonders and complexities of those remarkable feet they have fixed up than would have been the case if they had left the fixing to us.

Myles J. Schneider, D.P.M.
Mark D. Sussman, D.P.M.
Spring, 1980

2. How to Use This Book

You don't have to know anything about medicine to be able to use this book. The whole idea is to help you get relief for your feet (and in some cases your legs, hips or back) without the expense or inconvenience of going to a doctor.

Not all foot problems can be self-treated, however. To be sure that you are giving yourself the safest and most effective treatment possible, read all instructions carefully. Here is the sequence of steps to take:

1. Read the Guidelines to Treatment in this chapter. Take note of the kinds of conditions which require a doctor's attention, and *do not* attempt self-treatment on any of these. Notice that instructions are provided for various basic treatment techniques (such as icing and taping) which are prescribed in later chapters.

2. Also in this chapter, notice the "master list" of basic materials used in various treatments prescribed throughout the book. At the beginning of each chapter devoted to a specific condition to be treated, there is a list of "things you will need" for that condition. These "things" will be described in generic terms which may not always be familiar to you. For the names of familiar brands or inexpensive substitutes, turn to the master list in this chapter. For example, if the list of "things you will need" includes "soaking solution," the master list will show you that you can use either a solution of epsom salts or an inexpensive substitute—a solution of plain household detergent.

3. Once you have finished reading this chapter, look up the condition you wish to treat in the table of contents, and turn directly to the chapter indicated. Just in case you aren't sure what kind of condition you have, we have used descriptive names for our chapter titles. Each chapter starts off with a general description and sketch of the condition, which you should check carefully before proceeding any further.

4. Read through the entire chapter before beginning any treatment. If you do not understand the instructions, or if you are not certain what is wrong, or if you feel any reluctance to proceed with the treatment, see a podiatrist.

GUIDELINES TO TREATMENT

1. Contraindications (do not attempt self-treatment if you have any of the following):

A. Diabetes
B. Circulatory problems
C. Infection
D. Queasy stomach
E. Allergies or sensitivity to any of the recommended materials and medications
F. Poor eyesight
G. Unsteady hand

2. Precautions

A. Know your limitations. If you attempt a self-treatment and it does not improve the condition, see a podiatrist.

B. Follow directions for self-treatment as written. Do not overuse suggested medications or procedures.

C. Do not use any over-the-counter preparations other than those recommended in this book.

D. If during self-treatment you cause minor bleeding, apply a styptic as directed to control it. If bleeding is excessive, apply ice and compression to the area and see a podiatrist.

E. If you are instructed to use a heating pad for a specific problem, never use it in bed, and never at its highest setting.

F. Beware of frostbite: Don't use ice treatments for more than the recommended time periods.

3. *Preparedness*

A. Make sure any instruments you use are clean. Wash them in soap and water and rinse off with alcohol, Zephiran, Betadine, or some other recognized antiseptic.

B. Make sure all materials and suggested medications are clean and up to date. To sterilize any metal instrument, hold in a flame for a few seconds.

C. Scrub the entire foot thoroughly with warm soapy water and a terry wash cloth for at least one minute, and pat dry with a soft clean towel. For all of the self-treatments listed, this is sufficient preparation. However, if you care to, you may apply a mild antiseptic solution such as Zephiran chloride, Betadine, Phisohex, or any other similar preparation.

D. To prepare for soaking, dissolve any of the following in one gallon of warm water: two domeboro tablets; two tablespoons of epsom salts; or two tablespoons of a mild household detergent.

Techniques You May Need

Many of the treatments described in this book involve the use of ice, taping, elevation, and other simple techniques. These techniques are explained here, rather than repeated in full for each of the many chapters where they are used. We recommend that you familiarize yourself with these techniques before beginning any of the individual treatments described in later chapters.

Ice

How to make it up . . . .

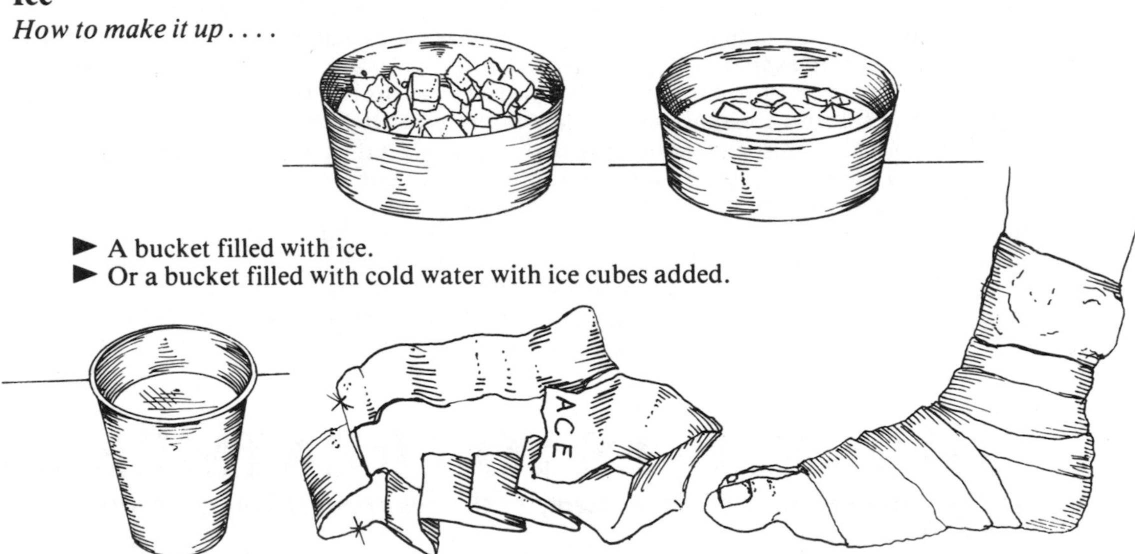

► A bucket filled with ice.
► Or a bucket filled with cold water with ice cubes added.

► Or fill a paper cup with water and freeze it into an easy-to-use ice applicator.
► Or soak an ace bandage in water and freeze it. Remove and put ice cubes over the painful area and wrap with the frozen ace bandage.
► Or if you have a home whirlpool, use cold water in it.
► Or soak a terry cloth hand towel in water, fold into a square and place in a plastic bag. Put it in the freezer until it hardens. The resulting ice pack can easily be used under an ace bandage.

How to use it . . . .

► Apply 30 minutes on and 30 minutes off for the first three to four hours after an injury.
► For the remainder of the first 48 hours after the injury, apply the ice at least 30 minutes three times each day.
► After two days, proceed to ice *therapy.* Ice the injured area for six to twelve minutes or until numbness occurs, massaging it with the paper cup, ice towels or ice whirlpools, etc. Put the injured part through range-of-motion exercises (as recommended for specific injuries) until the pain returns. If the pain does return, replace the ice for six to twelve minutes. Then repeat the motion exercises. If no pain returns after five to ten minutes of active exercise, then re-do the ice for six to twelve minutes and stop. Ice therapy should be started no earlier than 24 hours and no later than 48 hours after the initial injury. The normal sequence of events is *ice,* exercise, *ice,* exercise, *ice.*

Elevation and Compression

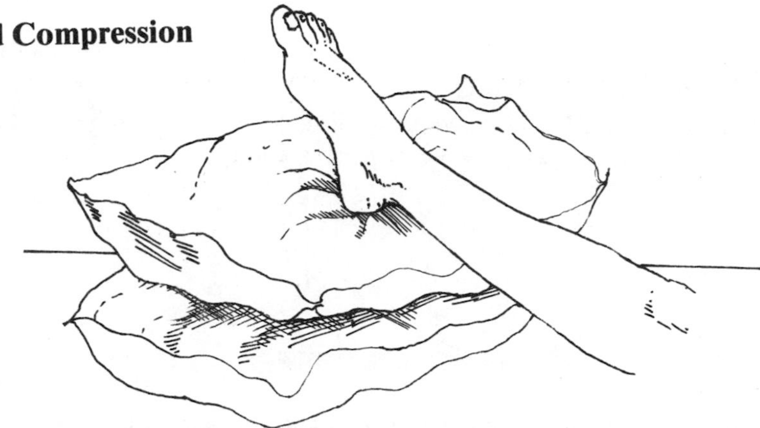

► Place the injured extremity on two pillows to keep it elevated above the level of the heart.

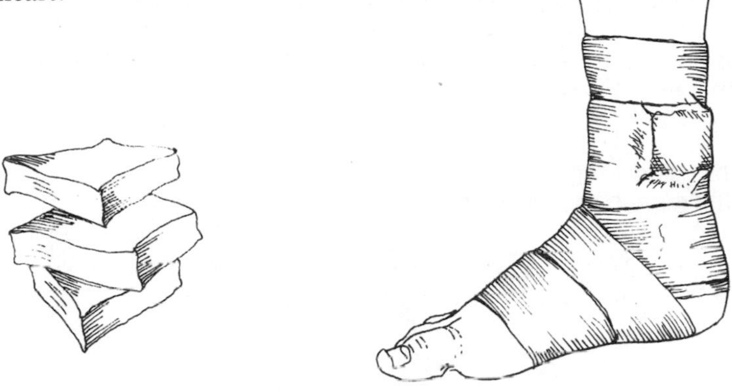

► Make a compression pad by cutting several thicknesses of foam rubber (approximately three inches square by one half inch thick). Place over the injured area and wrap snugly with an ace bandage.

► Place ice directly over the compression pad.

► If the injured area (or the foot on that side) becomes numb or begins to tingle, loosen the compression bandage until the numb part is comfortable again.

Moist Heat Applications

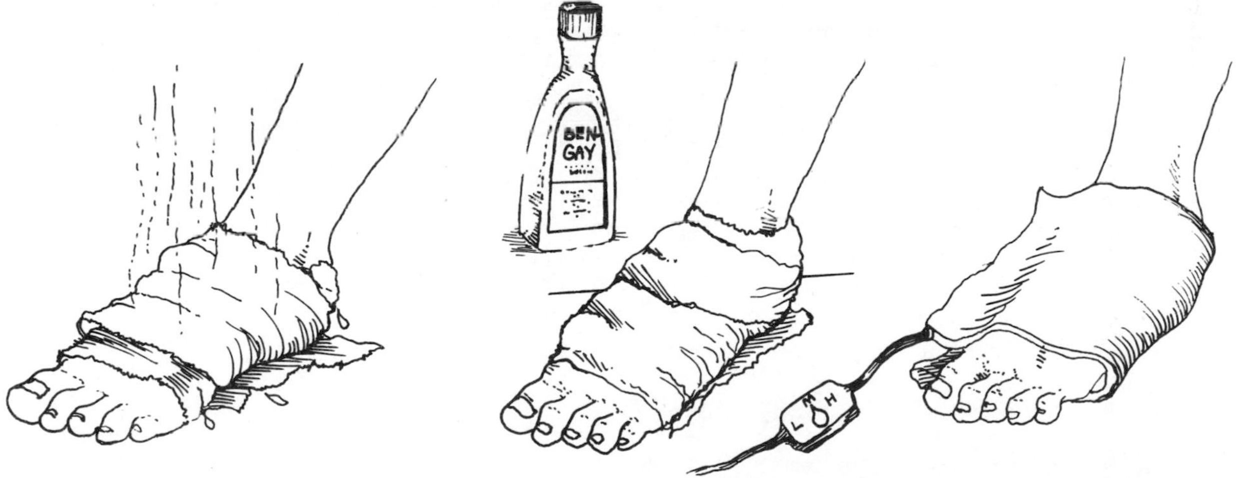

► Soak a towel in hot water and wrap it around the affected area for two to four minutes.

► Apply a heat-producing ointment like Ben-gay to the involved area, then soak a towel in hot water and wrap it around the area for two to four minutes.

► After the towel has cooled down, wrap a heating pad around the area for 15 to 20 minutes on medium heat.

► If you have a home whirlpool, use warm water, ninety to one hundred degrees Fahreheit for fifteen to twenty minutes as an alternative.

► Use heat applications two to three times a day unless otherwise specified.

Aspirin

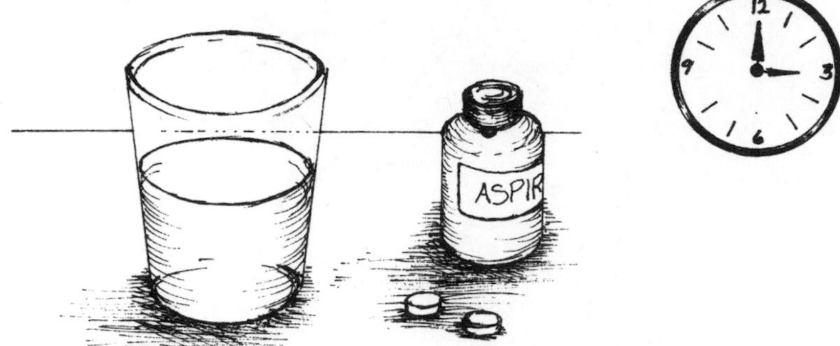

► To help eliminate inflammation and control pain, take two aspirin every four hours for two to three days and then two aspirin every six hours for up to a week thereafter, as needed.
► If you have an ulcer or an allergy to aspirin, or if you cannot take aspirin for any other reason, call your physician or podiatrist for an alternative method.
► Tylenol can be used to reduce the pain, but does not have the same anti-inflammatory properties as aspirin.

Taping

When using tape against the skin . . .
► Get yourself a good pair of scissors (bandage scissors are best).

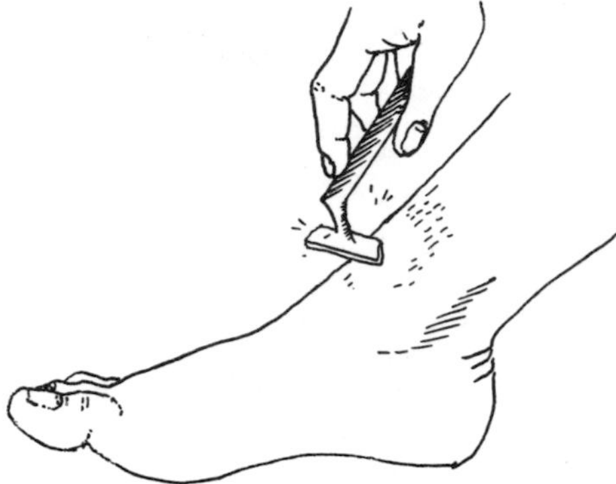

► Shave all hair from the area to be taped.
► Wash the area with soap and water before each application.
► Wipe the area thoroughly with alcohol on a cotton ball.

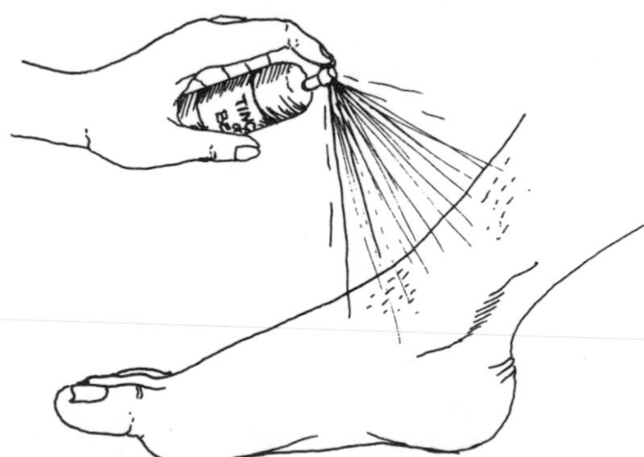

► Spray tincture of Benzoin on the skin to provide protection and help the tape adhere.

► Then apply tape as directed in the chapter which deals with your particular condition.
► After pads and tapings are in place, dust the taping liberally with powder to prevent sticking to socks and twisting of tape. As an alternative, rub a piece of paraffin over the tape.

► When you are using tape repeatedly, you can remove tape stains (the sticky greyish residue left when tape is removed) with hydrogen peroxide, nail polish remover, or acetone. Clean the nail polish remover or acetone off with rubbing alcohol, and wash with soap and water. This procedure will help to prevent skin irritation due to taping.

Exercise

► A *passive* exercise is one that is done without putting any weight on the part being exercised. It generally involves moving the foot or leg through a certain range of motion while sitting or lying down. An *active* exercise is one that is done while the part being exercised is actually bearing a full load as it normally would in walking or running. For example, in chapter 35, treatment #4, both of the illustrated exercises stretch the calf muscles. The one with the rope is passive; the other is active.

Rest

► In the treatment of athletic injuries, rest can be achieved in several different ways: It can mean pursuing all normal daily activities *except* those that put severe stress on the injured area (such as the stress of athletic training).

► It can mean *substituting* one activity for another (as in riding a bicycle or swimming instead of running).

► It can also mean putting *no* weight on the injured part (crutch walking). This type of rest would normally be prescribed by a doctor.

► In an extreme case, it can mean complete bedrest.

How to Remove Paddings and Tape

1. Soak in warm soap and water for five minutes to loosen.
2. Soak with baby oil.

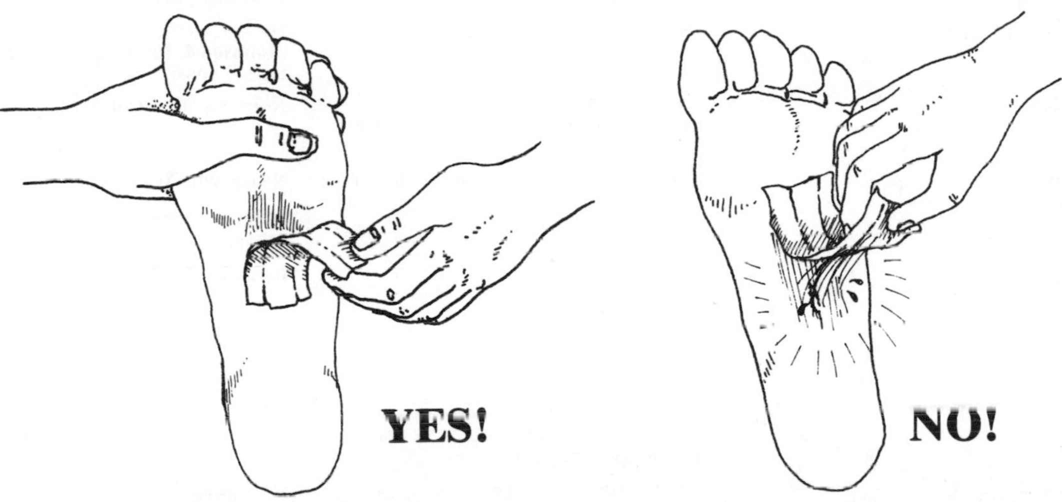

3. Always remove the tape slowly. When removing pads or tape on the bottom of the foot, *always remove in the direction of the heel*; otherwise you may tear the skin. With one hand, firmly grasp the skin just in front of the pad or tape; and with the other hand peel it slowly backward toward the heel.

► If you pull off pads or tape in the wrong direction and tear the skin, there will be bleeding and pain. If this occurs, do not be alarmed, but treat the wound as follows:

1. Do not cut skin away. Fold down in place.
2. Apply ice, compression, and elevation on two pillows for ten to fifteen minutes (see Elevation and Compression, above).
3. Once bleeding has stopped, apply an antiseptic cream. Cover with a 2"x 2" gauze pad and tape down. Remember, when removing *this* tape, pull it slowly *toward the heel* as suggested above!

Tape Allergy vs. Tape Reaction

Tape Allergy is a skin rash with itching, which will occur in susceptible individuals within a few hours after the first application of tape.

Tape Reaction is a skin rash with itching, burning, and blisters, which occurs only with repeated use of tape in certain individuals.

Treatment

1. Clean the affected area with soap and water. Pat dry with a terry cloth towel.
2. Apply Calamine or Caladryl lotion twice during the day and once just before bed.
3. Repeat step #2 until the skin reaction disappears.
4. If you have found that you are allergic to tape, remember to always use non-allergic tape in the future (and to tell any doctor who treats you that you have this allergy).

If the condition persists after three days of treatment, see a podiatrist. If severe itching, redness, warmth, blistering, and/or swelling occurs—or if pus formation occurs—see a podiatrist immediately.

MATERIALS LIST

At the beginning of each chapter we have listed the various materials and instruments needed for the treatment described in that chapter. Those materials are listed by generic names (rather than by familiar brand names) so that you can perform the treatment with maximum flexibility and at minimum cost.

For those who need information on brand names or inexpensive substitutes, we have provided the master Materials List below. This list covers the materials needed for all of the treatments described in the book. (*Example: if a particular chapter lists "soaking solution" and you don't have any epsom salts on hand, you can consult this list and see that any mild household detergent will serve as an acceptable substitute.)*

Item	Generic or Inexpensive form	"Top-of-line" form
ace bandage	store brand stretch bandage	**Ace bandage**
adhesive felt padding	homemade (felt backed with rubber cement)	**Scholl's**
adhesive foam padding	homemade (foam backed with rubber cement)	**Scholl's**
adhesive spray and skin protectant	tincture of benzoin	**Benzoin Spray**
adhesive tape	store brand adhesive tape	non-allergenic tape (**3M**) or "paper" tape (**Johnson & Johnson**) or porous adhesive tape (**Zonas**)
ankle brace	ace bandage or adhesive tape in figure "8" pattern (see chapter 36)	store-bought elastic ankle brace
antibiotic cream	a prescription item (may have around house)	**Neosporin Cream**
anti-fungal liquid	Tinactin liquid	**Tinactin liquid**
anti-perspirant	store brand	**Mitchum's**
antiseptic	Zephiran chloride, alcohol, or mer thiolate	**Betadine**
antiseptic cream	first aid cream	brand name
aspirin		
baby oil	castor or mineral oil	**Baby Oil**
bandaid	gauze and adhesive tape or store brand plastic bandage strips	Johnson & Johnson **Bandaid**
bed board	½" plywood cut to size	store bought
bunion shield	make your own (see chapter 16)	**Scholl's**
calfskin or kidskin leather		
callous file	home-made callous file (see chapter 8)	callous file available in drug stores
corn pad, non-medicated	cut your own out of moleskin, felt or foam (see chapter 6)	**Dr. Scholl's**
cotton	hank or roll of cotton	cotton balls
cotton material 1" by 18"	rope or rubber band	
cotton swab	home-made cotton swab (blunted tooth-pick and cotton) or store brand	**Q-tips**
desensitizing lotion	home-made paste (Baking soda and water or meat tenderizer and water) or **Calamine** lotion	**Caladryl lotion**
disinfectant spray	**Lysol**	**Desenex**
elastic adhesive bandage	non-elastic adhesive tape	**Elastoplast**
fabric for removal of dead skin	wash cloth or gauze pad	**Buf-Ped**
foot roller	soda bottle or rolling pin (do not subsequently use for pie)	custom hardwood foot rollers **Footsie Roller**
2"x 2" gauze pads	store brand pads, available in discount and chain drugstores	**Johnson & Johnson**
glue gun	soldering iron	glue gun
heating pad	electric cloth cover	electric rubber backed
heat ointment	liniment, mustard plaster	**Ben Gay**
heel cup	rubber or plastic store bought	**M-F Heel Protector**
ice bag	paper cup of water, frozen, or terry hand towel folded, soaked in water, put in plastic bag and frozen	chemical "ice" bag
knee brace	ace or elastic bandage	elastic knee brace

lamb's wool	wool shorn from your own lamb	store-bought lamb's wool
lipstick		
matches	matches	matches
material to inhibit odor	10% formaldehyde (as directed) solution	Johnson's "Odor-Eaters"
medicated foot powder	corn starch	**Tinactin or Aftate**
mildly abrasive tool	home-made abrasive tool (see chapter 6) or emery board	pumice stone
moleskin	**Dr. Scholl**	**Dr. Scholl**
nail brush	tooth brush	**Buf-Ped** or store-bought nail brush
nail file	emery board, mildly abrasive tool (see chapter 6)	store bought nail file
nail forceps, straight back	cuticle forceps, available in drug store	straight-back nail forceps available from medical supply house
nitrogen-impregnated foam innersole	store brand innersole	**Scholl Sponge Foam** or **Spenco innersole**
non-adhesive felt		
occlusive wrap	sandwich wrap	**Saran Wrap**
paper	plain drawing paper	graph paper
paper clip		
petroleum jelly	store brand petroleum jelly	**Vaseline**
pillow	2 pieces of material sewn and stuffed with feathers or foam	store bought pillow
pin, needle, or tweezers	sewing needle or straight pin	store bought tweezers
plastic wrap (air-tight dressing)	store brand	**Saran Wrap**
rubber seat cushion	1" thick piece foam rubber	storebought
Sacro-Illiac brace	elastic bandage and 6" x 6" to 8" x 8" square of 1" thick foam rubber	store bought
40% salicylic acid plaster	aspirin tablets crushed and mixed with water to make paste—applied to wart and covered with adhesive tape	store bought
scissors	any old pair	sharp, bandage type
slant board	home-made slant board (see appendix on Stretching)	**Flex-Wedge**
soaking solution	Epsom salts (in solution as directed on box) or mild household detergent (in solution)	**Domeboro** or **Bluboro** tablets or powder, as directed
soap & water	home-made soap (made with lye and left over fat from cooking	anti-bacterial soap (**Dial**)
softening agent (vegetable oil)	vegetable oil	olive oil
soft polyurethane foam	kitchen sponge	
sole patching material	tire repair kit	**Shoo Goo, Shoe Patch,** glue gun
sponge rubber heelpad or raise	scrap of indoor outdoor carpet cut to size,	store-bought heel cushions
tape measure	piece of measured rope, paper tape measure	fancy metal or wooden tape measure
tennis elbow brace	ace bandage	store bought tennis elbow brace
toothbrush	old toothbrush	new toothbrush
weights	old paint bucket or pocket book with padded handle, filled with rocks to desired weight	store bought ankle weights
wet heat	towel soaked in hot water, rubber heating pad over wet towel	hydrocollator or whirlpool bath

Part 1
Problems Anyone Might Have

3. Ingrown Toenail

(Onychocryptosis)

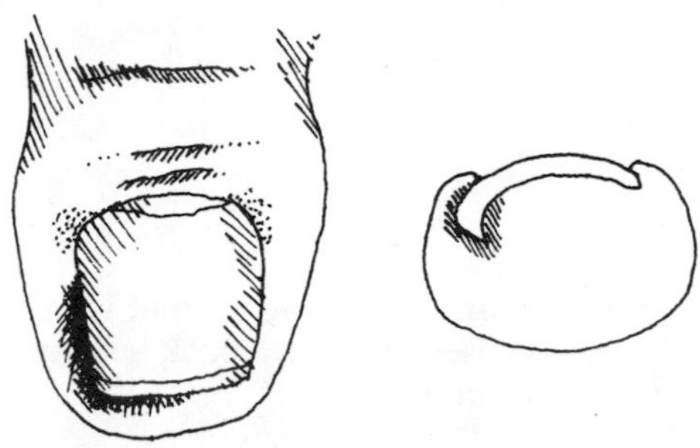

What is it?

An ingrown toenail occurs when the side of a toenail cuts through the surrounding skin. The area becomes very sensitive to pressure. Continued pressure may cause redness, swelling, and—eventually—infection. Nail pressure occurring over a long period of time may even lead to the formation of small painful corns in the nail groove.

Things you will need for this treatment

see chapter 2 "Materials List" for brand names and substitutes

soap & water
antiseptic
ice bag
nail forceps, straight-backed
2"x2" gauze pad
soaking solution
bandaid
antibiotic cream (if you have any)

Caution: ***Do not proceed with this treatment until you have read the Guidelines to Treatment in Chapter 2***

Preparation for Treatment

► Make sure any instruments you use are clean. Wash them in soap and water and rinse off with alcohol or some other recognized antiseptic.

► Make sure all materials and suggested medications are clean and up-to-date.

► Put two tablespoons of mild household detergent into ½ gallon of warm water. Dip your foot in the water and soak for ten minutes.

► Read through all the instructions which follow, and make sure you understand them before beginning treatment.

Treatment

The *only* way to solve the problem of an ingrown toenail is to remove the ingrown part. Soaks and antibiotics are otherwise useless. An ice pack held against the toe (for no more than five minutes) will provide some numbness.

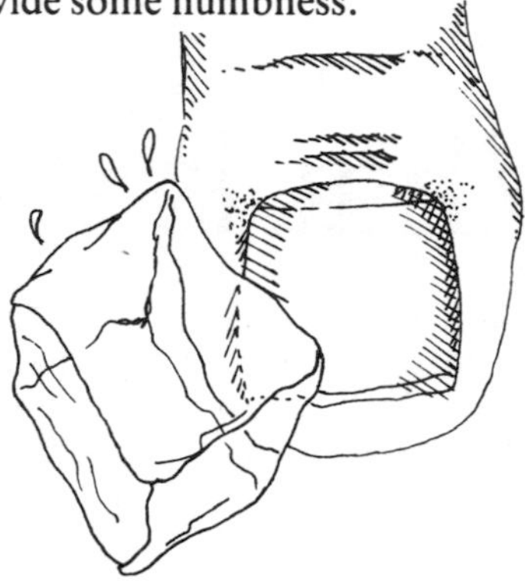

1. To remove the offending part of the toenail . . .

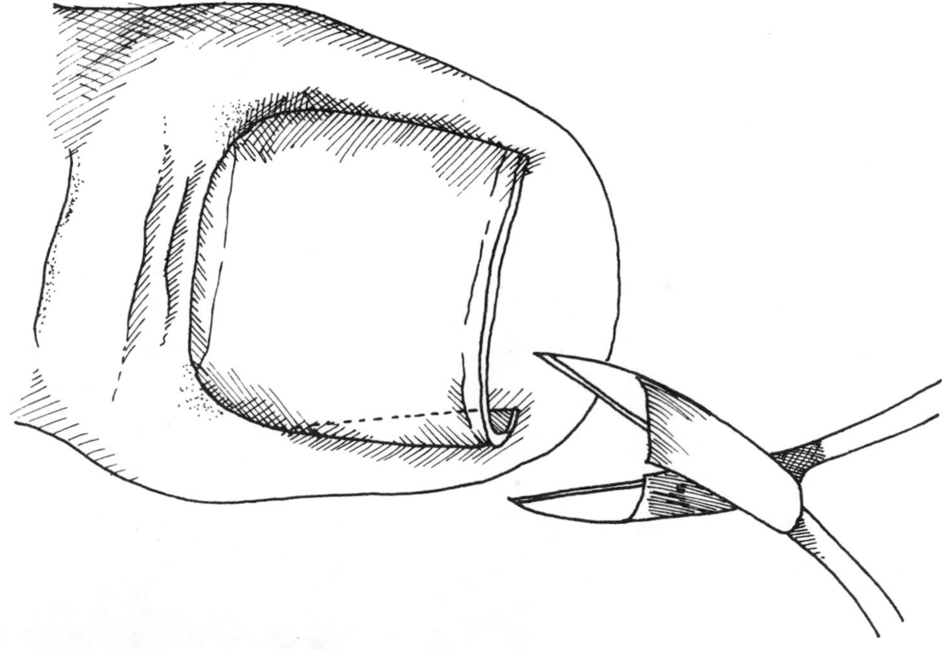

► Insert forceps under the nail border, as shown in the drawing.

► Clip out the ingrown toenail at a slight angle.

► Try not to cut flesh, by keeping the bottom of the clipper as close to the bottom of the nail plate as possible. *Hang in there!* It's normal for this to be a little uncomfortable.

► Try not to leave nail spicules (pointed fragments), as they will tend to start the ingrown process over again.

► Once the nail is cut, grasp the corner and gently pull it out.

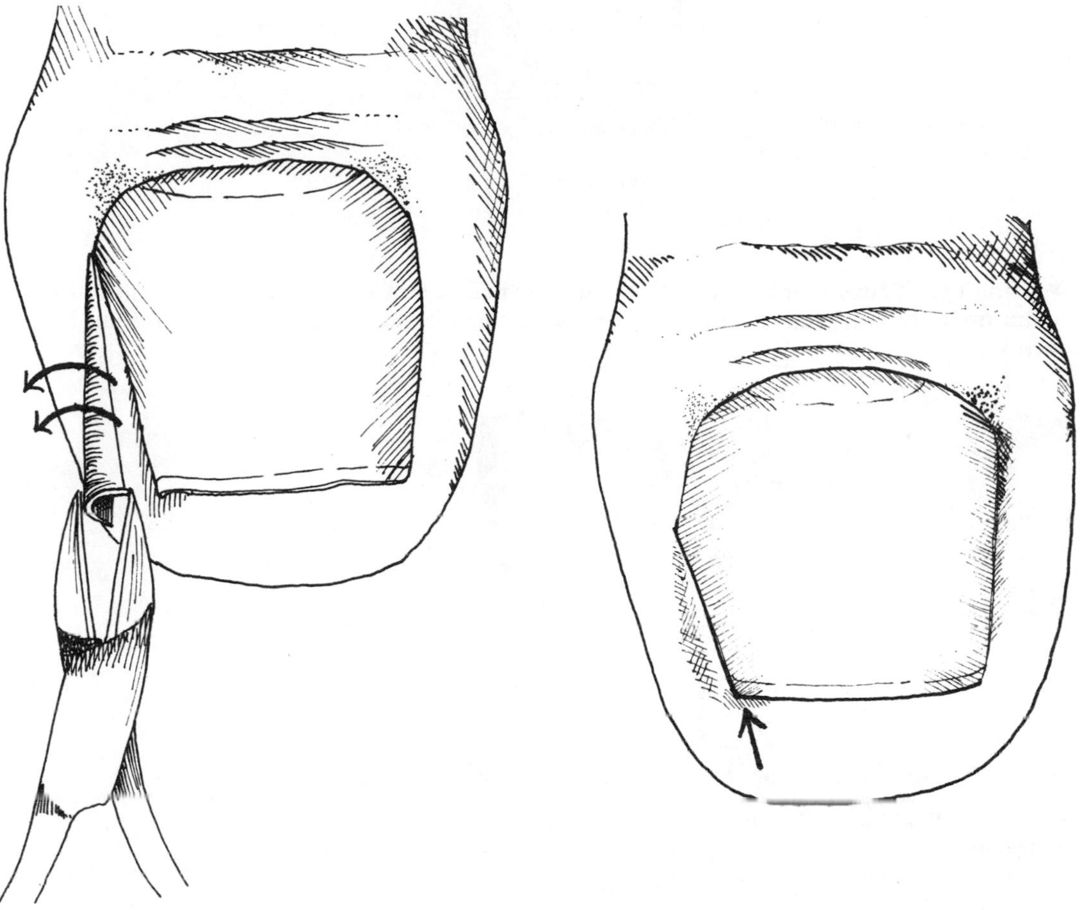

2. Wipe off the area gently with soap and water on a gauze pad.

   ► If there is bleeding, elevate the foot and apply an ice pack for ten minutes with light pressure. If bleeding is minor, you may use a styptic. If it is excessive, apply ice and pressure *and* see a podiatrist.

3. During the next few days...

   ► Until tenderness is gone, soak your toe for 20 minutes, twice a day, in one of the following:
   - Two domeboro tablets dissolved in one gallon of warm water
   or
   - Two tablespoons of epsom salts in one gallon of warm water
   or
   - Two tablespoons of a mild detergent such as Ivory Liquid, Tide, etc., in one gallon of warm water.

   After you soak, apply Merthiolate (which will act as a drying agent), a bandaid, and an antibiotic cream such as Neosporin (if you have any).

When to Call the Doctor

If pain is not reduced after one day, *or* if you have left a spicule (pointed fragment), *or* if you think you have an infection, see your podiatrist immediately. If the do-it-yourself treatment provides only temporary comfort and the problem soon returns, you can have the ingrown part of the toenail permanently removed by your podiatrist through a minor procedure that is done under a local anesthetic with very little pain and almost no disability.

DON'TS

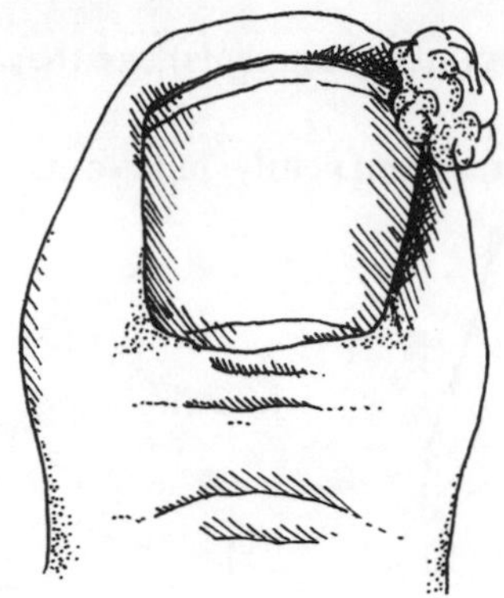

► Don't stuff cotton or anything else under the nail edge. Cotton hardens and will cause irritation to the nail groove This can give rise to corns in the nail groove, as well as to infection.

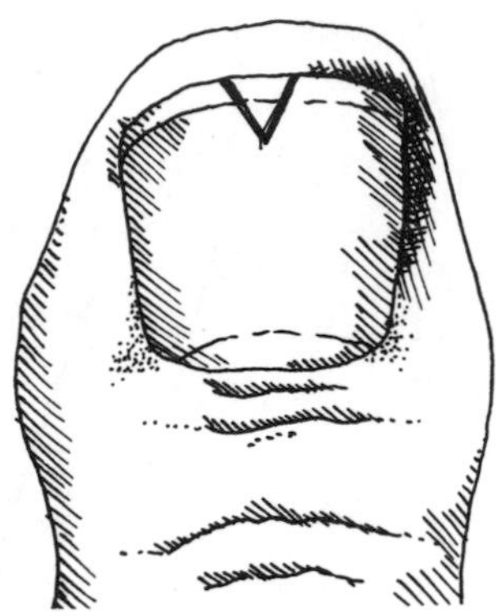

► Don't waste time cutting V's, S's, or any other design in the nail. It does not work.

► Don't use any over-the-counter preparations. They rarely work and may be dangerous.

Practical Pointers for Prevention

1. Keep your toenails clean.

2. Trim your toenails the way they are normally shaped, not necessarily straight across. Always leave the toenail a lit tle longer than you think it should be cut.

3. Watch out for excessive shoe pressure.

4. Do not wear improperly fitting shoes or socks. This advice is of particular importance for children who are used to receiving "hand-me-down" clothing and shoes from older brothers and sisters.

4. Thick Toenail

(Onychogryphosis)

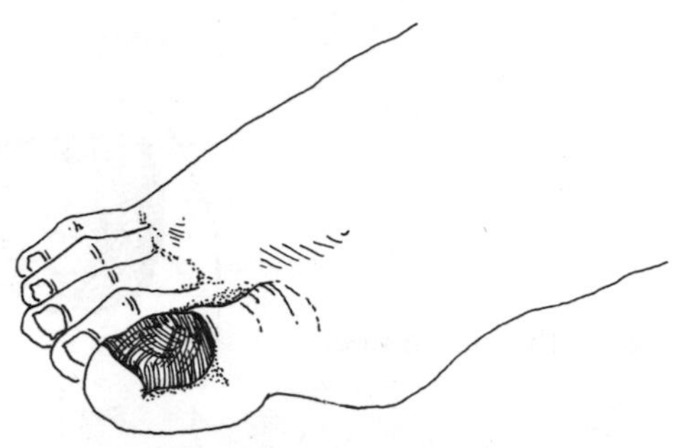

What is it?

A toenail may become thickened and/or discolored because of an injury or fungus infection. It will be dirty yellow or brown in color, with occasional blackened areas. There is usually a white or yellow crust that flakes off the toenail, and under or around the nail a cheesy substance with a strong odor may be present. The nail may be cracked and brittle. The most commonly affected nail is the large toenail.

Things you will need for this treatment

see chapter 2 "Materials List" for brand names and substitutes

ice bag
soap & water
soaking solution
antiseptic
softening agent
nail forceps-straight backed
cotton
nail file
forty percent salicylic acid plaster
nail brush
bandaids
antibiotic cream (if you have any)

Caution: *Do not proceed with this treatment until you have read the Guidelines to Treatment in Chapter 2*

Preparation for Treatment

► Make sure any instruments you use are clean. Wash them in soap and water and rinse off with alcohol or some other recognized antiseptic.

► Make sure all materials and suggested medications are clean and up-to-date.

► Put two tablespoons of mild household detergent into ½ gallon of warm water. Dip your foot in the water and soak for 10 minutes.

► Read through all the instructions which follow, and make sure you understand them before beginning treatment.

Treatment

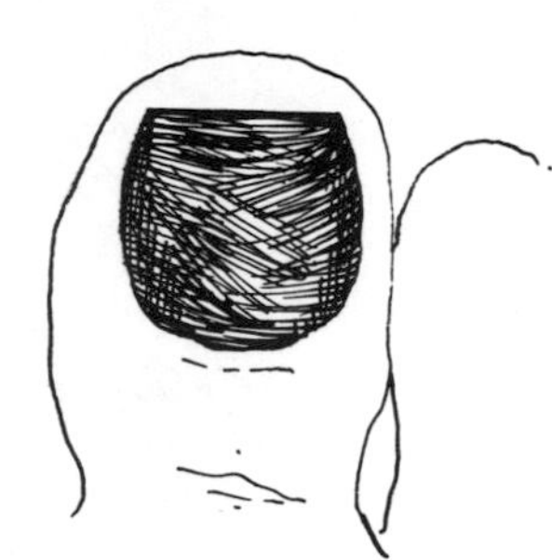

1. Cut the nail straight across with a nail nipper.

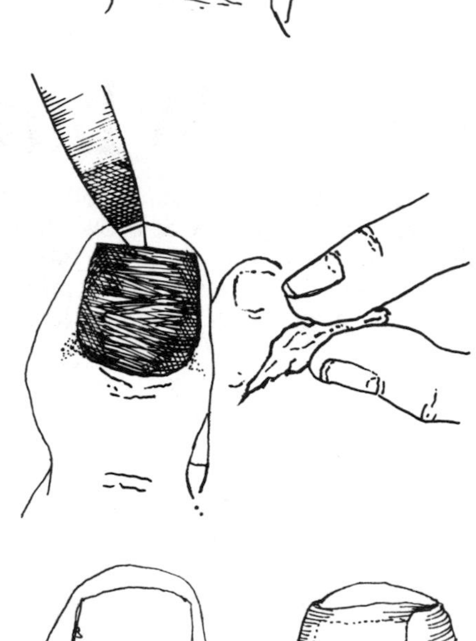

2. Take a clean nail file and a wisp of cotton, and clean out the debris under and around the sides of the toenail. You may have to do it in more than one sitting.

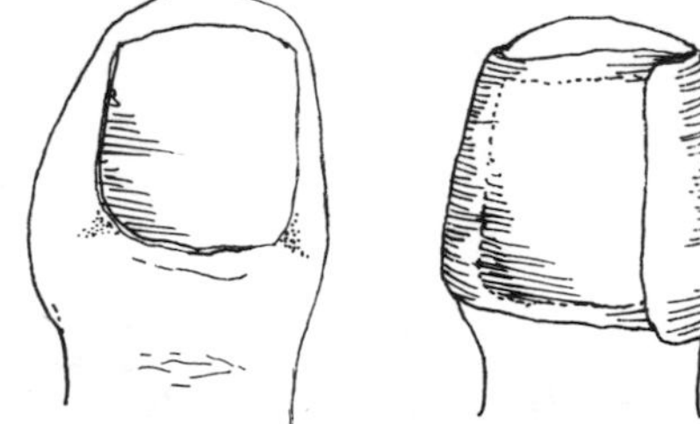

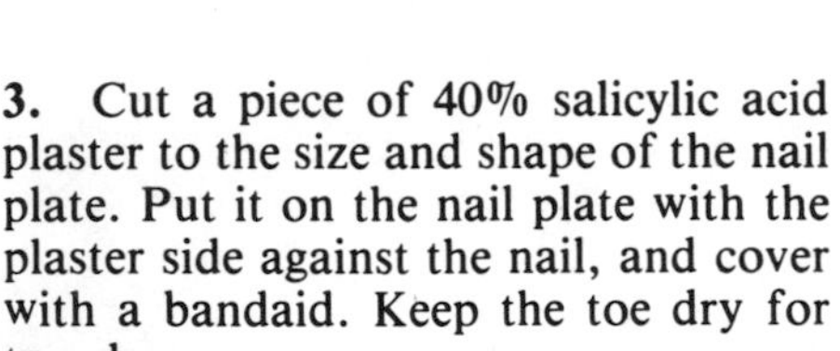

3. Cut a piece of 40% salicylic acid plaster to the size and shape of the nail plate. Put it on the nail plate with the plaster side against the nail, and cover with a bandaid. Keep the toe dry for two days.

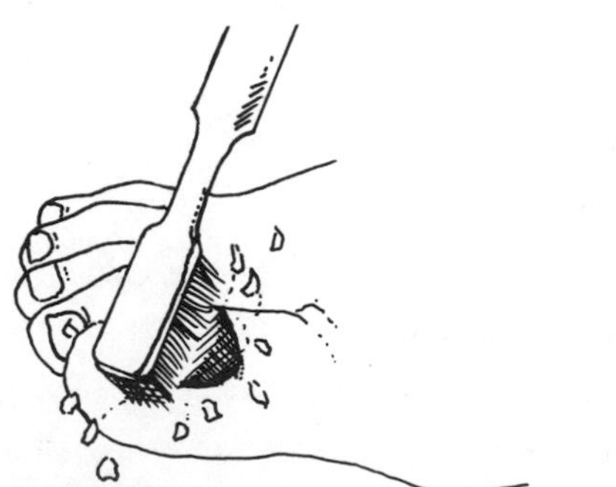

4. When you remove the plaster, take a nail brush or an old toothbrush and brush off as much flaky nail debris as possible. Then take your nail nipper and cut as much of the nail off as you can. File down any sharp points.

5. Thoroughly clean the area with warm, soapy water and put on an antiseptic solution like Merthiolate.

6. Repeat the salicylic acid treatment three to four times.

When to Call the Doctor

The salicylic acid treatment may cause a mild discomfort. However, if you have any severe pain, swelling or infection, see your podiatrist immediately. If the do-it-yourself treatment provides only temporary comfort and the problem soon returns, the podiatrist may suggest long-term medication therapy or permanent removal of the toenail (through a minor procedure done under local anesthetic with very little pain and almost no disability). It is important to note here that the toenails are appendages that were important in the early evolutionary development of man; but since the advent of protective shoe gear for the feet, the toenails have very little function.

DON'TS

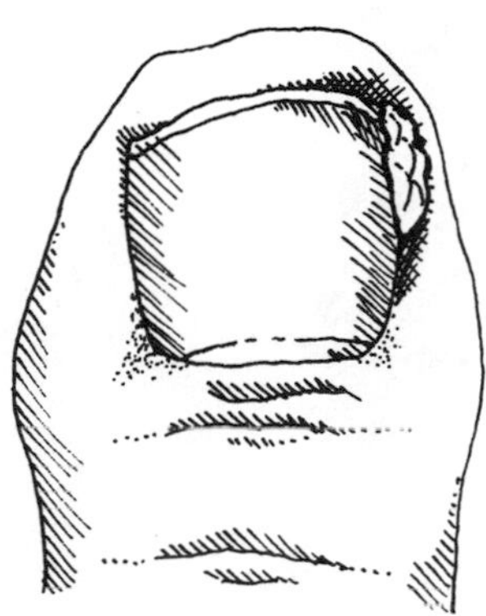

1. Don't stuff cotton or anything else under the nail edge. Cotton hardens and will cause irritation to the nail groove. This can give rise to corns in the nail groove, as well as to infection.

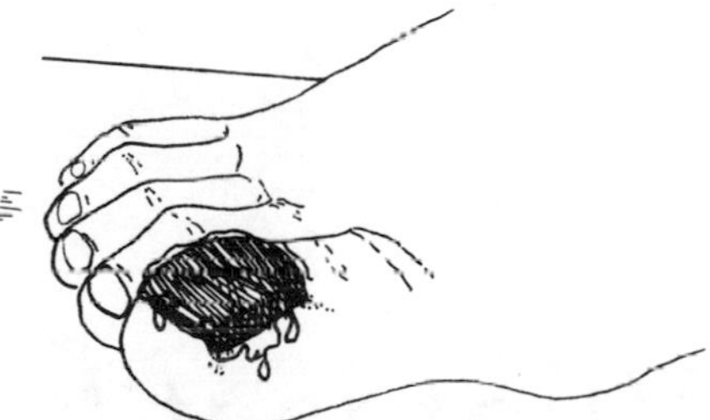

2. Don't use any over-the-counter preparations. They rarely work and may be dangerous.

Practical Pointers for Prevention

1. Keep toenails clean.

2. Watch out for excessive shoe pressure.

3. When working or doing anything where you might accidentally drop something on your toes, wear closed shoes to protect them.

4. Change shoes and socks daily, as excessive perspiration, darkness and warmth are the prerequisites for getting fungus infections of the toenails. You can't find a better environment than the inside of your shoes for creating these conditions.

5. Pain Under and Around Toenail

(Subungual exostosis or calloused nail groove)

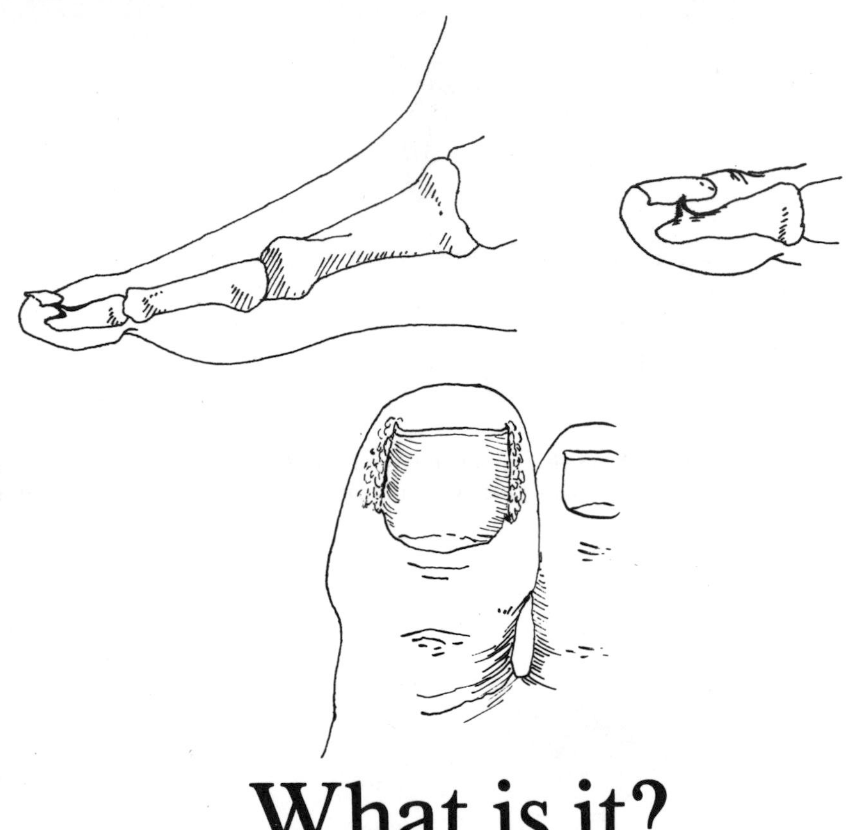

What is it?

There are two main causes of pain under and around the toenail, other than ingrown toenail (which is shown separately in Chapter 3). The two causes are (1) a bony projection, or spur, that forms on the big toe directly under the nail, resulting in painful upward pressure against the nail, and (2) a callous formation in the nail groove on either side of the nail.

Things you will need for this treatment

see chapter 2 "Materials List" for brand names and substitutes
soap & water
antiseptic
ice bag
nail forceps, straight-backed
2"x 2" gauze pads
soaking solution
bandaids
antibiotic cream (if you have any)

Caution: *Do not proceed with this treatment until you have read the Guidelines to Treatment in Chapter 2*

Preparation for Treatment

► Make sure all the materials you will be using are clean and fresh and that the forceps are clean, as discussed in chapter 2. Also make sure the foot itself is clean and dry.

► Read through all the instructions which follow, and make sure you understand them before beginning treatment.

► If you would like to numb the toe a little before beginning treatment, hold an ice pack against the toe—but not for longer than five minutes at a time.

► Put two tablespoons of mild household detergent into ½ gallon of warm water. Dip your foot in the water and soak for ten minutes.

Treatment of Callous Formation in Nail Groove

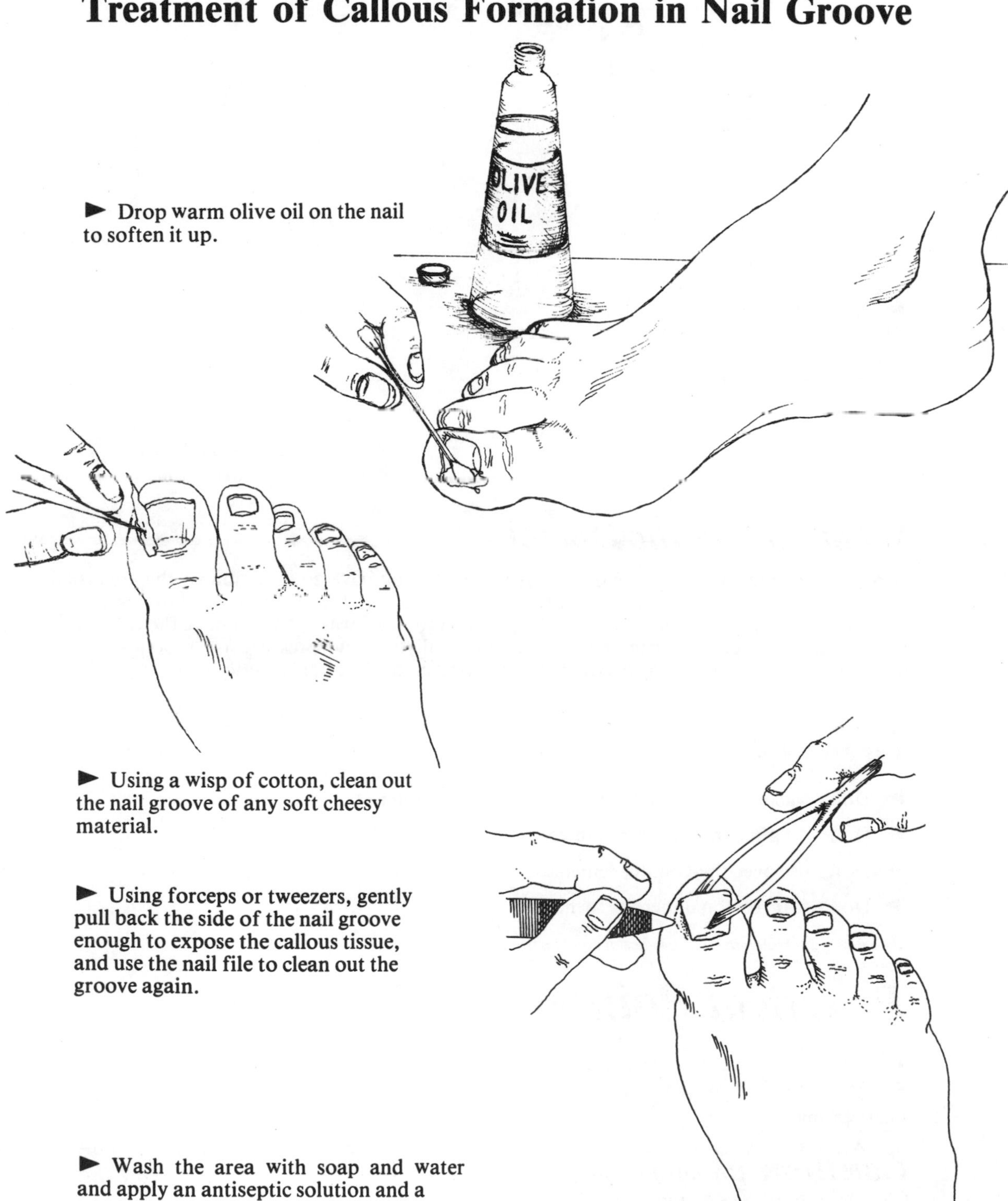

► Drop warm olive oil on the nail to soften it up.

► Using a wisp of cotton, clean out the nail groove of any soft cheesy material.

► Using forceps or tweezers, gently pull back the side of the nail groove enough to expose the callous tissue, and use the nail file to clean out the groove again.

► Wash the area with soap and water and apply an antiseptic solution and a bandaid.

Treatment of Pain Under the Toenail

Here the task is to reduce the pressure.

► First, note whether the nail is unusually thickened, as it often is in cases like this. If so, treat it as described in chapter 4.

► Second, when the nail is trimmed down to its proper thickness, if you still have pain when downward pressure is applied on top of the nail, make a pad by cutting a piece of moleskin, 1/8" felt, or 1/8" foam to the size of the toenail. Cut a hole in the pad large enough to surround the painful area caused by the downward pressure (chances are there is a bone spur under the toenail).

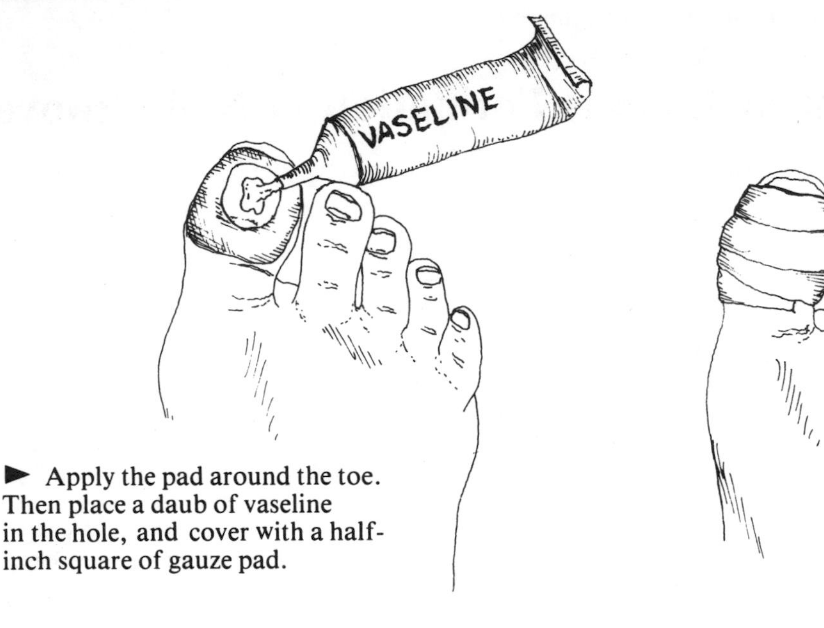

► Apply the pad around the toe. Then place a daub of vaseline in the hole, and cover with a half-inch square of gauze pad.

► Wrap the toe gently with bandaid or adhesive tape.

When to Call the Doctor

If pain is not reduced after one day, or if you think you have an infection (if the area is red, warm, or swollen), see a podiatrist immediately. If the do-it-yourself treatment provides only temporary comfort and the problem soon returns, you can have the callous part of the nail groove trimmed out professionally, or the pressure of a bone spur removed through a minor procedure that is done under local anesthetic with very little pain and almost no disability.

DON'TS

► Don't waste time cutting Vs in the toenail (see chapter 3)

► Don't wear narrow-toed or pointed shoes.

► Don't use over-the-counter remedies.

► Don't stuff cotton under the toenail.

Practical Pointers for Prevention

1. Avoid excessive shoe pressure.

2. Check shoes and socks for proper fit, especially pressure points or seams that could be irritating.

3. Always cut your nails as straight as possible, and do not let them dig down into the corners.

6. Corn on Top of Toe

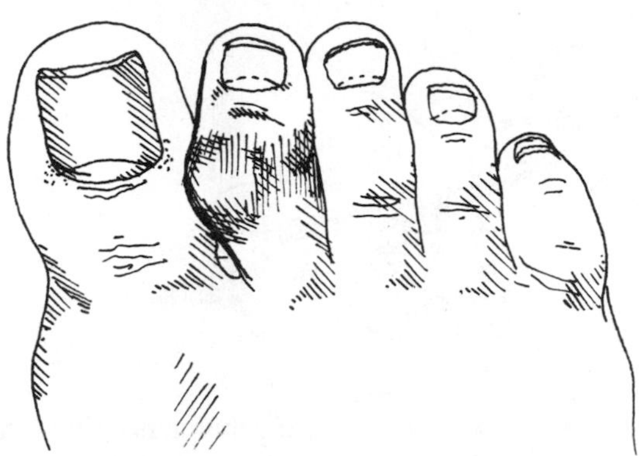

What is it?

Most corns on top of the toes are due to hammered (contracted, or claw-like) toes. The contracting usually occurs as a result of imbalances of bone structure or muscles, that make the toe stick up higher than normal and cause pressure, both from the bone inside the toe and from the shoe outside.

Things you will need for this treatment

see chapter 2 "Materials List" for brand names and substitutes

soap & water
softening agent
callous file or "mildly abrasive tool"
corn pads, non-medicated 1/8"
1/8" adhesive felt or foam or moleskin
petroleum jelly
2"x2" gauze pads
adhesive tape

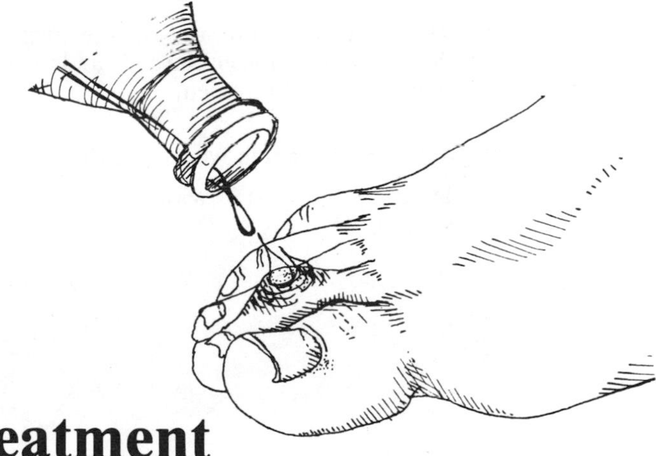

Preparation for Treatment

1. Make sure all the materials you will be using are clean and fresh as discussed in chapter 2. Also make sure the foot itself is clean and dry.

2. Read through all the instructions which follow, and make sure you understand them before beginning treatment.

3. Put two tablespoons of mild household detergent into ½-gallon of warm water. Dip your foot in the water and soak the corn for ten minutes.

4. Dry the foot and rub a few drops of cooking oil into the corn to further soften it.

Caution: *Do not proceed with this treatment until you have read the Guidelines to Treatment in Chapter 2*

Treatment

1. To provide temporary relief, remove the top layer of the corn.

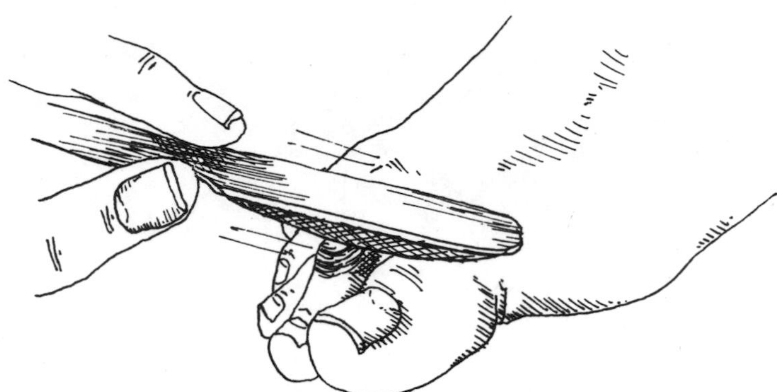

► Using a back-and-forth sawing motion, mechanically shave down the thick skin with a mildly abrasive pumice stone, sandstone, sandpaper, or callous file.

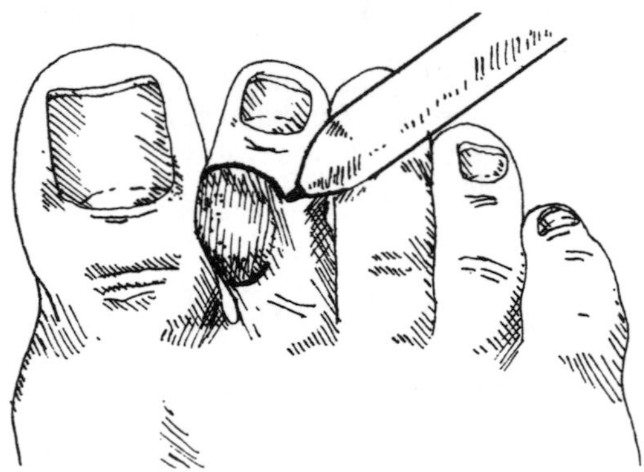

► Make sure you stay on the overlying thick skin. If you can't see the line of demarcation between the corn and the toe, it might be helpful to circle the corn with a ball point or felt tip pen.

2. After you have removed as much "top skin" as you can . . .

► Cleanse the area with soap and water, using a 2" x 2" gauze pad instead of a washcloth.

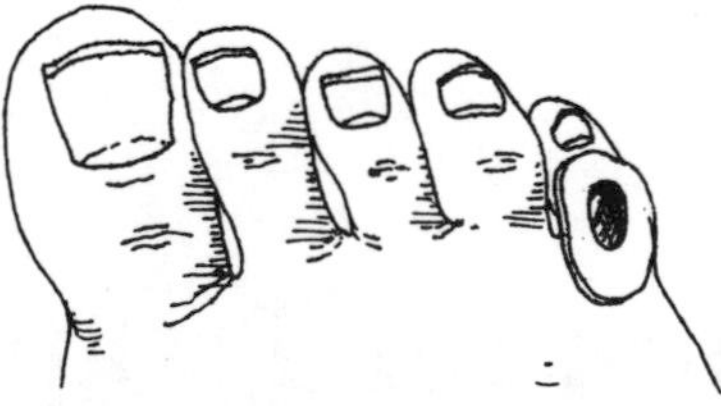

► Apply a commercially available *non-medicated* corn pad, making sure it is thick enough to cover the raised portion of the corn and that the pad overlaps the corn by at least 1/8 inch on all sides.

NOTE: To enlarge hole, gently tug from side to side and the material will usually stretch. Do this carefully, as the pad will easily tear.

To Make Your Own Pads:

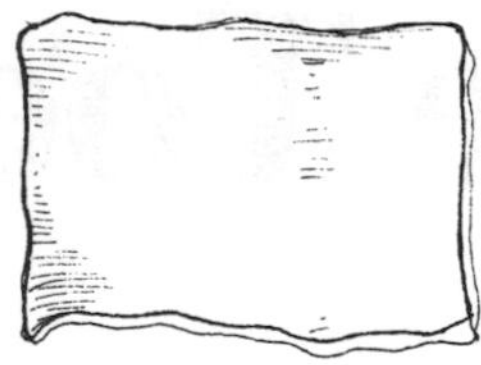 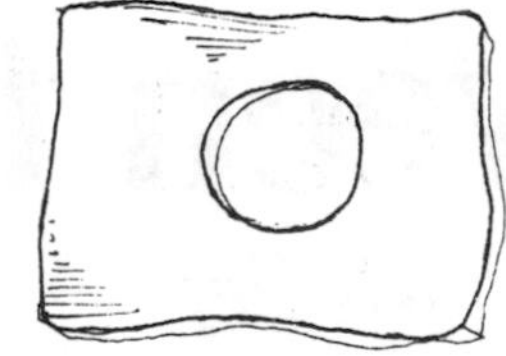 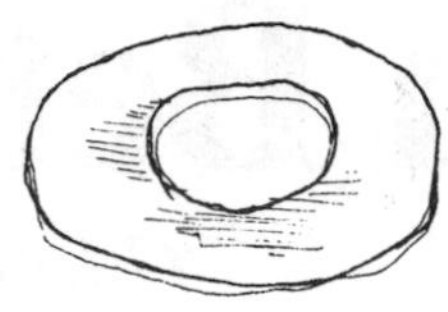 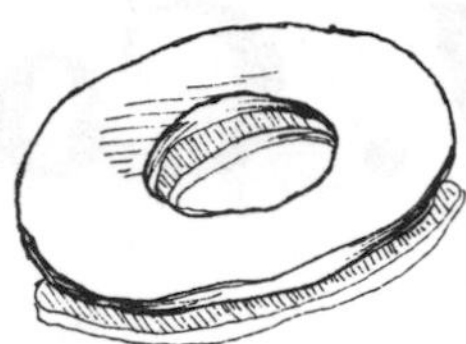

1. Take a piece of moleskin, 1/8'' felt, or 1/8'' foam. Cut a hole in it.

2. Trim to shape and stretch if necessary. Apply as many thicknesses as you need to remove pressure (usually one is enough).

► When the pad is in place, put a daub of vaseline ointment in the hole, then cover with a ½'' square of gauze pad.

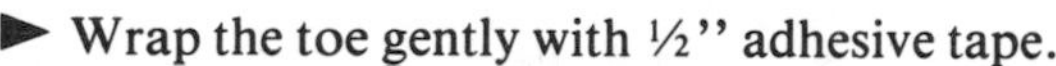

► Wrap the toe gently with ½'' adhesive tape.

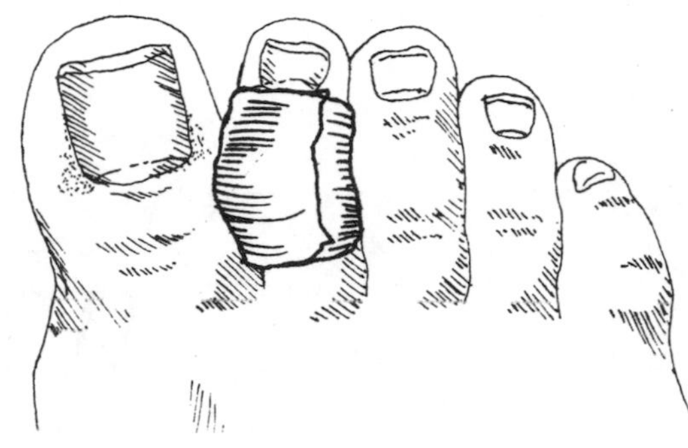

When to Call the Doctor

► If pain is not reduced in one day or you think you have an infection (if the area is red, warm, or swollen), don't touch it yourself! See a podiatrist immediately.

► This treatment provides temporary relief but does not remove the cause. Permanent correction may be available from a podiatrist, who can either keep the area trimmed down for you, or straighten the hammertoe using a procedure that causes only minor disability and has been highly successful in achieving permanent ''cure'' for corns of this type.

DON'TS

► Don't use razor blades

► Don't use any other sharp objects

► Don't use medicated corn pads. (They contain acids and can cause burns and infection in normal skin surrounding the corn).

► Don't put pads directly on top of a corn. This will only increase pressure and pain.

Practical Pointers for Prevention

► To relieve pressure, stretch the shoe at the spot where it covers the corn. To do this, put a broom handle into the toe box and pull the shoe downward so that the end of the handle pushes the fabric at the appropriate spot. Hold for ten minutes (see ''Running Shoes'' section in the appendix on shoes).

► To soften leather on new shoes, polish with Meltonian© shoe polish of proper color.

7. Corn Between the Toes

(Heloma Molle)

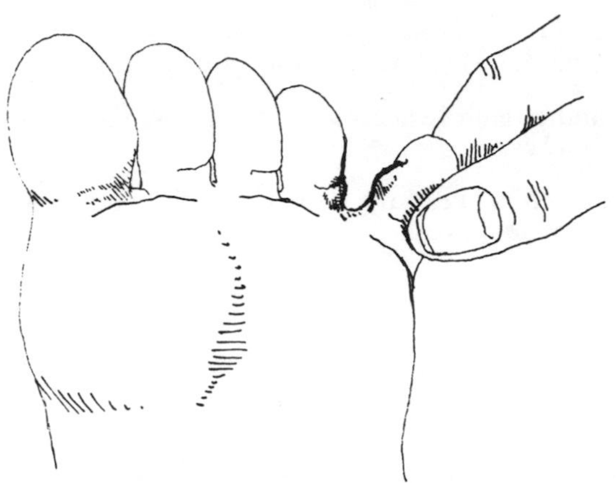

What is it?

A soft corn forms between two toes when a bony prominence in one toe becomes "attracted" to a bony prominence on the adjacent part of the toe next to it. Over a period of time, with side-to-side pressure they "hug" each other and a corn develops over each prominence. The moisture between the toes keeps the corns "soft." Initially, these soft corns must be differentiated from any early fungus infection (see chapter 14).

Things you will need for this treatment

see chapter 2 "Materials List" for brand names and substitutes

soap & water
softening agent
callous file or "mildly abrasive tool"
2"x2" gauze pads
petroleum jelly
lamb's wool

Preparation for Treatment

► Make sure any instruments you use are clean. Wash them in soap and water and rinse off with alcohol or some other recognized antiseptic.

► Make sure all materials and suggested medications are clean and up to date.

► Put two tablespoons of mild household detergent into ½ gallon of warm water. Dip your foot in the water and soak for ten minutes.

► Read through all the instructions which follow, and make sure you understand them before beginning treatment.

Caution: *Do not proceed with this treatment until you have read the Guidelines to Treatment in Chapter 2*

Treatment

1. Remove the "top layer" of the soft corn to give temporary relief.

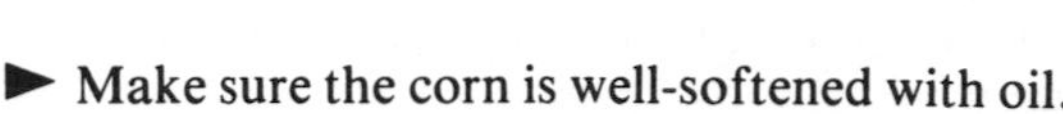

► Make sure the corn is well-softened with oil.

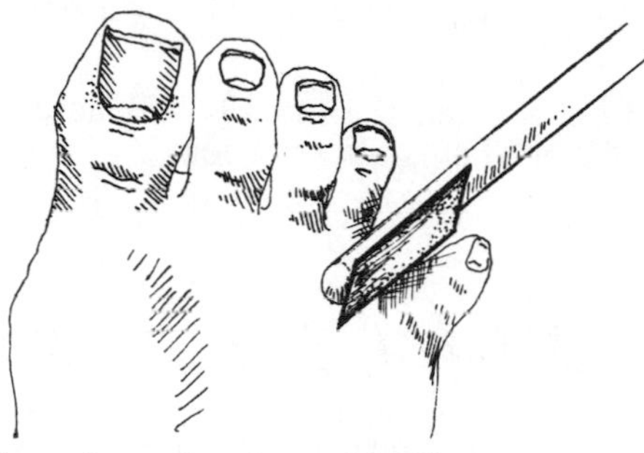

► Using your emery board or abrasive tool, file away the top layer of dead skin from the corn.

► Try to touch only the corn, keeping the abrasive tool away from the toe web (deep between the toe). If the corn is so large that it is located in the web itself, the best you can do is to skip the filing and go directly to step 2, below:

2. After you have removed as much "top skin" as you can . . .

► Cleanse the area with soap and water on a 2"x 2" gauze pad.

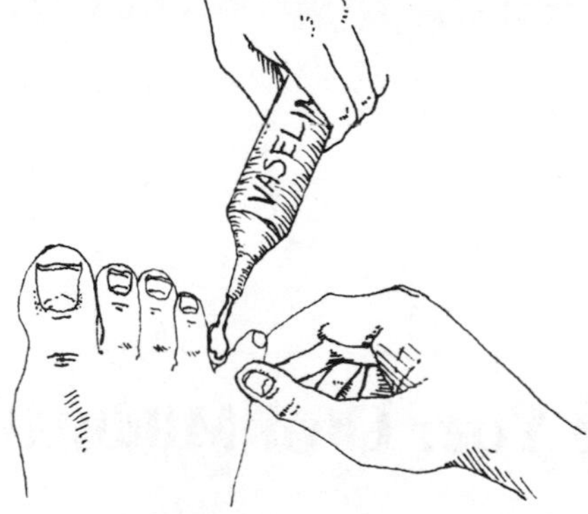

► Rub vaseline ointment into the areas you have just finished working on.

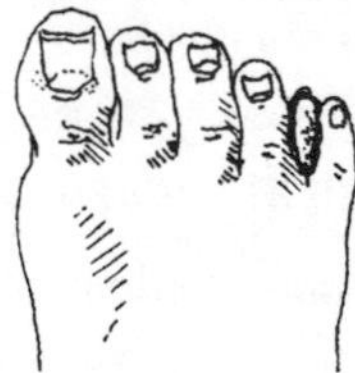

► Insert a plug of lambswool about the size of a ball of cotton between the toes.

► Use vaseline and lambswool daily to keep buildup under control.

When to Call the Doctor

► If pain is not reduced in one day, or if you think you have an infection (if the area is red, warm, or swollen), don't touch it yourself! See a podiatrist immediately.

► In many cases, this treatment will give temporary relief but will not remove the cause. A podiatrist can keep the area trimmed down for you, or may be able to provide a permanent correction by removing the bony prominences which caused the corn initially. This removal is usually done with a local anesthetic and a minimum of discomfort. In many cases, this procedure causes no disability and no loss of time from work.

DON'TS

► Don't use razor blades.

► Don't use any other sharp objects.

► Don't use medicated corn pads. (They contain acids and can cause burns and infection in normal skin surrounding the corn.)

► Don't put pads directly on top of a corn. This will only increase pressure and pain.

► Don't ever stick cotton between the toes. It will harden and cause increased irritation—just the opposite of what lambswool does.

Practical Pointer for Prevention

► Make sure shoes fit properly with plenty of room for toe comfort. You should be able to freely wiggle your toes in your shoes.

How to Make Your Own Mildly Abrasive "Tool"

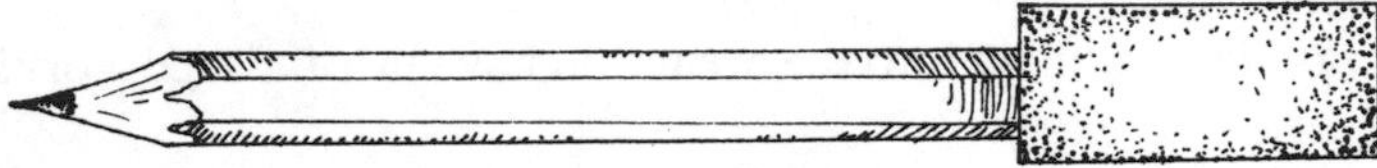

► Find a thin, clean piece of wood such as a tongue depressor, thin dowel, or a pencil.

► Glue a 1" by ½" strip of medium grade sandpaper around its end.

► Allow to dry.

8. Callous

(On the Ball of the Foot)

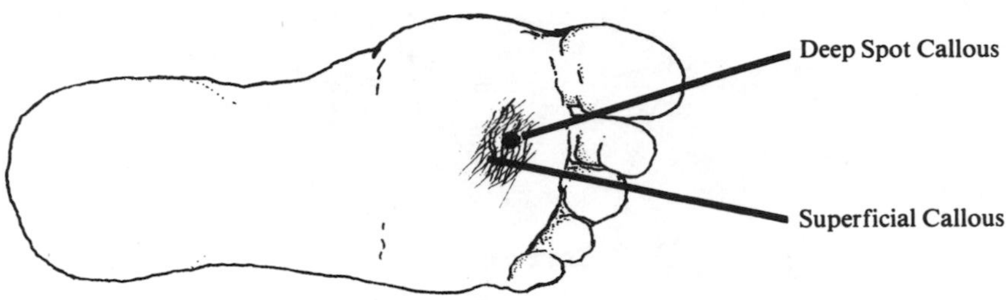

What is it?

A callous is a buildup of thickened skin that usually occurs in areas of extreme friction and pressure—such as under the bony areas on the ball of the foot.

Usually a foot that is not aligned properly, or not mechanically sound, will "wear out" under continuous stress. What happens to the foot is like what happens when you drive a car with a poorly aligned front end, causing the tires to wear excessively in certain areas. The difference is that the foot protects itself by developing extra thickness in the skin in those spots where the skin might otherwise wear right through.

A "spot" callous is a deep, plug-like area of corny consistency located in the center of a more superficial, more spread-out callous. It is severely painful, and can cause a limp in many cases. This particular corn-within-a-callous, as it is sometimes referred to, is caused by an abnormally depressed metatarsal head, or an overlong metatarsal bone. Since all the metatarsal heads should bear an equal share of the weight load, if one is "too low" in the foot it will produce a pinpoint pressure point and a much greater stress in the skin of the bottom of the foot. You could achieve the same result from the outside-in, if you taped a pebble on the bottom of your foot and walked on it all day long!

CAUTION: If you are a diabetic or have circulatory problems, refer only to the parts of this chapter concerned with relief of pressure. It is also important to be sure that what you are treating is indeed a callous, or a corn in a callous. Sometimes a wart, an ulcer, or a foreign substance (splinter, glass, etc.) can resemble a deep callous in appearance and symptoms.

Things you will need for this treatment

see chapter 2 "Materials List" for brand names and substitutes

soaking solution
softening agent
callous file
moleskin
petroleum jelly
adhesive tape
2"x2" gauze pad
adhesive spray and skin protectant
adhesive foam or felt 1/8"

Caution: *Do not proceed with this treatment until you have read the Guidelines to Treatment in Chapter 2*

Preparation for Treatment

► Make sure all materials and suggested medications are clean and up to date.

► Thoroughly scrub the entire foot with warm soapy water and a terry wash cloth. Pat dry with a soft clean towel.

► Read through all instructions that follow, and make sure you understand them before beginning treatment.

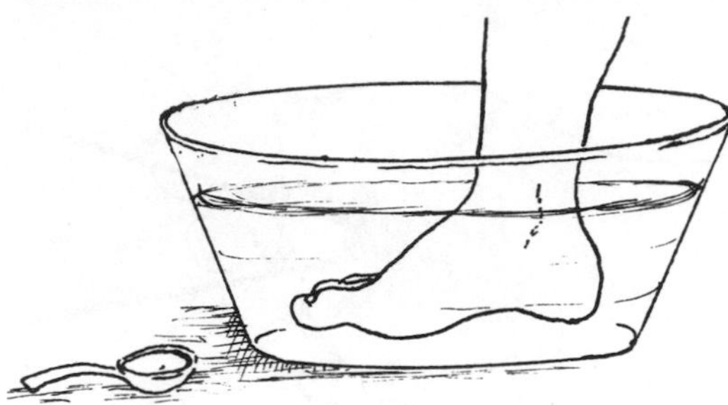

► Put two tablespoons of mild household detergent into half a gallon of warm water. Soak for twenty minutes.

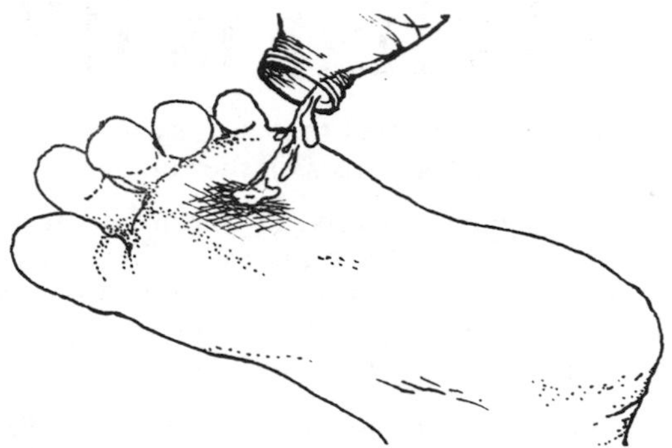

► Rub about 5 drops of cooking oil into the callous to soften it further.

Treatment

The same *general* treatment is recommended for all types of callous, but a few special suggestions will be given for each of the different types discussed in this book.

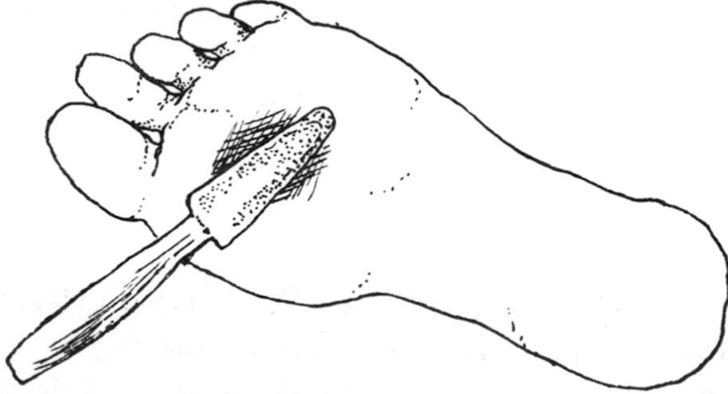

1. **Filing down the callous.**
   ► Using a back and forth sawing motion, remove the thick skin with a pumice stone, sandstone, mildly abrasive sandpaper, or callous file.
   ► Make sure you stay on the thickened skin.

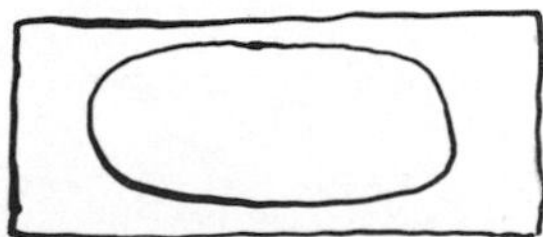

2. After filing down the callous, wipe off the area gently with soap and water on a gauze pad.
   ► Take a piece of 1½" by 1½" moleskin, bend in half with sticky side up, and cut a hole in it. The hole should be wide enough to go around the filed-down callous, leaving 1/8" border of good skin between the callous and the pad.

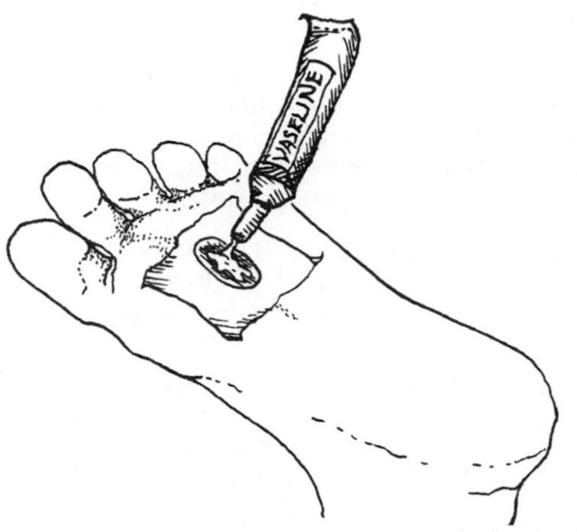

3. After the pad is properly placed on the foot, place Vaseline in the hole.

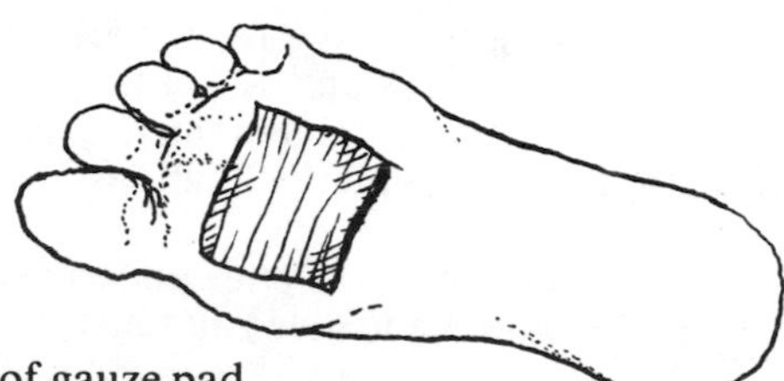

► Cover with a ½'' square of gauze pad.
► Cover this with a strip of 1'' adhesive tape.

4. Once you have trimmed and medicated the callous, it is very important to pad pressure away from it. You will need the following additional materials: A ''stick'em,'' such as tincture of Benzoin; 1/8'' foam or felt.

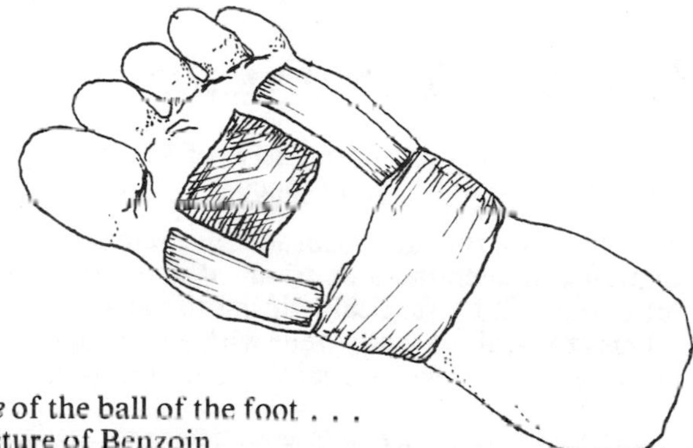

If your callous is in the *middle* of the ball of the foot . . .
► Prepare area with tincture of Benzoin
► Cut 2 strips of foam or felt ½'' wide and 2'' long.
► Cut 1 strip 2'' wide by 2'' long.

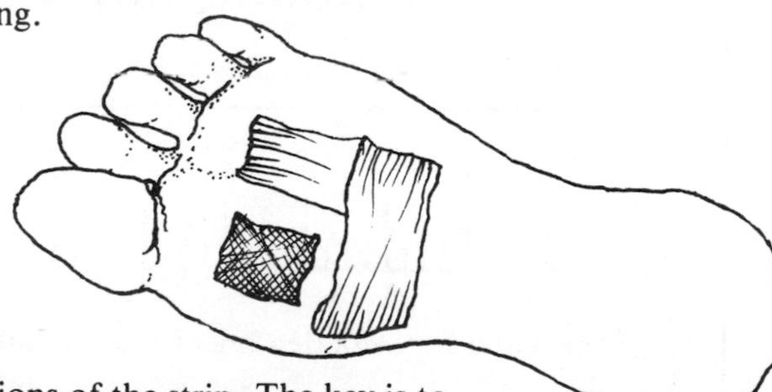

For isolated callouses, use combinations of the strip. The key is to redistribute the weight of the body away from the painful callous.

NOTE: For treatment of the heel, no pads are used. Heel callous is discussed separately (see chapter 9).

5. Keep pads completely dry for one full day, after which it is OK to get them wet. We don't recommend total saturation with wetness, however. Don't swim or take baths, and confine your bathing to quick showers as long as the pads are on. You may use a hair dryer to blow them dry after your shower.

► After wearing these pads for five days, *carefully* remove them by pulling tape from the toes toward your heel. To avoid pulling skin off the foot, peel very slowly and gently (see chapter 2).

► Apply powder liberally when dry.

NOTE: If you are allergic to adhesive tape, ask your druggist for non-allergenic paper tape.

6. For longer relief between home treatments, you can make a balanced inlay for your shoes to keep pressure off your callouses all day long.

► Go to a drug store or athletic shoe shop and pick up a pair of Dr. Scholl's full length foam rubber insoles or Spenco insoles.

► Wear them for one week, and your callouses will leave impressions on the insole, locating the areas of greatest stress and showing you the spots *around which* the insole needs to be built up to even out the pressure.

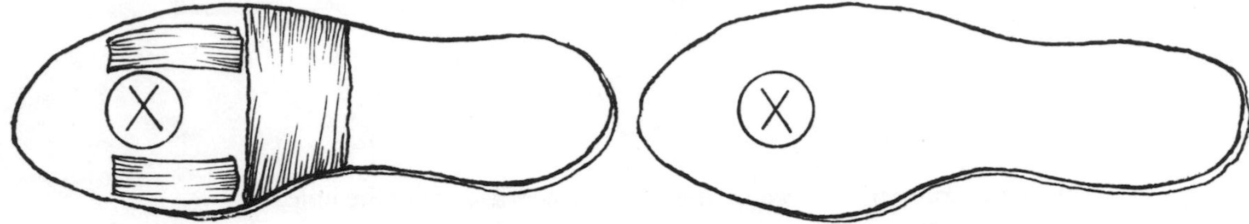

► Or, instead of wearing the insole for a week, try holding it against your foot to feel where the callous hits. Mark an "X" at the spot. Push in hard on that "X" until you feel your finger on the bottom, and make a large circle around your finger. Glue your strips of foam or felt around the "callous" area (circle) just as you did on your foot.

► With the insole in your shoe, the pads underneath the insole will redistribute your weight away from the callous and give you relief.

If you are flatfooted or pronate (roll foot from the outside inward) excessively, you will probably have more friction and pressure on the ball of your foot—and may be more likely to have callouses (see appendix on Foot and Leg Structure). To reduce this excessive pressure, fit a Spenco inlay to your shoe and attach to it a varus wedge long enough to extend from the heel to the arch (see appendix on Shoe Inserts You Can Make).

When to Call the Doctor

► If pain is not reduced in one day, or if you think you have an infection (if the area is red, warm, or swollen), don't touch it yourself! See a podiatrist immediately.

► In many cases, this treatment will give temporary relief but will not remove the cause. A podiatrist can keep the area trimmed down for you, or may be able to provide a permanent correction by surgically lifting the abnormally depressed or overlong matatarsal bone. This removal is usually done with a local anesthetic and a minimum of discomfort. In many cases, this procedure causes no disability and no loss of time from work.

To make your own callous file:

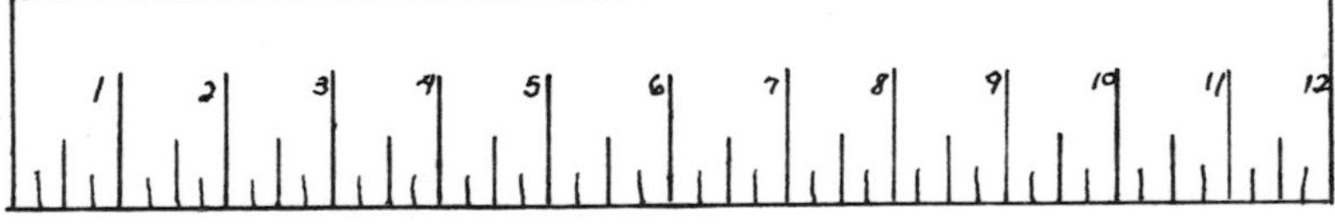

1. Take a one-foot wooden ruler (or any similar smooth-finished piece of wood)...

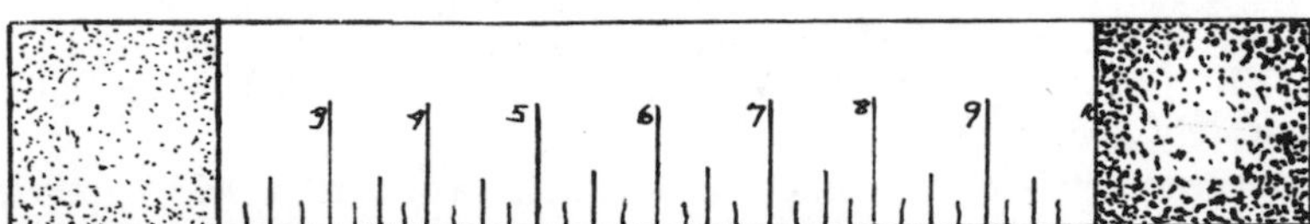

2. Glue a 2"x 2" piece of mildly abrasive grade sandpaper on one end and a 2"x 2" piece of "fine" sandpaper on the other end.

3. Begin treatment using mildly abrasive paper and finish with fine paper.

9. Heel Callous and Fissures

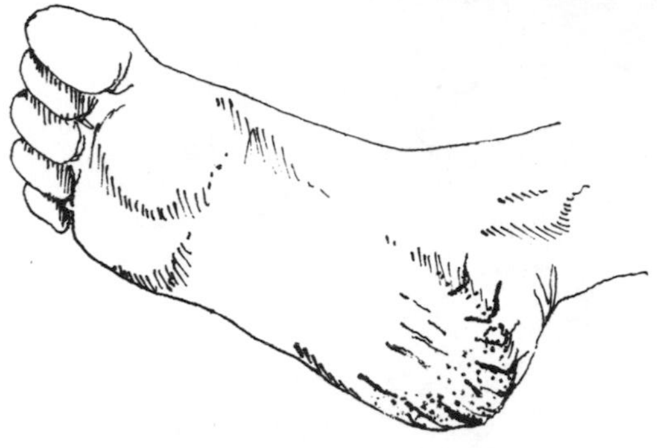

What is it?

A heel callous is a build-up of thickened skin caused by excessive friction between the skin of the heel and the sock or shoe. For example, a foot that is not properly aligned causes excessive movement of the heel bone against the shoe. When this happens, the skin which is caught between the bone and leather has to thicken to protect itself from irritation. Open backed sandals, slingback shoes, and "mule" type step in shoes and slippers can aggravate this problem by slapping against the heel with each step and moving in the opposite direction of the foot. This causes especially rapid build-up of callous. Thick callouses will sometimes crack and split through to the uncalloused skin. These deep cracks, or fissures, may bleed and become quite painful. If not treated, they may even become infected.

Things you will need for this treatment

see chapter 2 "Materials List" for brand names and substitutes

soap & water
soaking solution
softening agent
callous file or "mildly abrasive tool"
petroleum jelly
heel cups
medicated foot powder

Caution: *Do not proceed with this treatment until you have read the Guidelines to Treatment in Chapter 2*

Preparation for Treatment

1. Make sure all the materials you will be using are clean and fresh as discussed in chapter 2.

2. Put two tablespoonfuls of mild household detergent into a half gallon of warm water. Soak for twenty minutes.

3. Read through all the instructions which follow, and make sure you understand them before beginning treatment.

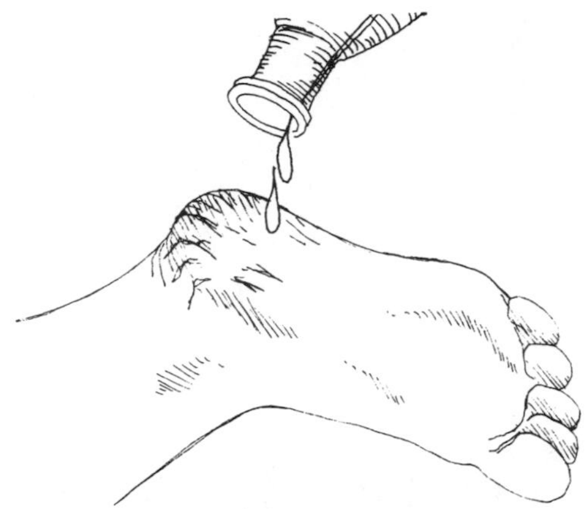

5. Rub about 5 drops of cooking oil into the callous to soften it further.

Treatment

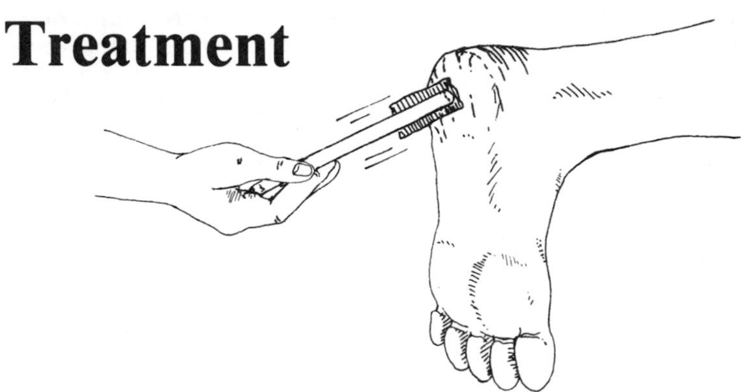

► Using a back-and-forth sawing motion, remove the thick skin with a pumice stone, mildly abrasive sandpaper, or callous file. (You can make your own file by gluing sandpaper to a wooden ruler (see chapter 8).

During the next two weeks . . .

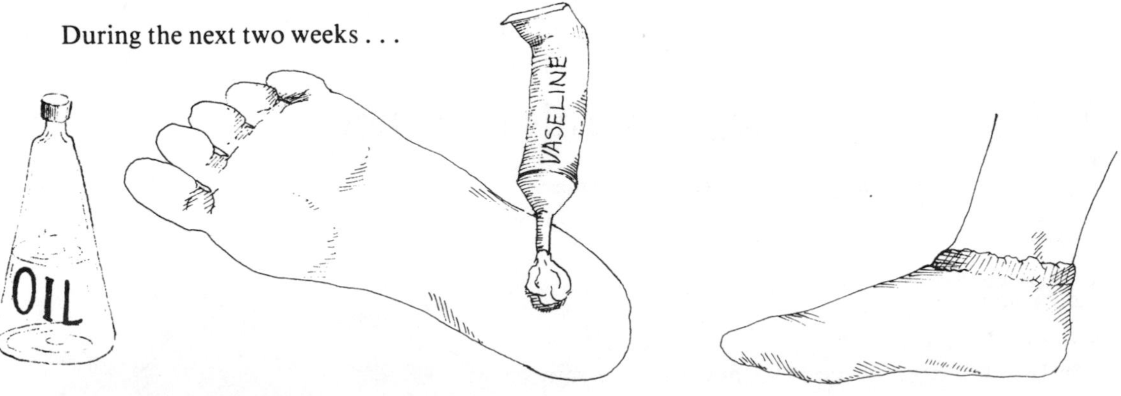

► Before going to bed, rub in some cooking oil, cover with vaseline, and put on a pair of white cotton socks for the night.

► Continue this procedure for two weeks.

► After two weeks, repeat this procedure once a week for two or three more weeks.

If you are a runner or weekend athlete:

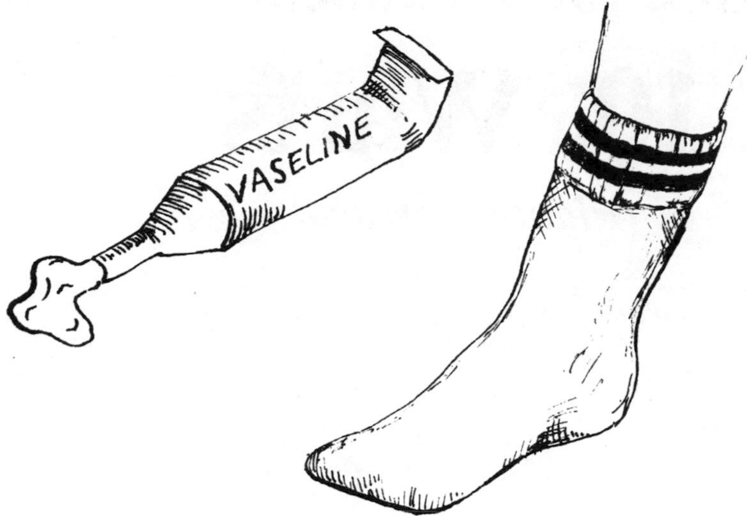

- Coat the area with vaseline before running
- Put a "ped" on the foot, and a cotton sock over the ped.

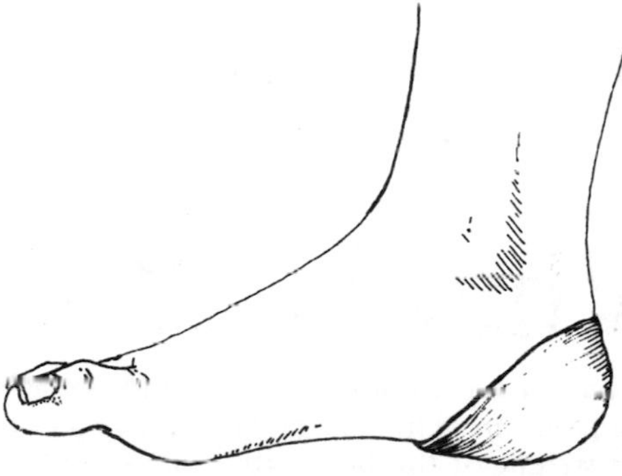

- Try using a heel cup (available in drug and sporting goods stores).

When to Call the Doctor

If you have tried the recommended treatment for several weeks and the condition is still present, or if the heel is red and hot, you need professional care.

DON'TS

- Don't wear the same shoes two days in a row, so they will dry out.
- Don't wear open back or sling back shoes.
- Don't go barefoot or wear shoes without socks.

- If you perspire excessively, see chapter 13.

10. Warts

(Plantar verruca)

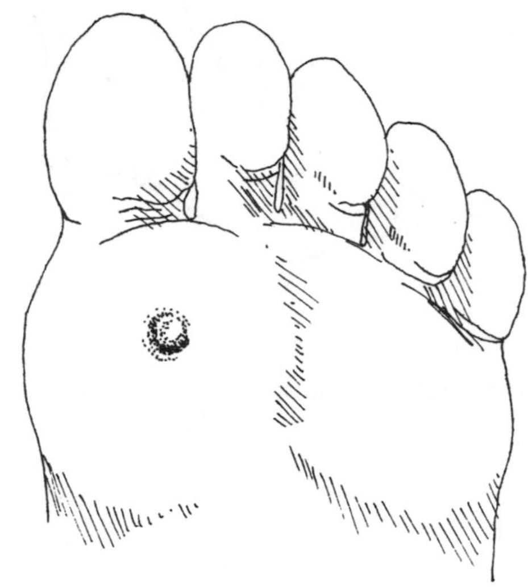

What is it?

A wart is a virus infection that can occur anywhere on the body. It usually looks a little like a tiny cauliflower projecting from the skin, except when it occurs on the bottom of the foot. Then, due to the constant weight of the body, the wart grows "into" the foot instead of "out" of it. Although warts are sometimes confused with corns and callouses, if you look at them closely you can see a well-defined border and little dark spots resembling blood vessels running all through them. They are also more sensitive to side-to-side pressure, while corns are more sensitive to direct pressure. Warts occur both singly and in clusters. They are contagious, and are especially prevalent in the fall and spring. Children are more susceptible than adults.

Things you will need for this treatment

see chapter 2 "Materials List" for brand names and substitutes

soap & water
scissors
40% salicylic acid plaster
toothbrush
bandaid or adhesive tape

Caution: *Do not proceed with this treatment until you have read the Guidelines to Treatment in Chapter 2*

Preparation for Treatment

► Make sure all the materials you will be using are clean and fresh as discussed in chapter 2.

► Put two tablespoons of mild household detergent into ½ gallon of warm water. Dip your foot in the water and soak for ten minutes.

► Read through all the instructions which follow, and make sure you understand them before beginning treatment.

Treatment

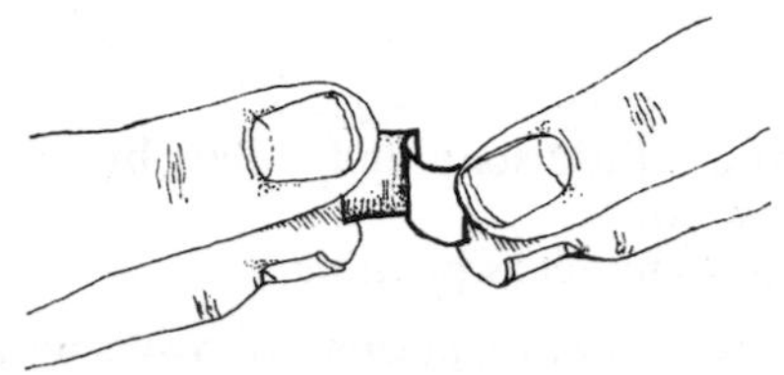

1. Cut out a square of 40% salicylic acid plaster (about the size of the wart) and remove backing to expose the self-stick surface.

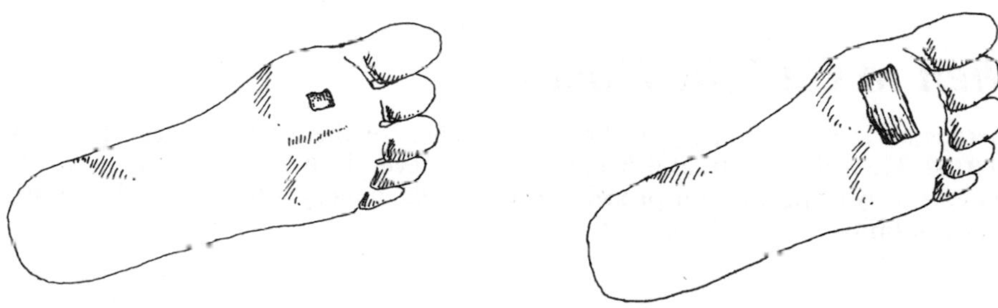

2. Apply sticky side directly onto the wart. Push down and cover with bandaid or tape.
3. For the next two days . . .
   ► Keep the plaster on and dry
4. After two days . . .

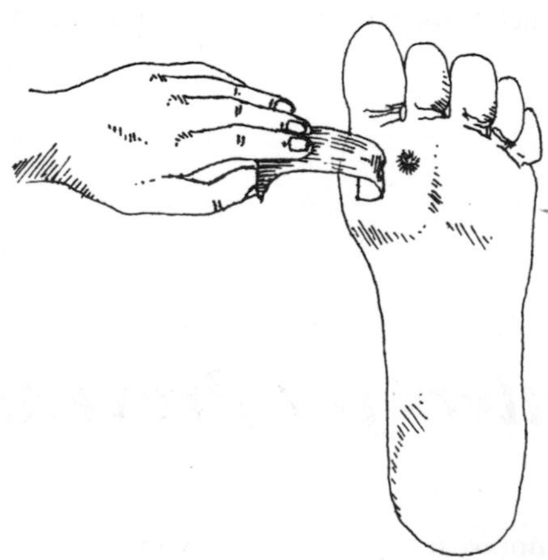

► Carefully remove the bandaid, tape and plaster. The wart will have a whitish appearance.

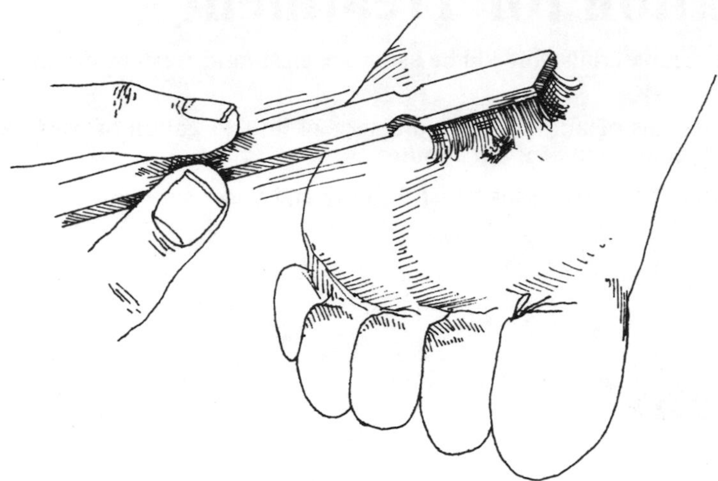

► Using the toothbrush and a little soap and water, brush the wart vigorously for one minute twice a day for two days.
► Expose the wart to the air as much as possible.

5. Repeat the entire process—two days of plaster followed by two days of brushing—for a period of two weeks.

When to Call the Doctor

If there is no improvement, or if the pain increases or the wart or warts spread, see your podiatrist. He will either treat it over a period of several weeks with different medications, or remove it by using a minor procedure that results in very little pain and only slight temporary disability.

DON'TS

- ► Don't use razor blades, knives or any other sharp objects on the wart!
- ► Don't use any drug store remedies except as directed here.
- ► Don't let the salicylic acid touch ''normal'' skin, if you can help it.

Practical Pointers for Prevention

1. Do not go barefoot.

2. Change shoes every day. Do not wear the same shoes daily.

3. If your feet perspire excessively, you may be prone to warts (see chapter 13).

4. Children are prone to this condition. Check their feet periodically, especially during fall and spring months. Early treatment is a good prevention for spread and contagiousness.

11. Needles, Glass, and Splinters

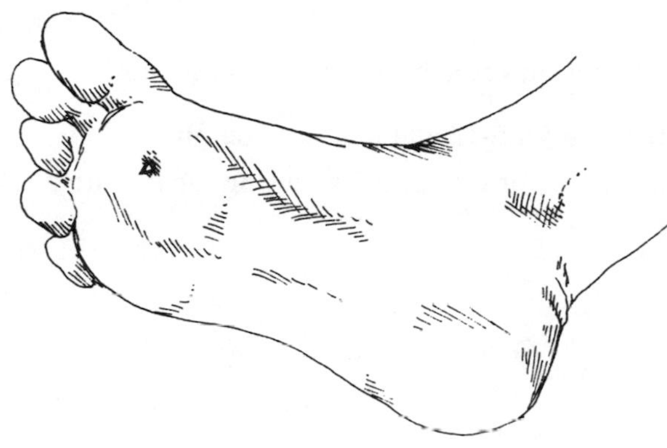

This treatment can be used whenever a foreign body becomes imbedded in the foot. A "foreign body" is anything that gets stuck in the foot and doesn't belong there—most often, a splinter of wood or a sliver of glass.

Things you will need for this treatment

see chapter 2 "Materials List" for brand names and substitutes

soap & water
antiseptic
ice bag
softening agent
2"x2" gauze pads
soaking solution
bandaid
antibiotic cream (if you have any)
pin, needle or tweezers
match

Caution: *Do not proceed with this treatment until you have read the Guidelines to Treatment in Chapter 2*

Treatment

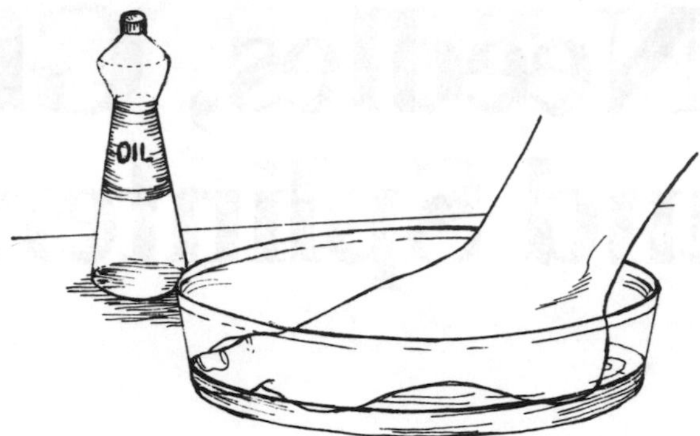

1. Soak the injured part in vegetable oil for a few minutes.

2. Apply ice to the area for 6-12 minutes, until numb.

3. Sterilize a pin, needle, or tweezers, by putting the tip into a flame of a match or dipping it in alcohol.

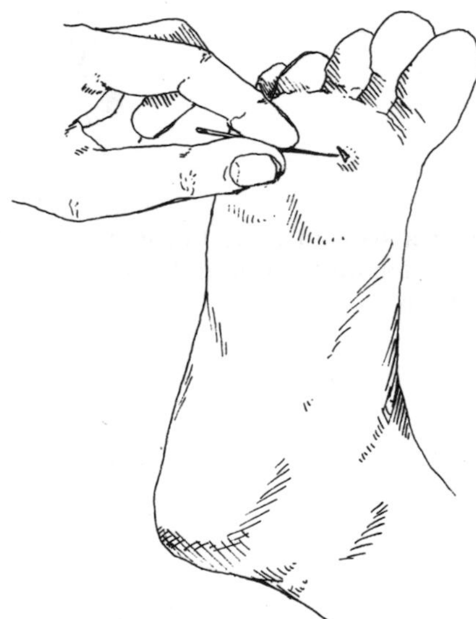

4. Use the pin to try to move the foreign body out. After soaking in oil, the foreign body should be loose and easy to remove.

5. Once the foreign body is removed, clean the area with soap and water and dry with gauze pads.

6. Apply Merthiolate or antibiotic cream and cover with a bandaid.

7. Once a day for two weeks, soak the injured part in a solution of Domeboro or epsom salts.

When to Call the Doctor

If there is any persistent redness, swelling, or drainage from the area, or if you can't remove the object yourself, see a podiatrist immediately.

NOTE: If you can't easily get to the injured area of your foot, have someone else follow these instructions for you.

12. Bee Sting

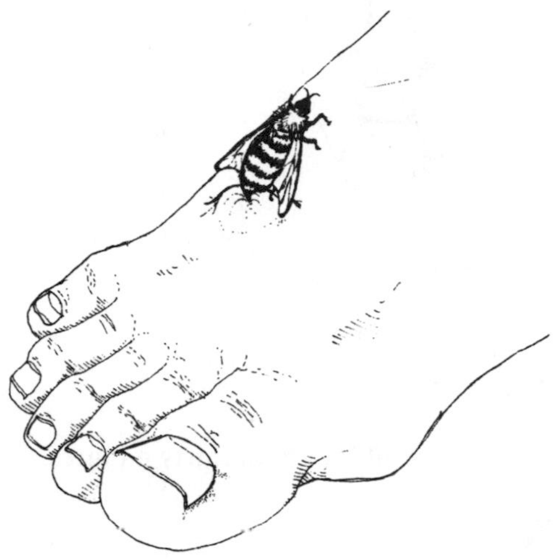

In most cases, the stings of bees and other insects are not very serious. In many cases, no treatment is necessary. However, for people who are allergic to bee stings, treatment is of urgent importance. This type of allergic reaction is usually caused by the sting of a bumble bee, hornet, wasp, or yellow jacket. It may also be caused by the bite from an ant or spider. Stings are usually painful, and sometimes itchy. They often result in swelling and heat.

CAUTION. If chills, fever, nausea, vomiting, cramps and/or breathing difficulties occur within minutes after a sting, call a rescue squad. *A severe, immediate reaction signifies a medical emergency.* If these symptoms occur later but within 24 to 48 hours, contact a doctor. Such symptoms usually indicate an allergic reaction. If the reaction is severe and you are on your way to a doctor or emergency room, place ice around the area to slow the absorption of venom.

If the reaction is localized, swelling and itching due to multiple bites in an area might last 24 to 48 hours before starting to subside. If you show any unusual allergic reaction at all to your very first sting, stay away from areas where these insects are prevalent and make proper arrangements with your physician for the handling of any future sting.

Things you will need for this treatment

see chapter 2 "Materials List" for brand names and substitutes

soap & water
ice bag
softening agent
pin, needle or tweezers
desensitizing lotion

Caution: *Do not proceed with this treatment until you have read the Guidelines to Treatment in Chapter 2*

Treatment

1. Put ice on the area for 15 to 30 minutes to numb it and help reduce the swelling.
2. Wash the area with soap and water.

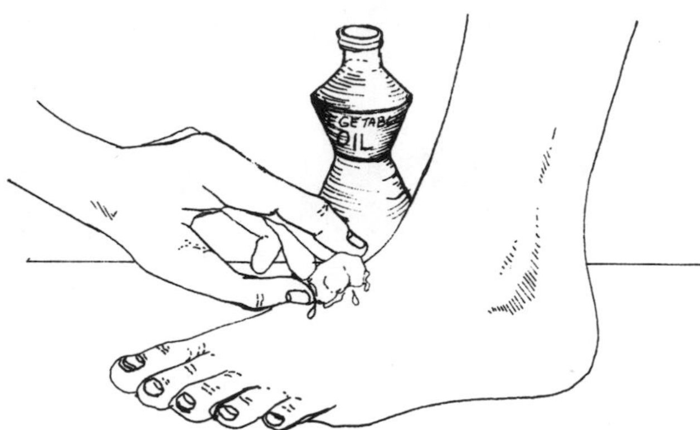

3. Coat the wound with vegetable oil for about thirty minutes.

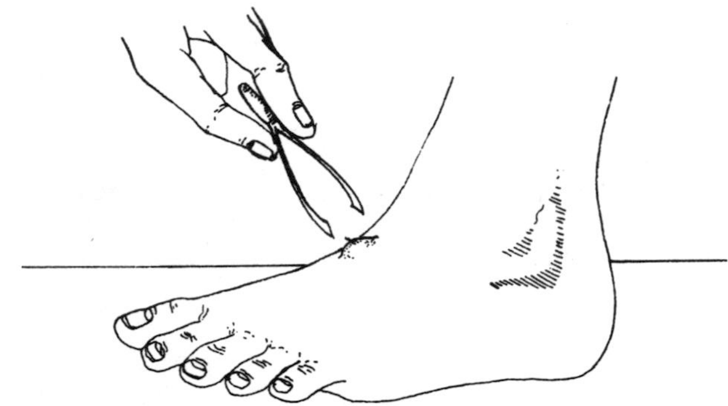

4. If a stinger is visible in the wound, try to remove it with sterilized tweezers.
5. Repeat the ice treatment (or soak in cold water) for about 15 minutes.

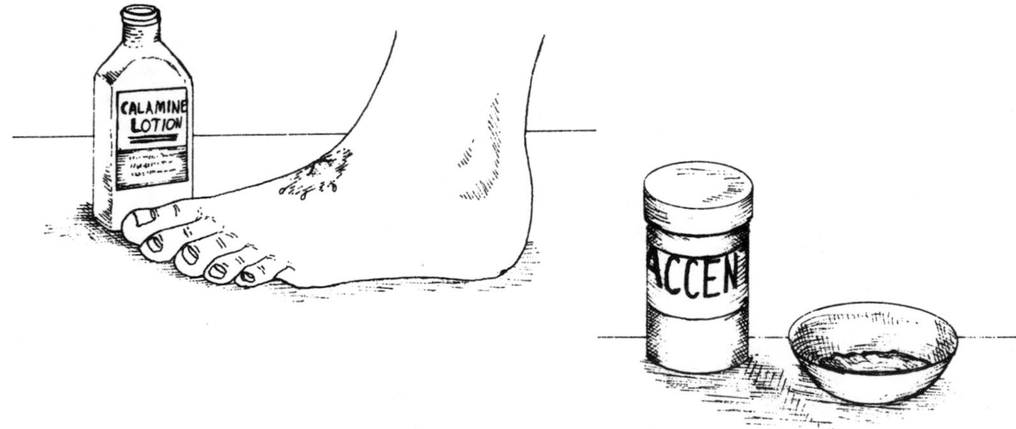

6. If there is any itching, put Calamine lotion on the area every few hours, or make a homemade paste out of half a teaspoonful of meat tenderizer and two teaspoonfuls of water, and place on the area. Baking soda is effective also and may be substituted for the meat tenderizer.

When to Call the Doctor

If the swelling does not go down within 24 to 48 hours and severe pain remains (or if the stinger cannot be removed), consult a podiatrist. If you can't do this treatment yourself, have someone else follow the instructions and do it for you.

13. Sweaty and Smelly Feet

(Hyperhidrosis and Bromhidrosis)

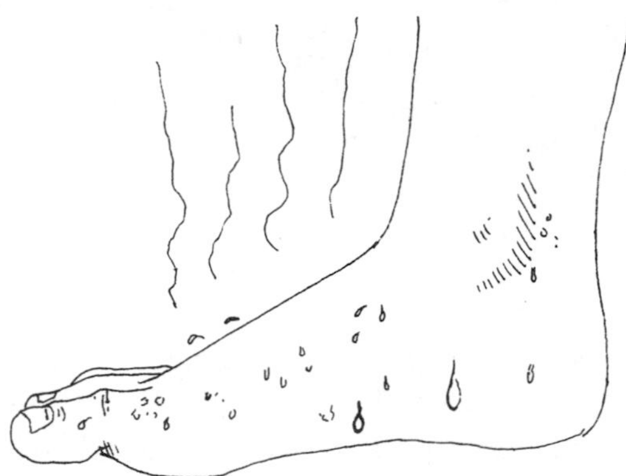

Excessive perspiration occurs when feet sweat too much due to overactivity of the sweat glands. It is a common problem for children and young adults.

The problem of smelly feet—not "normally" smelly feet, but those with an unusually foul odor—is usually caused either by bacteria which decompose skin by-products, or by localized fungus infections (see chapter 14). The problem of odor is especially common in feet that perspire excessively.

Things you will need for this treatment

see chapter 2 "Materials List" for brand names and substitutes

soap & water
fabric for removal of dead skin
medicated foot powder
disinfectant spray
material to inhibit odor
antiperspirant
occlusive wrap
cotton swab

Treatment

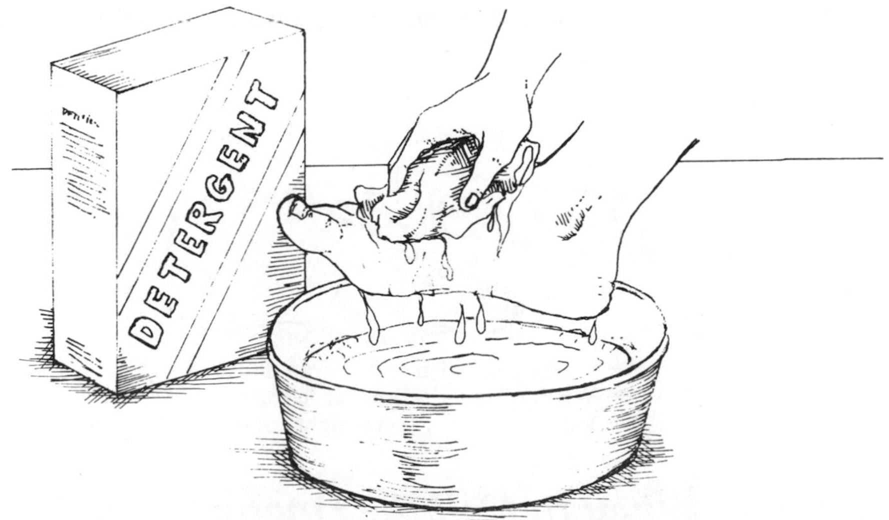

1. Thoroughly scrub the feet with a warm solution of laundry detergent. Use a wash cloth to wash and remove the dead skin.

2. Rinse feet thoroughly and dry with soft clean towel.

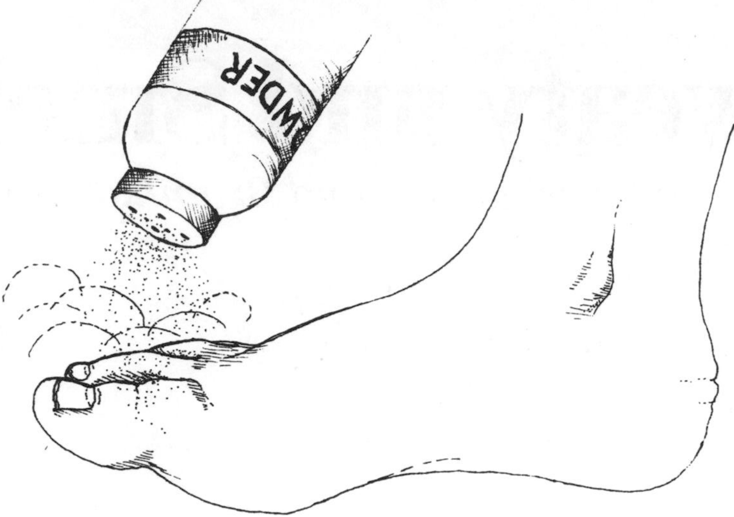

3. Powder feet liberally with medicated foot powder, and be sure to get it in between the toes. Tinactin powder and Aftate powder are two good commercial products for this.

4 If steps 1-3 don't do the job after a few days, try Mitchum's deodorant. Use it as follows:

- ► Wash foot thoroughly with rubbing alcohol.

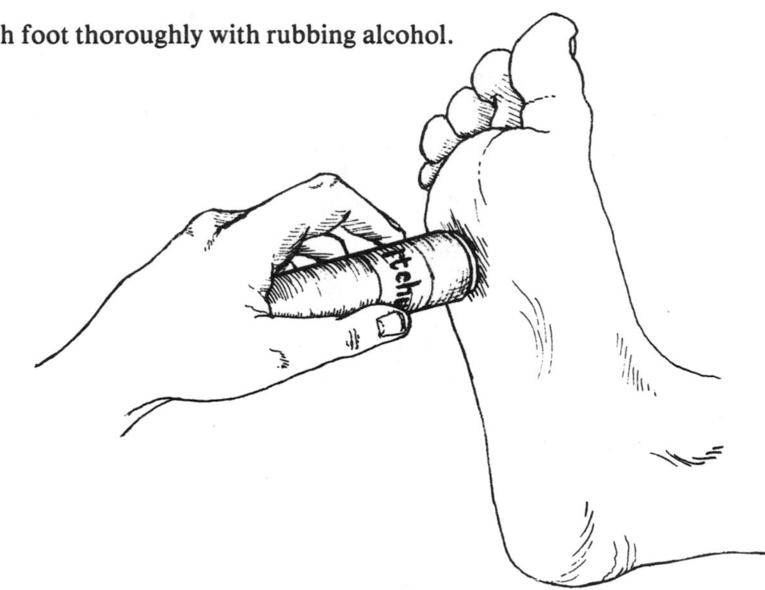

- ► Apply Mitchum's deodorant over the bottom of the foot at bedtime.

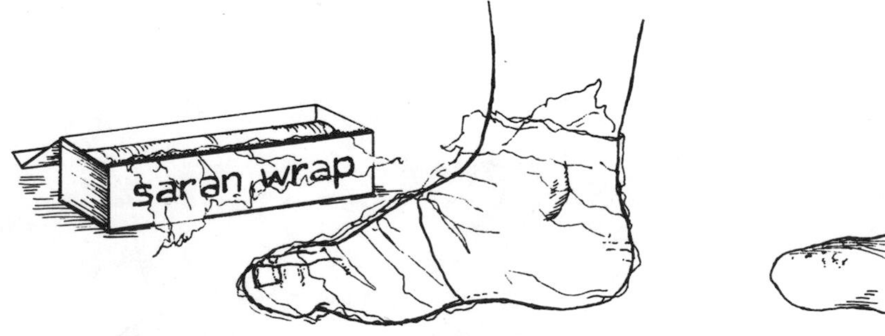

- ► Cover foot with saran wrap and sock.
- ► Wash off excess powder in the morning.
- ► Repeat process every night for one week, then once or twice a week as needed.

When to Call the Doctor

Sometimes excessive sweating and foot odor are caused by a mechanically unsound foot or an underlying fungus infection (Athlete's Foot). In these cases—or in any case where the treatment does not work within a few days—it is appropriate to consult a podiatrist.

DON'TS

- Don't wear the same shoes for two or more consecutive days.
- Don't wear shoes made of synthetics or leather substitutes which don't have pores and don't breathe well (see appendix on shoes).
- Don't use synthetic or nylon socks.
- Don't wear shoes without socks, especially in sports.

Practical Pointers for Prevention

1. Use the right kind of shoes for each of your activities.

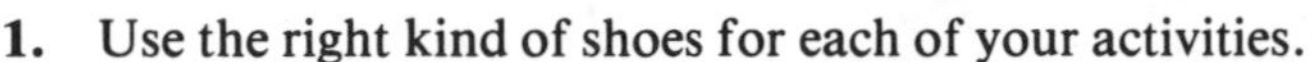

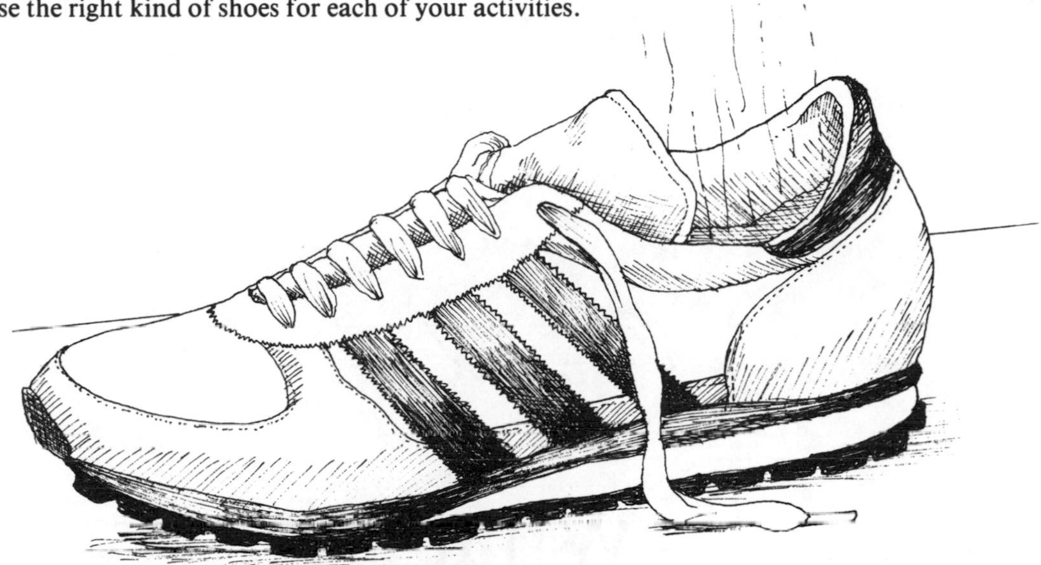

2. Air shoes out after use. It takes 24 hours for a shoe to dry out and reshape after using.
3. Use clean, absorbent cotton socks.
4. Change socks daily.

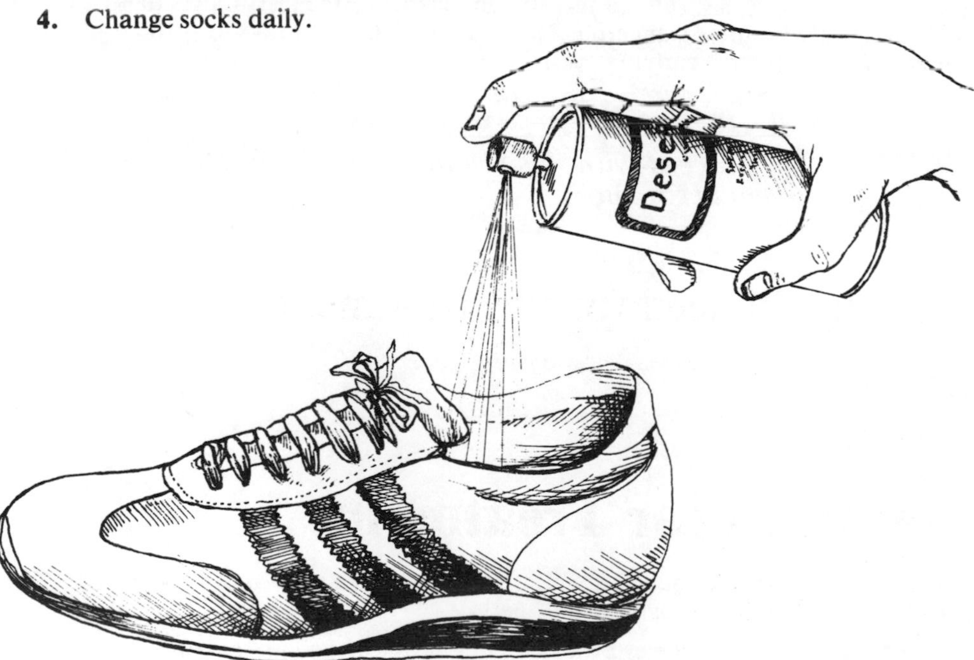

5. Spray shoes daily with Desenex or disinfectant before use.
6. Powder feet and socks liberally each day.

14. Athlete's Foot

(Tinea Pedis)

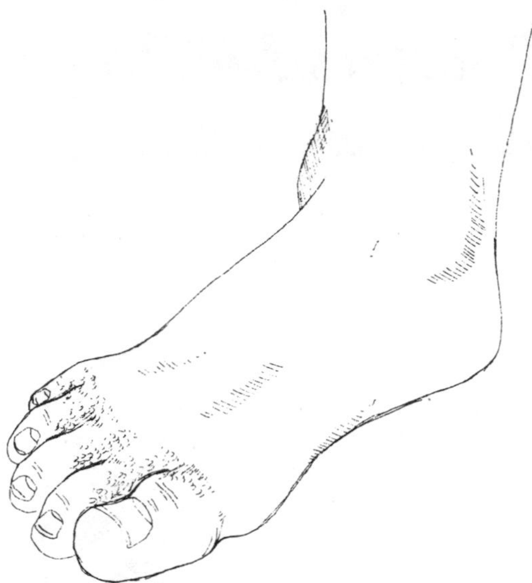

What is it?

Athlete's Foot (also called Ringworm) is a superficial fungal infection of the skin of the feet. It is a very common affliction, especially among males. In the early stages, fluid-filled blisters occur on the soles, sides or in-between the toes of the feet. Later, these areas become red, dry, scaly fissures. Dangerous secondary infections can occur if the primary (fungal) infection is not treated early.

Caution: *Do not proceed with this treatment until you have read the Guidelines to Treatment in Chapter 2*

Things you will need for this treatment

see chapter 2 "Materials List" for brand names and substitutes

soap & water
antifungal liquid
medicated foot powder

Preparation for Treatment

► Make sure any instruments you use are clean. Wash them in soap and water and rinse off with alcohol or some other recognized antiseptic.

► Make sure all materials and suggested medications are clean and up to date.

► Thoroughly scrub the entire foot with warm soapy water and a terry wash cloth. Pat dry with a soft clean towel.

► Read through all the instructions which follow, and make sure you understand them before beginning treatment.

Treatment

1. Minimize heat and sweating (see chapter 13).

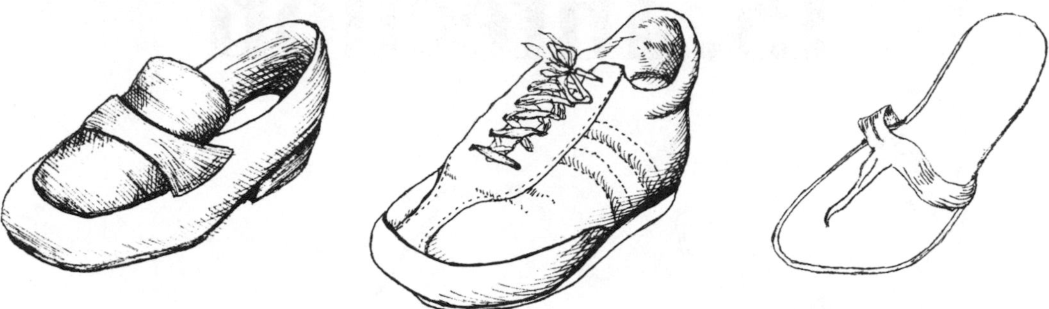

2. Wear well-ventilated shoes or sandals. Avoid using rubber or plastic shoes or boots (which prevent proper breathing).
3. Wear white cotton socks.
4. Apply Tinactin liquid twice during the day and once at bedtime.
5. Use an anti-fungal dusting powder such as Aftate or Desenex. Dust between the toes daily.
6. Continue treatment for two weeks after you think the condition has cleared.

CAUTION: If the area becomes red or swollen, or if it is draining, or isn't considerably improved within 2-3 weeks, see a podiatrist.

Practical Pointers for Prevention

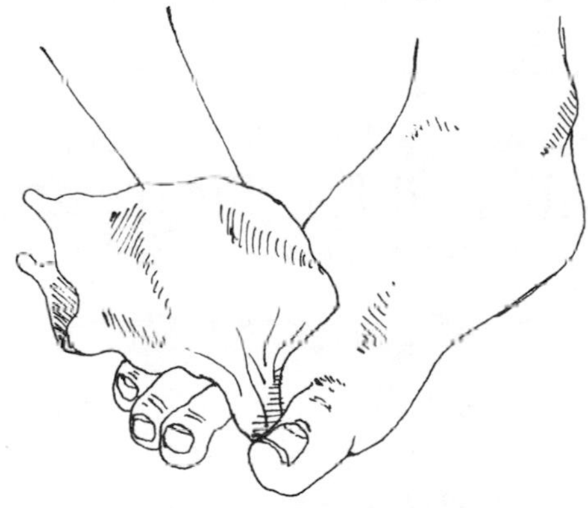

1. Wash the feet daily with mild soap and water, using a wash cloth or soft brush. Make sure you get between the toes.
2. After washing, dry thoroughly—especially between the toes.
3. If you are susceptible, use an anti-fungal powder daily and apply liberally between the toes and into the socks.
4. Wear cotton socks.
5. Avoid sweat socks and socks of synthetic materials, as they are good absorbers of heat—and therefore conducive to the environment in which fungi thrive.
6. Wear open-toed shoes or leather shoes of good quality that breathe properly. Be sure to change shoes and socks daily.
7. Always wear socks or stockings when wearing shoes.
8. Do not go barefooted.
9. When removing your shoes after a day's wear, air them out for 24 hours and spray them with an antiseptic spray such as Desenex before wearing again.
10. Avoid becoming overweight, as excessive weight leads to foot strain and excessive perspiration.

15. Infection

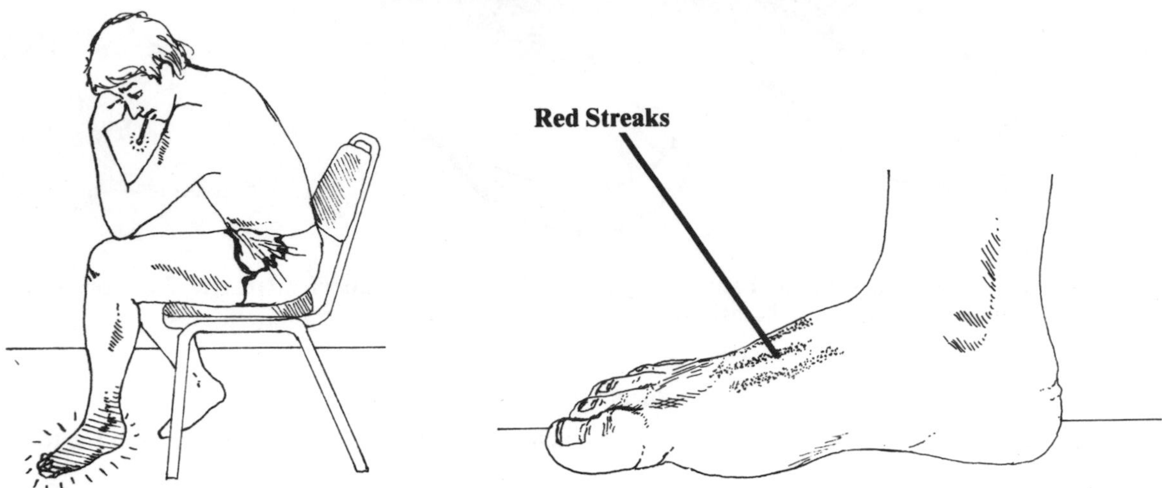

This chapter deals with infections of the skin, which are usually accompanied by redness, heat, swelling, pain and pus.

CAUTION: ***If you develop a temperature or notice red streaks or get chills, or if the symptoms of infection do not subside within 48 hours after you start treatment, see a podiatrist.*** Do not proceed with this treatment until you have read the Guidelines to Treatment in chapter 2.

Things you will need for this treatment

see chapter 2 "Materials List" for brand names and substitutes

soap & water
soaking solution
antiseptic
2"x2" gauze pads, sterile
antibiotic cream (if you have any)
adhesive tape

Preparation for Treatment

1. Make sure all the materials you will be using are clean and fresh as discussed in chapter 2.

2. Read through all the instructions which follow and make sure you understand them before beginning treatment.

Treatment

1. Clean the area well with soap and warm water.

2. Soak for 20 minutes in warm water with Domeboro or epsom salts added, two to three times daily.

3. Rest and keep pressure off the area by padding around it when possible.

4. Put an antiseptic solution on the infected area after each soak, and then cover with antibiotic cream and 2x2 sterile gauze pads.

5. To control pain and/or fever, take two aspirin every four hours.

16. Bunions

(Bursitis of the first or fifth metatarsophalangeal joint)

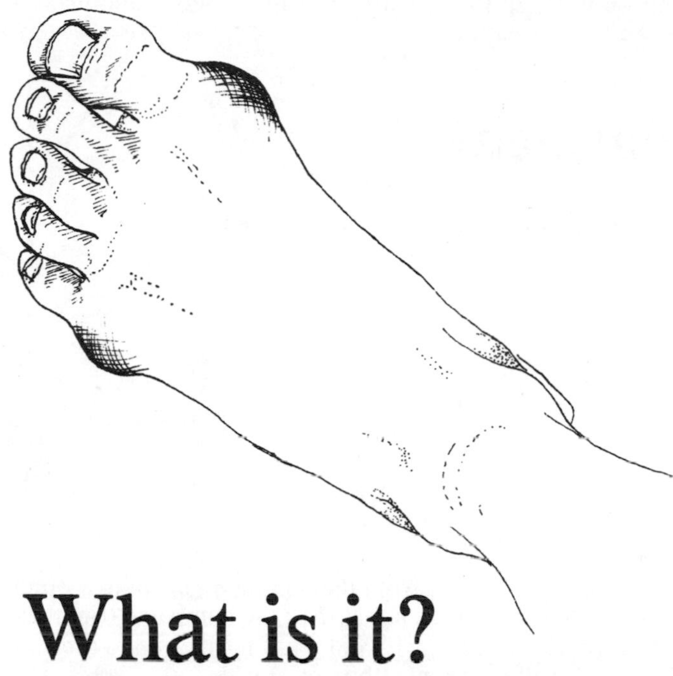

What is it?

A bunion is an inflammation which can occur either on the outside of the big toe joint or the outside of the little toe joint. A "big toe" bunion is an enlargement of the outside of the head of the first metatarsal bone. The big toe may be straight, but is sometimes angled or pointed toward the small toe, subjecting the bony bump to a great deal of irritation. The skin and soft tissue around this bump become irritated and inflamed. The area may become red, hot, and swollen, and very painful. Continued pressure on this area can lead to the development of infection or the formation of corns over the bump. The small toe bunion, or Tailor's bunion, is an enlargement of the outside of the head of the fifth metatarsal bone. The little toe is sometimes pointed in toward the big toe, causing irritation to the enlargement. This area may also become red, hot, swollen, and very painful. Continued pressure on this area can also lead to the development of an ulcer, infection, or the formation of corns over the bump.

Things you will need for this treatment

see chapter 2 "Materials List" for brand names and substitutes
soap & water
adhesive spray and skin protectant
adhesive foam or felt 1/8" and 1/4"
2"x2" gauze pad
adhesive tape 1"
moleskin or elastic adhesive bandage 3" square
heating pad
ice bag
aspirin
soft polyurethane foam 1/4"
cotton material 1" by 18"
nitrogen-impregnated foam innersole
bunion shield

Caution: *Do not proceed with this treatment until you have read the Guidelines to Treatment in Chapter 2*

Preparation for Treatment

► Make sure any instruments you use are clean. Wash them in soap and water and rinse off with alcohol or some other recognized antiseptic.

► Make sure all materials and suggested medications are clean and up to date.

► Thoroughly scrub the entire foot with warm soapy water and a terry wash cloth. Pat dry with a soft clean towel.

► Read through all the instructions which follow, and make sure you understand them before beginning treatment.

Treatment

1. Apply tincture of benzoin to the irritated area.

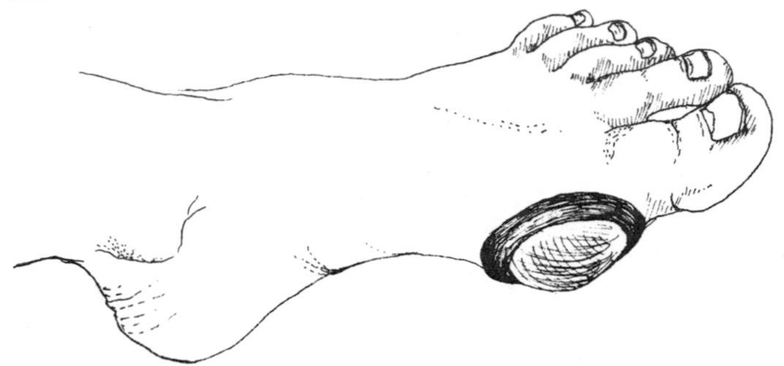

2. Remove the irritation from the bunion by padding around it with 1/8'' adhesive felt. Cut a hole in the felt a little larger than the bump and trim the circumference of the pad so that there is 1/8'' to 1/4'' width of padding all around the bump. An alternative here is to use a commercially available ''bunion shield.''

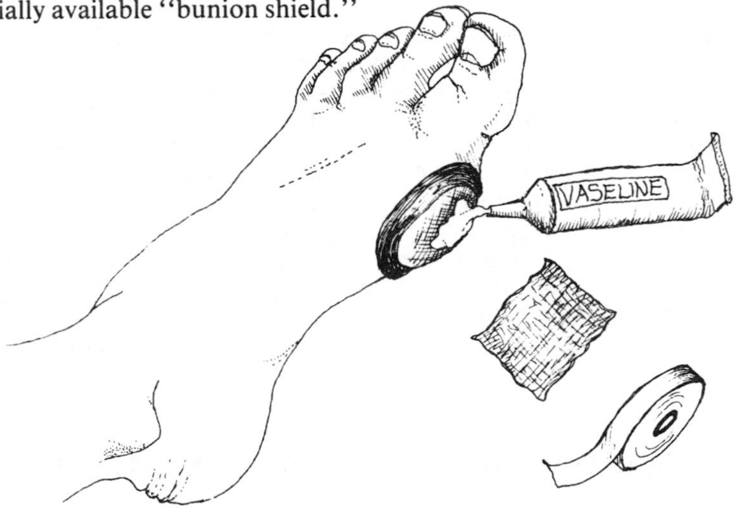

3. Apply vaseline into the hole, cover with gauze and tape down.

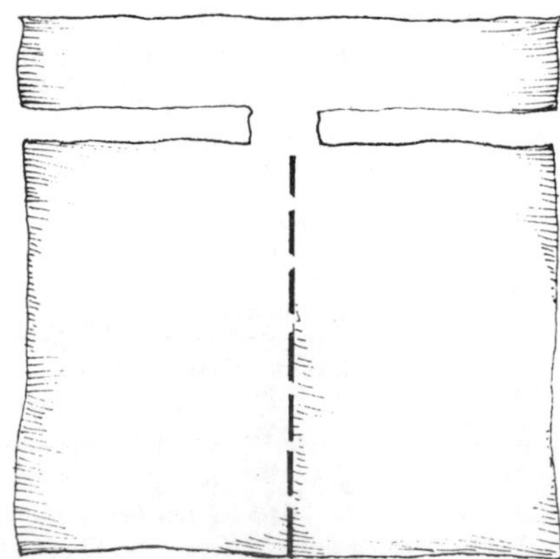

4. Make a ''prehensile strap'' as follows:

► Take a piece of 3''x 3'' adhesive tape, Elastoplast©, or moleskin and fold it in half, sticky side up.

► Cut it into a ''T'' shape.

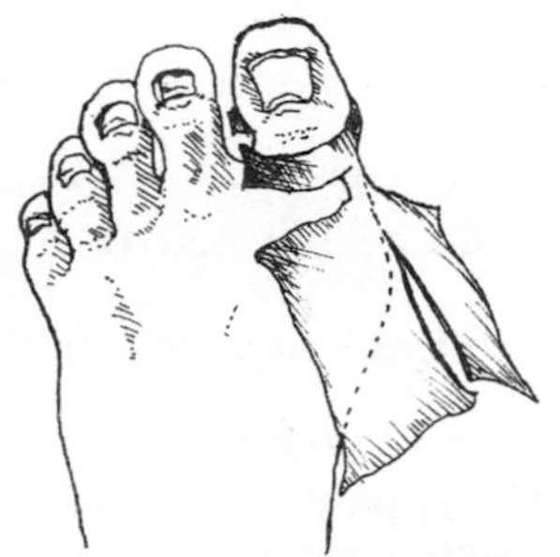
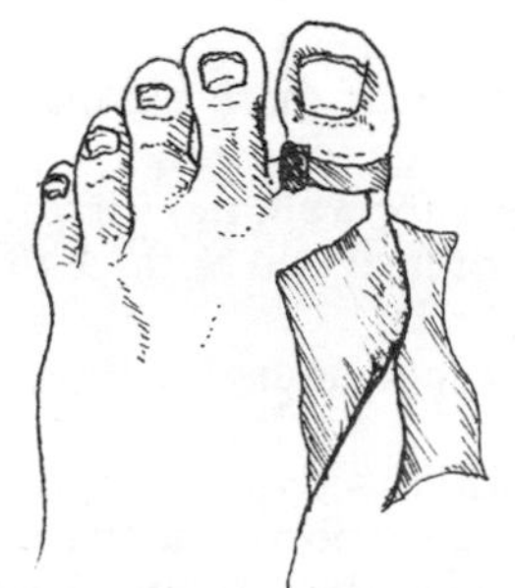
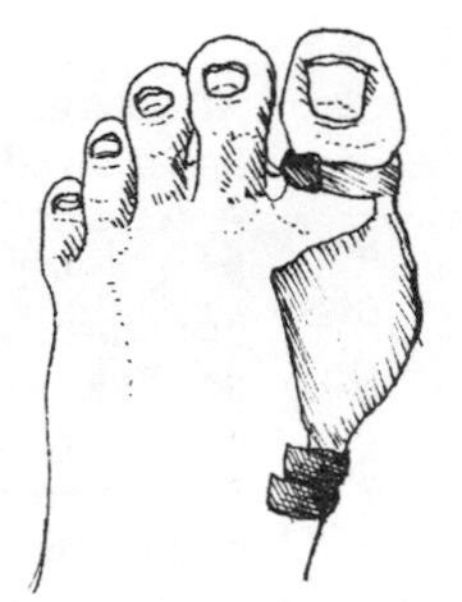

► Apply the top of the "T" around the base of the big toe and lock with tape. Pull the two bottom "T" flaps into place, covering the bunion. The strap will spread the pressure of the shoe against the foot so that it is not concentrated on the bunion.

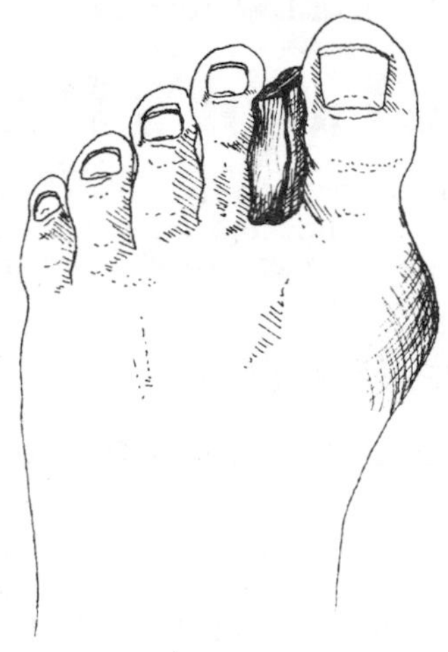

5. For further relief from pressure against the bunion joint, insert a piece of ¼" thick foam or polyurethane foam between the first and second toes.

6. Wear shoes that have proper width and depth in the toe box. If necessary, change shoes until you find a pair that won't irritate the sore area (see appendix on shoes).

7. If you can't find a comfortable pair of shoes, take one of the pairs you have and slit it or cut a hole in it to relieve the pressure.

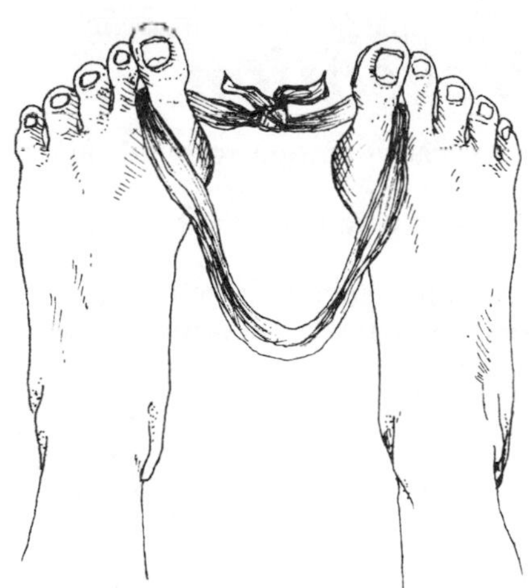
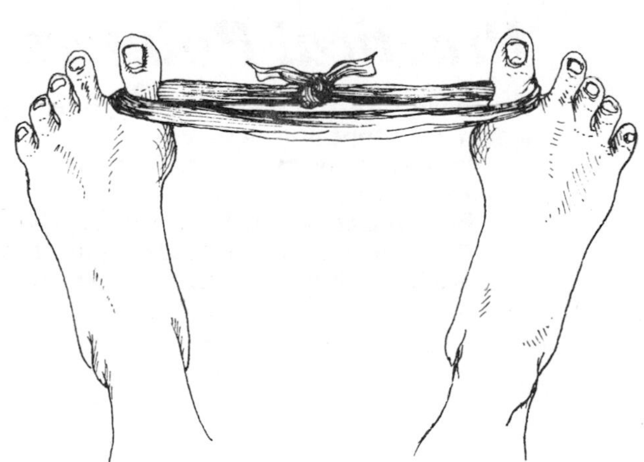

8. Make an exerciser that you can use every morning to loosen up the bunion joint and make it more mobile.

► Take a 1" by 18" piece of cotton material or thin rope.
► Tie a loop and place one end around each large toe.
► Keep heels on a flat surface, pull toes apart, and hold for five seconds. Start by doing this pull ten times a day, and increase one time each day until you get to 25 pulls a day.

9. After you have tried steps 1-8, if there is pain deep in the bunion joint, or if there is redness or swelling around it, try the following:

- ► Get off your feet (except for walking) for a few days.
- ► Use local applications of heat two or three times a day, with a heating pad, or with hot water soaks (see chapter 2).
- ► Take two aspirin every four hours for three days, then two every six hours for up to one week.
- ► When you resume normal activities, apply an ice pack for 15-30 minutes at the end of the day. If partaking in sporting activities or long walks, apply an ice pack for 15-30 minutes before and after the activity. Discontinue this step when pain is gone.

10. Once the acute stage is over, you may want to fit your shoes with a Spenco inlay.

- ► Make a varus wedge long enough to extend from the back of the heel to the arch (see appendix on making your own inserts).
- ► If you also have a callous present on the bottom of the ball of your foot, incorporate bi-plane padding made out of 1/8'' foam onto the Spenco inlay (see chapter 8).

If you have a Tailor's Bunion . . .

If your bunion is on the side of the little toe, follow steps 1, 2, 3, 6, 7, 9, and 10 above. For step #2, the bunion pad, vaseline and 2x2 gauze can be all held down by a piece of moleskin cut out in an egg shape and anchored with two or three strips of ''1'' adhesive tape.

When to Call the Doctor

If severe swelling, redness, heat and pain persist for two days with no relief, or if you see a break in the skin and/or are running a fever, see a podiatrist.

NOTE: The treatments recommended in this chapter are aimed at providing relief from the pain and discomfort of a bunion. To actually get rid of a bunion, see a podiatrist. In most cases, the surgical procedures can be performed in the podiatrist's office.

DON'TS

1. Don't wear a shoe with a narrow toe box.
2. Don't wear high heeled shoes, especially when the bunion is in an acute (painful) stage.
3. Don't wear socks or stockings that are too tight.

Practical Pointers for Prevention

1. Make sure you wear properly fitted shoes, paying special attention to width and length. (See appendix on shoes).
   - ► If you are an athlete, make sure you use athletic shoes with good toe box width and depth.
   - ► If you are a runner, get running shoes with good forefoot shock absorption.
   - ► Once the pain is under control, you may wish to purchase a commercially available ''bunion shield'' to wear daily.

17. Pain in Front of Foot

(Morton's Neuroma)

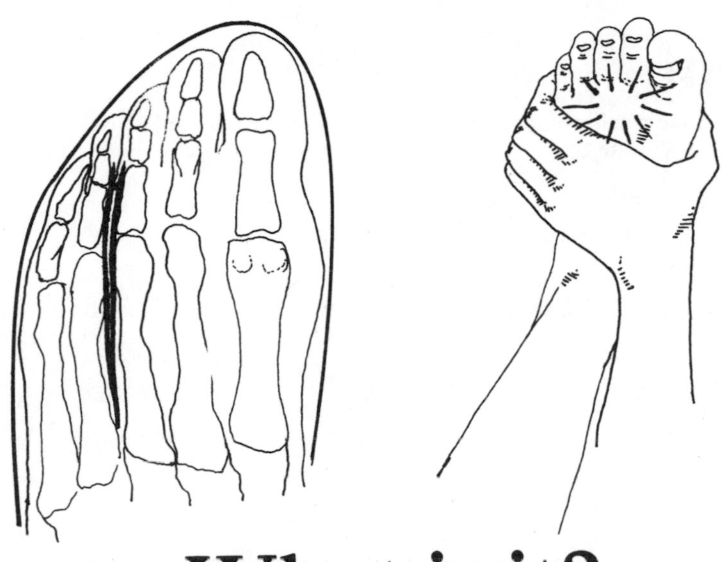

What is it?

Occasionally one of the small nerves in the front of the foot gets pinched between two metatarsal bones, causing tingling, numbness and/or pain extending from the adjacent toes into the front of the foot. This pain is especially noticeable if you squeeze the front part of the foot from side to side. This condition most commonly occurs between the third and fourth toes.

CAUTION: A painful burning sensation in the feet can be caused by many local (foot) as well as general (body) conditions. Local pain can be caused by poor circulation in the foot, athlete's foot (chapter 14), or a pinched nerve or neuritis such as Morton's neuroma (described above). However, a general burning sensation can also be caused by diabetes, anemia, thyroid disease, alcoholism, and other conditions. Therefore, if you do not get relief with what is suggested, see a podiatrist or a physician immediately.

Things you will need for this treatment

see chapter 2 "Materials List" for brand names and substitutes

wet heat
adhesive felt 1/8"
nitrogen-impregnated foam innersole
aspirin
ice bag

Caution: *Do not proceed with this treatment until you have read the Guidelines to Treatment in Chapter 2*

Preparation for Treatment

1. Make sure that all the materials and medications you will be using are clean and fresh as discussed in chapter 2.

2. Read through all the instructions which follow, and make sure you understand them before beginning treatment.

Treatment

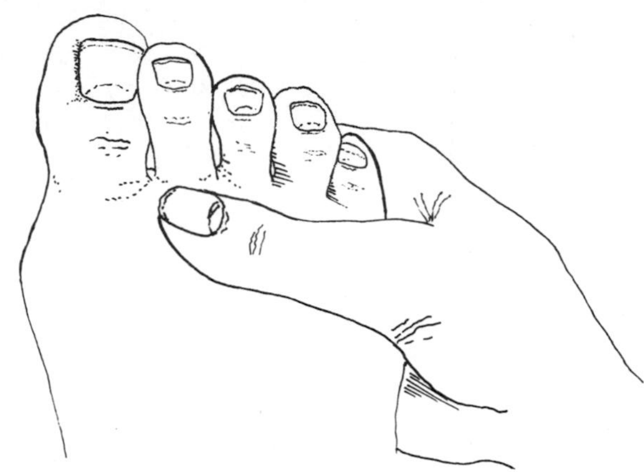

1. When the burning sensation occurs, remove the shoe and massage the toes and front of the foot. Move the toes gently up and down.

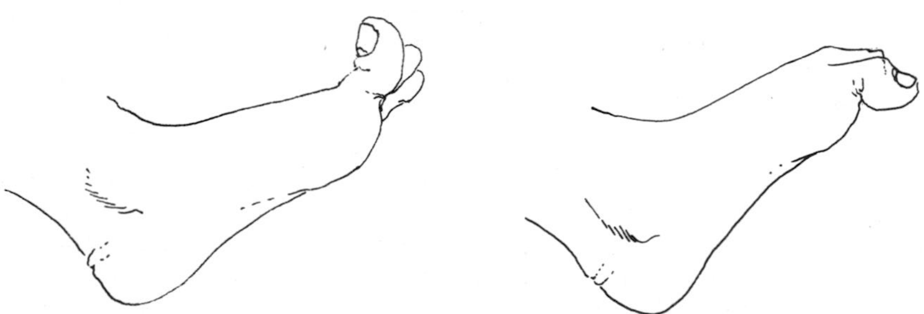

2. Do toe stretching exercises as illustrated.

3. Wrap a heating pad around the foot two times daily for twenty minutes each time on the medium setting. If you have a home whirlpool bath, use it with warm water.

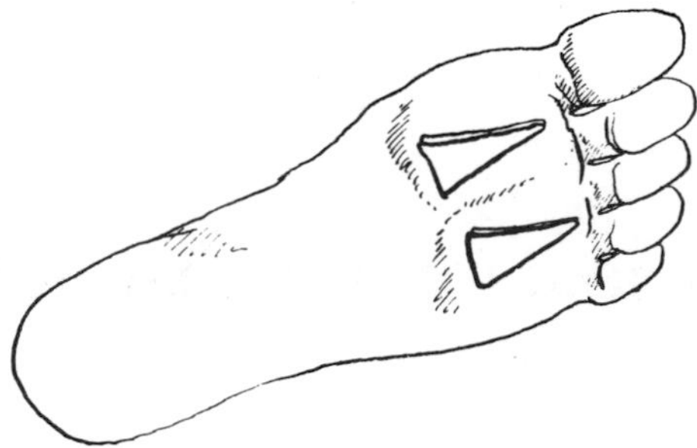

4. Place a triangular shaped pad cut out of 1/8'' felt on the bottom of a Scholl or Spenco inlay to keep the bones which are irritated separated (see the section on callouses in chapter 8, and the appendix on Shoe Inserts You Can Make). You can also put this pad directly on the bottom of your foot.

5. Take two aspirin every four to six hours (for up to one week) to diminish inflammation and pain.

Practical Pointers for Prevention

1. Wear shoes that have these features:
   ► A large toe box, giving the foot plenty of room in the front. (A narrow toe box will increase irritation.)
   ► Low heels, to keep pressure off the ball of the foot.
   ► Laces, buckles, or straps that permit adjustment of width.

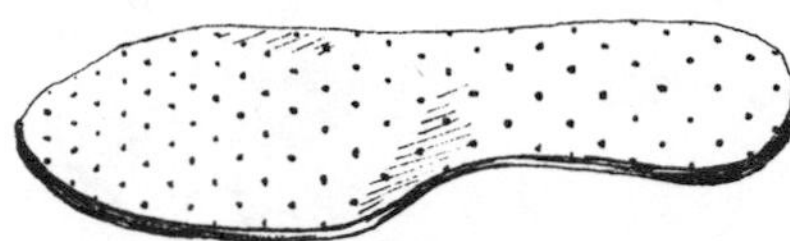

   ► Thick, shock-absorbent soles. (For thin-soled shoes, you can try a Dr. Scholl's cushion sole or Spenco innersole—but make sure the insert doesn't cramp the toes. You may be able to stretch the shoe to accommodate the insert by filling a sock with sand, stuffing it into the toe box, and wrapping the shoe with a wet towel. Let it dry out over the next 24 hours. Repeat once or twice if needed.

2. If you are an athlete:
   ► Add plain Spenco innersoles to running or athletic shoes to aid in forefoot shock absorption. Two pairs of Spencos, one on top of the other, will provide even more shock absorption.
   ► Wear shoes with the widest possible toe box and the best possible forefoot shock absorption (see appendix on running shoes).
   ► Ice the area down for 5-10 minutes after running, then apply heat later as previously discussed.

18. Arch Pain

(Plantar fasciitis)

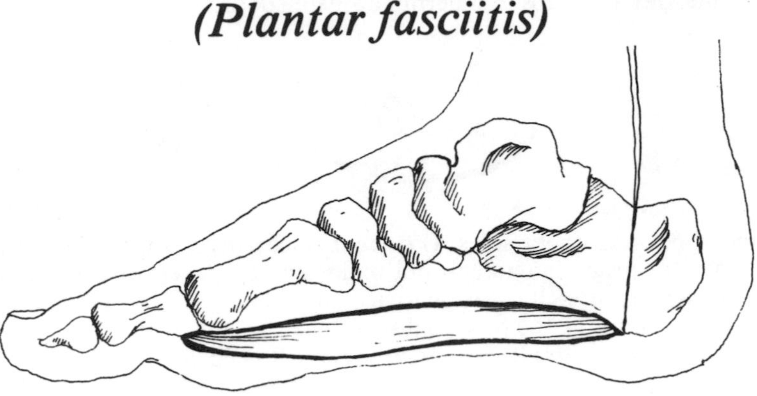

What is it?

The strongest ligament in the body is the plantar fascia, a fibrous band of tissue that starts on the bottom surface of the heel bone and extends forward on the bottom of the foot to just behind the toes. Its function is to protect the softer muscles and tissues on the bottom of the foot from injury, as well as to help maintain the integrity of the foot structure itself. For pain along the outside arch on the bottom of the foot, the treatment is basically the same.

CAUTION: If the fascia becomes stretched or strained, or in some cases actually torn, the arch area becomes tender and swollen. This inflammation, called plantar fasciitis, is likely to be painful from the heel through the arch. In the early stages, there may be swelling and a feeling of rigidity (stiffness) in the arch.

Do not proceed in this treatment until you have read the Guidelines to Treatment in chapter 2.

Things you will need for this treatment

see chapter 2 "Materials List" for brand names and substitutes

soap & water
ice bag
foot roller
adhesive tape 1" and 1½"
adhesive spray and skin protectant
nitrogen impregnated foam innersole
adhesive felt ¼"
soft polyurethane foam
aspirin

Preparation for Treatment

1. Make sure all the materials and medications you will be using are clean and fresh as discussed in chapter 2.

2. Read through all the instructions which follow, and make sure you understand them before beginning treatment.

3. Thoroughly scrub the entire foot with warm soapy water and a terry wash cloth. Pat dry with a soft clean towel.

Treatment

1. Apply ice for intervals of 30 minutes (on for 30 minutes and off for 30 minutes) for as long as possible during the first 24-48 hours, to reduce the swelling and spasm.

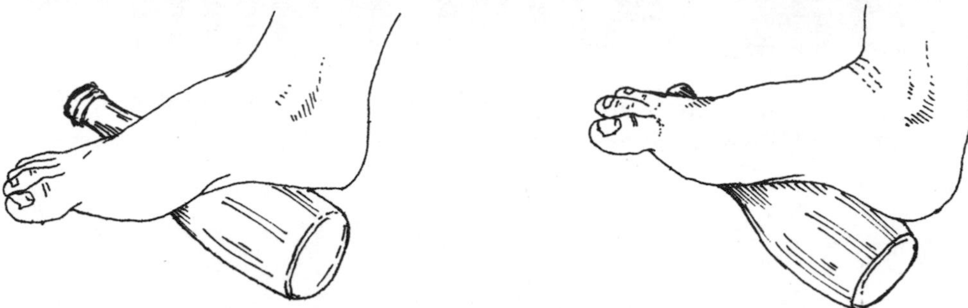

2. During the "off" periods, place a soda bottle on the floor, place your foot on top of it, and move the bottle back and forth from heel to toe. Do this for 2-5 minutes, three times daily, to help alleviate the swelling and spasm.

3. Rest, with very limited weight on the feet for 24-48 hours. After 48 hours, if you still feel pain, do not walk any more than necessary or participate in sports. When you are off your feet, elevate them.

4. Strap the foot as instructed below, to relieve pressure:

► Spray or paint tincture of Benzoin over the area of the foot to be taped.
► Cut three or four pieces of 1½" to 2" adhesive tape, each five to six inches long.

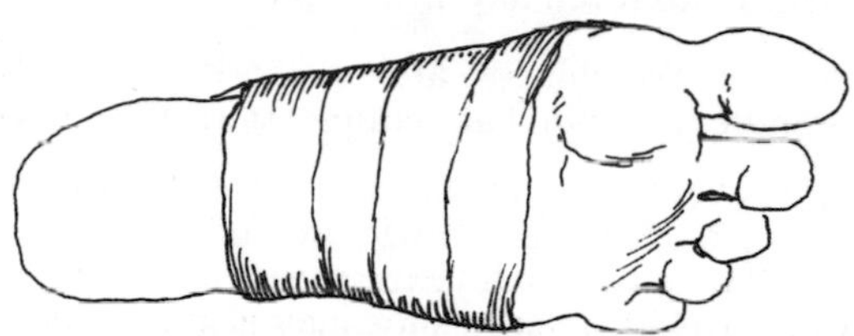

► Anchor each piece along the outside border of the foot and pull inward and upward with plenty of tension to support the arch. Start with the first piece of tape about one inch in front of the heel.

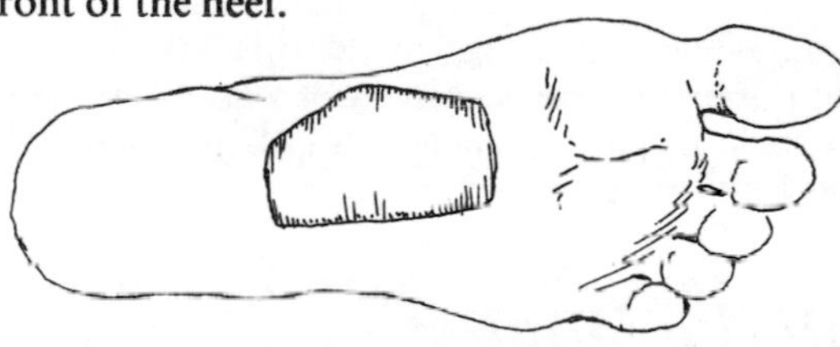

► If the tape alone does not seem to help enough, try using ¼" foam or felt padding cut to the contour of your arch as illustrated:

5. If this type of strapping does not provide enough support, carefully remove the tape (see chapter 2) and try using "retention" straps, as follows:

► Spray or paint tincture of benzoin over the area of the foot to be taped.
► Cut three strips of one inch tape approximately 8-12 inches long, depending upon your foot size.

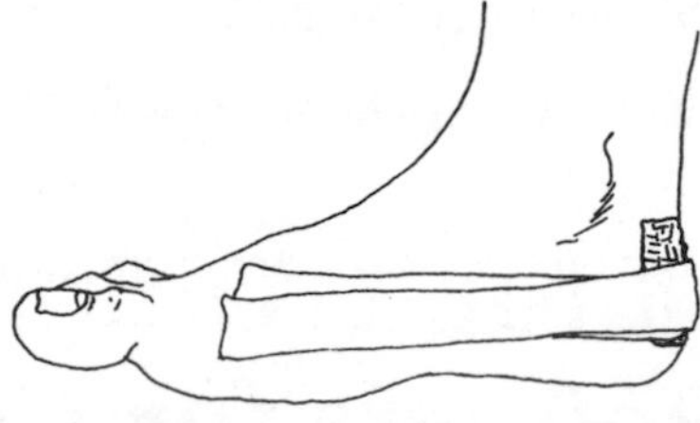

► Place one end of the tape along the outside border of the foot about one inch behind the little toe. Following the outside border of the foot, take the tape behind the heel and around to the other side of the foot, ending about one inch behind the large toe. (Before placing the tape down on the foot, point your toes downward to raise your arch up, then smooth the tape down. To avoid irritation at the back of the heel, before taping, place some vaseline over the heel and cover with a piece of gauze).

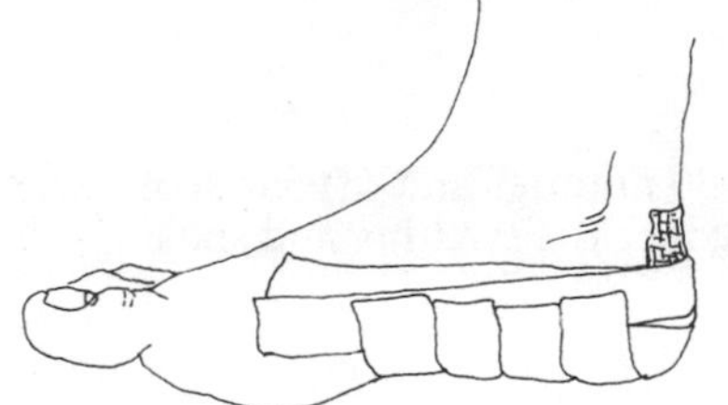

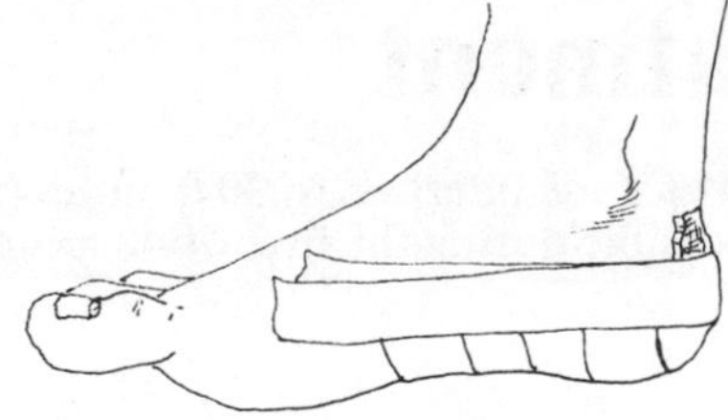

► After two retention straps are on, place the arch straps as described in step four. Then apply the third long retention strap the same way as the first two.

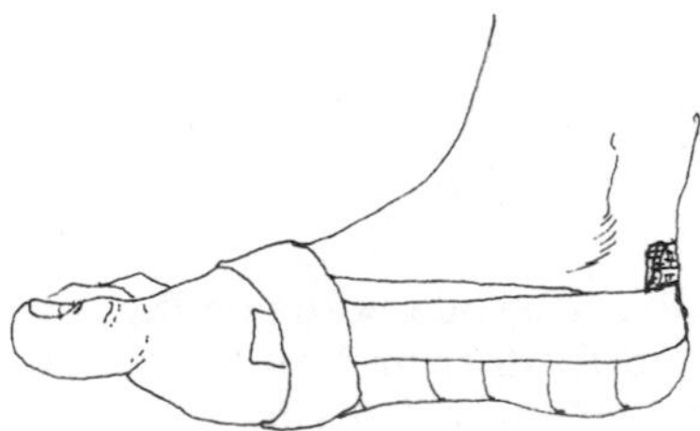

► All of this is finally anchored securely by placing one or two strips of 1½'' or 2'' wide adhesive tape on the top of the foot and ending underneath the arch on each side.

6. If pain is along the outer arch area, apply two retention straps and one ''ankle eight'' strap as described in chapter 36. As long as pain and inflammation continue, take two aspirin every four hours (for up to seven days).

7. If you are an athlete, when returning to athletic workouts, apply ice before and after the workout for twenty minutes and again at bedtime, until all the pain is gone.

8. After the severe stage is over (this may take one to two months of strapping), keep the condition controlled by using a Spenco insole with an arch build-up attached to its underside, and if you pronate (roll in at the ankle) excessively, a ''varus wedge'' in the shoes. If you have a high arch, a ¼'' heel lift in each shoe may also be beneficial (see appendix on Shoe Inserts You Can Make).

9. Shoes with flexible soles should be worn for all activities, especially athletic workouts.

10. Excessive toe movement may aggravate this condition. To cut down on toe movement for at least the first six weeks after you've got this condition under control, try using an extra pair of socks or placing Spenco or polyurethane foam in the toe box of your shoes to make the toes fit more snugly.

When to Call the Doctor

If the pain and inflammation persist for more than five days after all of this treatment, or if you cannot bear weight on your foot, consult a sports medicine podiatrist.

DON'TS

► Don't go barefoot.

► Don't wear high-heeled shoes (over 1½ inch).

► Don't wear clogs, exercise sandals or negative-heeled shoes.

► Don't wear loafers.

► Don't run on the balls of your feet if you are prone to pain in the arch.

Practical Pointers for Prevention

1. Once the pain is gone and the problem is under control, use regular stretching exercises. Exercises which help to prevent recurrence include the wall push, push-ups on the toes, heels down on stairs, and rope pulls (see appendix on stretching).

2. If you are a runner, avoid speedwork and hills until the condition is gone.

19. Pain in Bottom of Heel

(Calcaneal spur, bursitis, or neuritis)

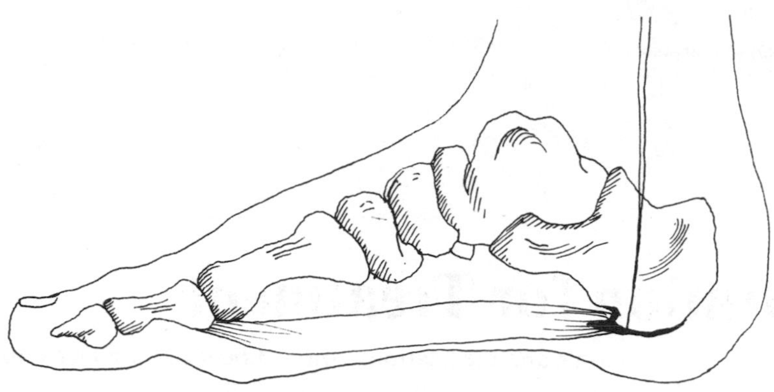

What is it?

Discomfort in the heel which is more than skin deep can have any of several causes.

- ► A *bone bruise* or *contusion* is an inflammation of the covering of the heel bone. It is painful in either walking or running.
- ► A *stone bruise* is a sharply painful injury caused by the direct impact of a hard object or surface against the foot (see chapter 21).
- ► *Plantar fasciitis* is an inflammation of the fibrous tissue band where it originates at the bottom of the heel bone. The pain often extends to the inside of the arch area and if you are a runner, is usually more severe when you are running faster or more on the ball of your foot (see chapter 18).
- ► *Nerve irritation* or *inflammation* is a condition which often afflicts the nerve just on either side of the heel bone extending down to the bottom of the heel.
- ► A *heel spur* is a shelf of bone, usually the entire width of the heel bone, formed by the continuous tearing away of the lining of the heelbone by the pull of the strong plantar fascia. Every time the lining tears, it heals forming a layer of new bone (calcium deposit) which eventually thickens to form 'The Bony Shelf.' This prominence digs into and irritates the surrounding tissue, usually giving rise to a *heel bursitis.*
- ► *Heel bursitis* is the formation of a protective sack of fluid, called a bursa, resulting from irritation caused by the spur. When this bursa becomes inflamed, it is called bursitis.

The latter two conditions, heel bursitis and heel spur, are often accompanied by pain and stiffness in the bottom of the heel, especially when you are getting out of bed in the morning. They often feel better after you have been walking on them for a few minutes. If you are a runner, you may also find that they are painful at the beginning of a run but start to feel better as the run progresses.

If swelling persists or recurs after a few days of rest, see a podiatrist. Similarly, if redness and heat are present, see a podiatrist. Remember, the problems covered here are the most common causes of pain in the bottom of the heel, but there are other possibilities—including conditions such as fractures, which should be treated by a podiatrist.

Caution: *Do not proceed with this treatment until you have read the Guidelines to Treatment in Chapter 2*

Things you will need for this treatment

see chapter 2 "Materials List" for brand names and substitutes

soap & water
antiseptic
ice bag
aspirin
a rope
adhesive felt or foam 1/8" and 1/4"
adhesive tape 1", 1½" or 2"
adhesive spray and skin protectant
nitrogen-impregnated foam innersole

Preparation for Treatment

1. Make sure all the materials and medications you will be using are clean and fresh as discussed in chapter 2.

2. Read through all the instructions which follow, and make sure you understand them before beginning treatment.

3. Thoroughly scrub the entire foot with warm soapy water and a terry wash cloth. Pat dry with a soft clean towel.

Treatment

The following treatment is designed for the heel spur syndrome, which can include at one time or another all of the different types of heel pain discussed above.

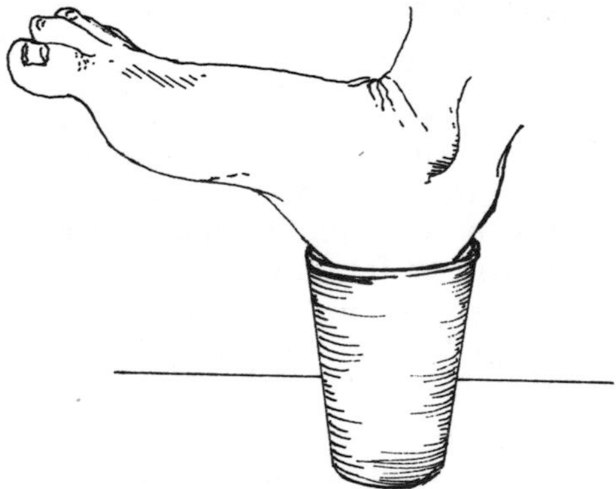

1. When you first have pain, apply ice to the bottom of the heel for 30 minutes.

2. Repeat the ice treatment at least two more times during the day, allowing 30 minutes for each application.

3. If swelling is present, elevate the leg (place the foot on two pillows above the level of the heart) as much as possible until the swelling diminishes. Plan on at least two days of rest from excessive standing, walking and/or running once the swelling has disappeared. If you swell up again when you try to run, double the amount of rest.

4. Use aspirin to help reduce inflammation. Take two aspirin every four hours for two to three days, then two aspirin every six hours for up to seven more days.

5. Pad the bottom of the heel to help take stress off the spot where the pain is. This padding can go directly inside the shoes. You can use heel cushion pads, sponge rubber heel pads, ¼" felt, or a piece of indoor/outdoor carpeting cut to the shape of the heel. Whenever you add a heel raise to an inlay or a shoe, you should do so for *both* feet, unless you are compensating for a leg length difference. The pad may be more comfortable if it is shaved down so the front part is a bit thinner (lower) than the back.

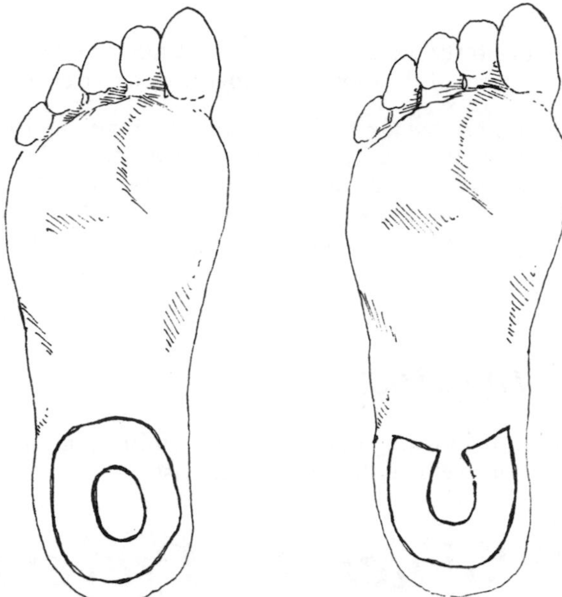

6. Note the specific spot where you feel pain, and cut a hole in the pad, making it a "donut." When in place, it will take direct pressure off the painful area. If there is discomfort because of the depression of the hole in the donut pad, then you can make it into a horse-shoe shape by cutting off the front part of the donut as shown.

7. If the problem is acute (occurred suddenly), it may be beneficial to tape the arches. Wash the feet first with soap and water and then clean them with rubbing alcohol. Apply tincture of Benzoin to all areas to be taped. Strap the area as instructed in chapter 18, steps 4 and 5.

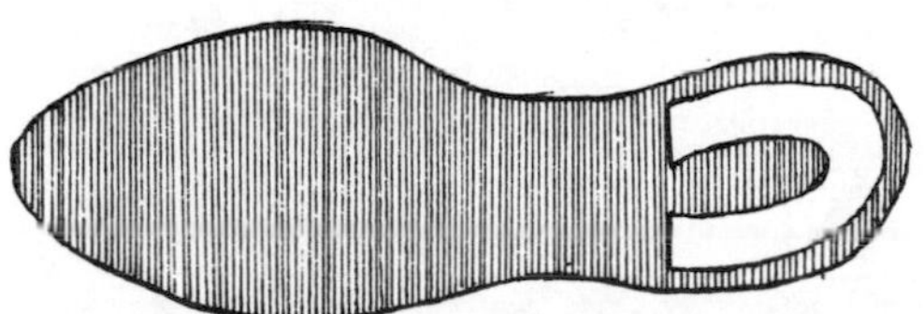

8. If the tape irritates your skin, purchase a pair of Spenco inlays. Put felt padding on the bottom surface of the Spenco inlays (chapter 18, #4), and from time to time, add to or replenish the felt build-ups as they wear down. You can also glue the heel pads you are using onto the bottom of the Spencos, so that they can easily be moved from one pair of shoes to another.

9. If you are bow-legged or have excessive shoe wear on the outside heels of your shoes, add a tilt of up to ¼" adhesive felt to the inside of the heel of your foot or to the Spenco inlay (see appendix on Shoe Inserts You Can Make). You can also put felt directly into the inside of your shoes, in the form of an arch pad, heel pad or "varus wedge" previously described.

10. If the pain is present on walking, keep the foot taped all day or wear the built-up Spenco inlays in all of your shoes. Other commercial insoles and inlays (such as Dr. Scholl's) are occasionally helpful, but making your own by applying felt build-ups onto the Spenco inlays is the most effective.

11. An additional aid to use with or without the various insoles discussed would be a plastic or rubber heel cup.

12. While convalescing, do not walk or run on your toes, as this will definitely irritate the condition. If you have a dull pain when you begin to walk or run but the pain goes away after a little while, you can continue to do so. If the pain gets worse as the walk or run goes on, stop!

13. Do the following series of stretching exercises daily. If they irritate the problem, they should be stopped or done with less intensity. As a rule, do the stretches slowly. Avoid bouncing or making jerky motions. If you feel burning in the back of the leg or bottom of the feet, you may be stretching too far and should ease off a little.

► Sit on the floor with your legs stretched out straight. Grasp your toes with your hands and pull slowly for 30 seconds. Repeat. Do another two 30-second stretches, using a rope around the bottom of the foot for a better stretch (see chapter 35, treatment #4).

14. If you think that you are having heel spur syndrome pain and have tried all of the recommended treatments without results, the problem could be an entrapment of cutaneous nerve branches below the inside of the ankle. For this condition, the appropriate treatment would be to use a heating pad two to three times daily for twenty minutes on medium heat and a varus wedge in your shoes (see appendix on Shoe Inserts You Can Make).

When to Call the Doctor

If you have followed all or most of these recommendations and are still having trouble with pain, redness, heat, or swelling, then see a podiatrist.

Practical Pointers for Prevention

1. Wear athletic shoes with good rearfoot shock absorption, a good heel counter for motion control, and good flexibility in the sole.

2. Make sure the shoes do not have excessive sole wear in the heel area.

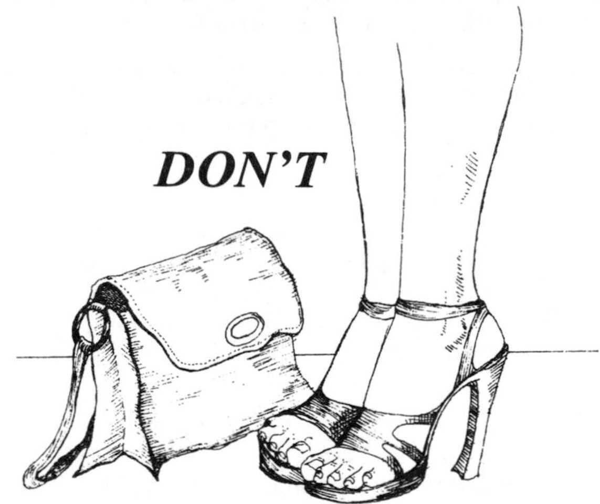

3. Don't use everyday shoes of more than 1½'' in heel height; they can cause havoc with your feet. If you have a heel problem and are stretching the back of the legs in order to alleviate it, the use of built-up heels in your walking shoes will work against everything you are trying to accomplish with your stretching.

4. If you are overweight, lose weight.

20. Back-of-Heel Pain

(Retrocalcaneal spur or *Haglund's Deformity)*

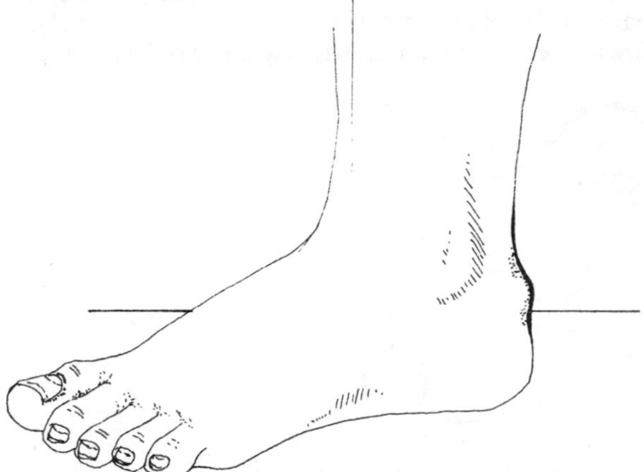

What is it?

A heel spur is a hard, usually painful area at the back of the heel where the achilles tendon attaches itself to the heel bone. When you squeeze this area you feel hard bone rather than the soft suppleness of the achilles tendon. Typically, the pain is not associated with any redness or blistering and is not brought on by squeezing the achilles tendon itself. The pain is usually located right below the achilles tendon where it attaches to the heel bone.

A Haglund's Deformity (pump bump) is an enlargement of the back of the heel bone. In many cases the pain in the heel is due to a bursitis which was in turn caused by the spur or Haglund's Deformity. The following treatment is applicable to all conditions associated with pain in the back of the heel, except blistering (chapter 21).

Things you will need for this treatment

see chapter 2 "Materials List" for brand names and substitutes
soap & water
ice bag
aspirin
rope
slant board
adhesive felt 1/8" to 1/4" or adhesive foam
nitrogen-impregnated foam innersoles
adhesive spray and skin protectant
heel cup

Preparation for Treatment

1. Make sure all the materials and medications you will be using are clean and fresh as discussed in chapter 2.

2. Read through all the instructions which follow, and make sure you understand them before beginning treatment.

3. Thoroughly scrub the entire foot with warm soapy water and a terry wash cloth. Pat dry with a soft clean towel.

Caution: *Do not proceed with this treatment until you have read the Guidelines to Treatment in Chapter 2*

Treatment

1. Rest (keep off your feet as much as possible) for 24-48 hours. Use ice and elevation at least two or three times a day for 15 to 30 minutes each time.

2. Take two aspirin every four hours for two days, then every six hours for the next seven days (or until pain subsides).

3. After 48 hours begin ice therapy and the following exercises. Ice the back of the heel for six to twelve minutes or until the area is numb. Then do the exercises. Repeat the *ice*-exercise-*ice*-exercise-*ice* routine at least once and preferably two or three times daily, until there is no more pain. Take each stretch as far as you can—but if you reach the point where you feel a burning sensation, let up slightly and hold the stretch.

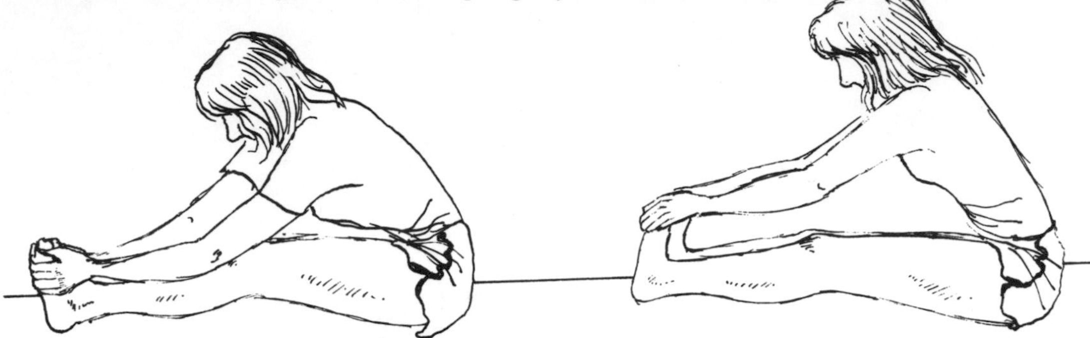

► Sitting down with the legs straight, grasp your toes and pull your feet slowly toward you. Hold for 30 seconds, then repeat.
► Do wall pushes with the back knee bent, then the back knee straight, two times each for 30 seconds. Only do this up to the point of pain (see appendix on stretching).
► Do stair stretches for 30 seconds, twice.
► Do slant-board stretches for 30 seconds, twice (see appendix on stretching).

4. Place heel raises in your shoes, starting with 1/8" and going as high as possible to try to take some of the stress off the back of the heel. A donut pad of foam rubber can be applied directly over the bump. See chapter 19, treatment #6.

5. If you are bow-legged or have excessive wear on the outside heel of your shoes, try placing a varus wedge on the inside of the heels of the shoes (see appendix on Shoe Inserts You Can Make).

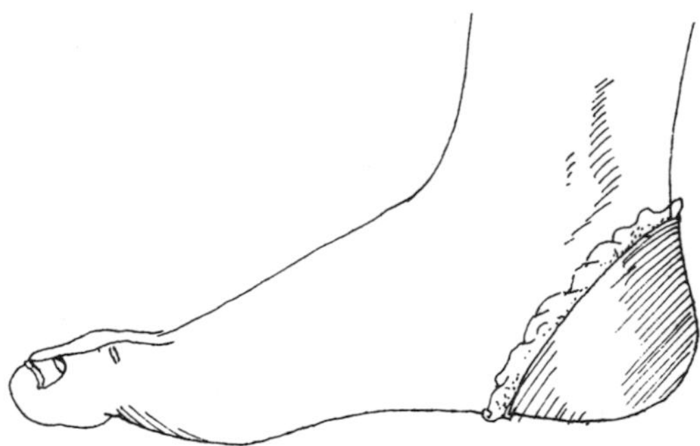

6. A plastic or rubber heel cup can be placed in the shoe to protect the spur or bump. It may be helpful to add a piece of 1/8" foam to the inside of the heel cup.

7. If you feel any pain when you walk or participate in sporting activities, ice down for 15 minutes after exercising. Repeat later on that night. Once the pain is gone, discontinue icing.

8 Do not walk or run on your toes while convalescing, as this will definitely irritate the condition. If you are a toe runner, use a heel raise made of ¼" felt thinned down in front.

9. If a dull pain occurs when you begin to walk or run, but disappears after a few minutes, you may continue. If the pain gets worse as you go on, stop!

When to Call the Doctor

If you have followed most of these recommendations and are still having trouble and there is pain, redness, or heat, then see a podiatrist. After four days, if the heel is swollen, see a podiatrist.

21. Blistering in Back of Heel

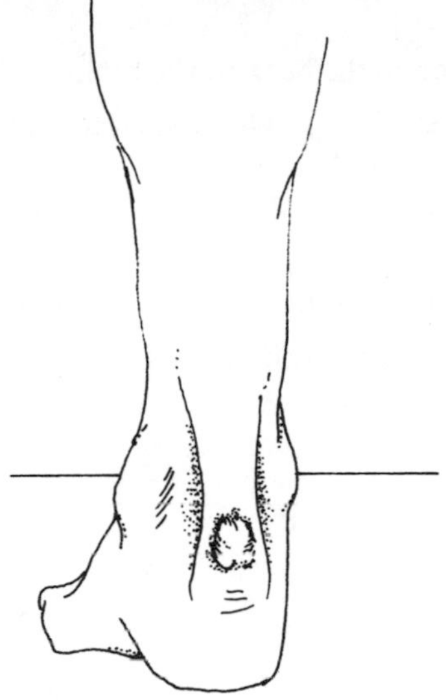

What is it?

Blistering in the back of the heel is a condition that can lead to painful retrocalcaneal bursitis and eventually to heel spurs on the back of the heel (chapter 20), if irritation is prolonged. It occurs when the skin at the back of the heel is caught between the pressures of the shoe counter (the back of the shoe) and the side-to-side motion of the heel bone. Immediate treatment may help to prevent progression to these more serious chronic conditions.

Things you will need for this treatment

see chapter 2 "Materials List" for brand names and substitutes

soap & water
ice bag
adhesive felt 1/8" and 1/4"
petroleum jelly
2"x2" gauze pads
adhesive tape 1½"
nitrogen-impregnated foam innersoles
adhesive spray and skin protectant
slant board
sole patching material
glue gun
rubber tips

Caution: *Do not proceed with this treatment until you have read the Guidelines to Treatment in Chapter 2*

Preparation for Treatment

1. Make sure all the materials and medications you will be using are clean and fresh as discussed in chapter 2.

2. Read through all the instructions which follow, and make sure you understand them before beginning treatment.

3. Thoroughly scrub the entire foot with warm soapy water and a terry wash cloth. Pat dry with a soft clean towel.

Treatment

1. Apply ice and compression to the back of the heel.

2. Take a sterile pin (or the sterile tip of a scissors) and puncture the blister several times around its outer edges (see chapter 31).

To sterilize the pin or scissors' tip (a) place a lighted match to the tip, or (b) dip it into alcohol.

3. Squeeze the fluid out of the sides by applying gentle pressure to the top of the blister.

4. Leave the roof intact and clean with alcohol or soap and water, and pat dry with a soft clean towel.

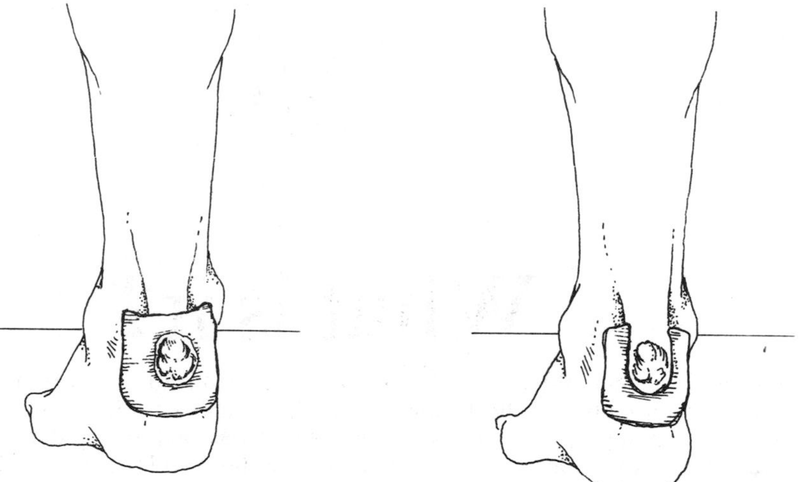

5. Cut a piece of 1/8'' felt into a donut or ''U'' shape a little larger than the blister.

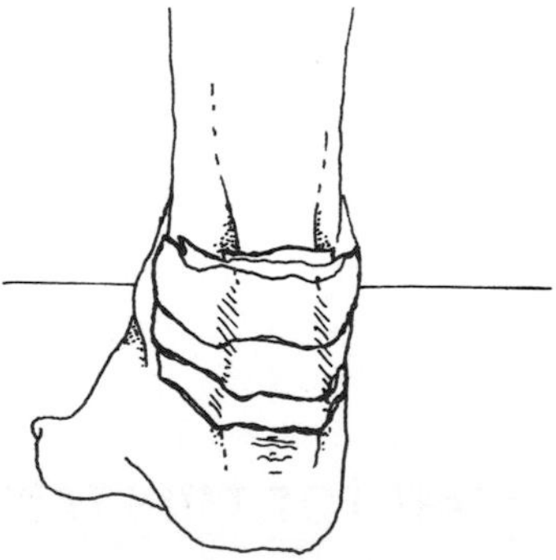

6. Lubricate the heel with vaseline or A&D ointment. Cover with gauze and tape down. Leave in place (replace if necessary) for about a week.

7. Check to see if there is a seam on the inside part of the heel counter of the shoe that is causing this irritation to the back of the heel. If there is, cover it up with a piece of moleskin or tape, or get new shoes if necessary.

8. Repeat puncture and drainage procedure once a day if the fluid build-up recurs.

9. Sometimes heel blisters are caused by shoes which fit too loosely. If this is the case, add a layer of moleskin onto both sides of the back of the heel to make for a snugger fit. If the shoes are *very* loose, you can use 1/8'' adhesive foam for this purpose, although it is preferable to purchase a new pair of shoes (see running shoe section of appendix on shoes).

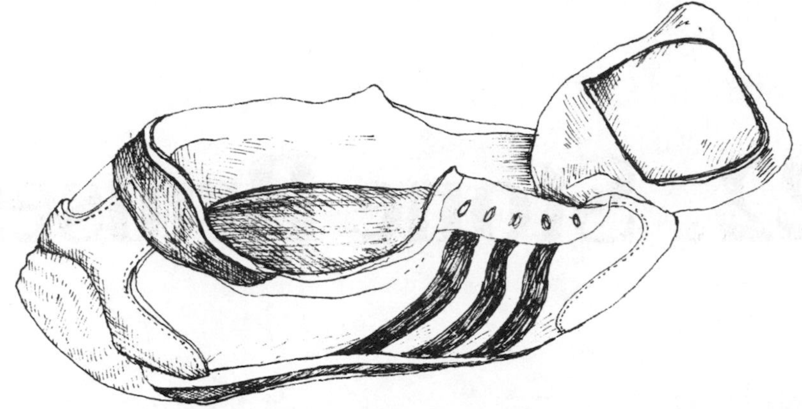

10. You can also try attaching 1/8" self-adhesive foam or felt to the underside of the tongue, if the shoe style allows.

11. If irritation persists, add a pair of Spenco insoles to raise or change the position of the heel against the inside of the counter of the shoe. You can use a heel raise to elevate and change the position of the back of the heel in relation to the heel counter. Make sure you do the same to both shoes, so that you do not cause an imbalance. The heel raise should be made out of 1/8" to ¼" felt (depending upon how high you need it), and placed directly in the shoe. It should be beveled down so that the front part is thinner.

12. As an alternative, glue the felt heel raise to the under portion of the Spenco inlay, so that the heel raise can be moved conveniently from one pair of shoes to another.

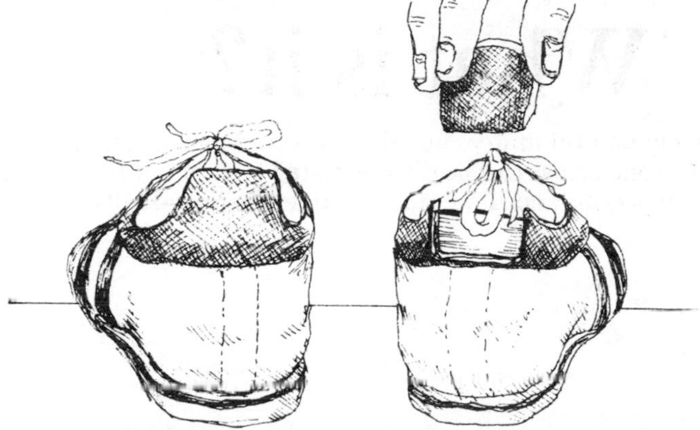

13. If the condition is severe, you can try cutting out the back of the shoe and sewing a piece of an ace bandage to the back of the shoe where you cut the counter out. Any elastic material will do if you do not have an ace bandage. A backless shoe also is helpful.

14. Try inserting a "varus wedge" in the heel of your shoe (see appendix on Shoe Inserts You Can Make). As an alternative, place this wedge on the bottom of a Spenco inlay instead of putting it directly in the shoe, so you can easily move it from one pair of shoes to another.

15. Do the following stretches each day before and after any extensive walking or athletic activity (see appendix on stretching).

- ► Wall pushes with back knee straight two times for 30 seconds each time.
- ► Wall pushes with back knee bent, two times for 30 seconds each time.
- ► Slant board stretches, two times for 30 seconds each time.

16. Once you get the inflammation calmed down, 15 minutes of icing before and after extensive walking or athletic activity should help keep the problem under control. Discontinue icing once pain free.

When to Call the Doctor

If you think you have an infection (if the area is red, warm, or swollen), don't touch it yourself. See a podiatrist immediately.

Practical Pointers for Prevention

1. Make sure your athletic shoes do not have excessive sole wear in the heel area. If they do, you can repair them with shoe goo or shoe patch, or have the shoe resoled or replaced.

2. Make sure your shoes are properly fitted. If they are too loose in the heels, build up the insides of the shoes as described in Treatment sections #9 and #10.

22. Stone Bruises

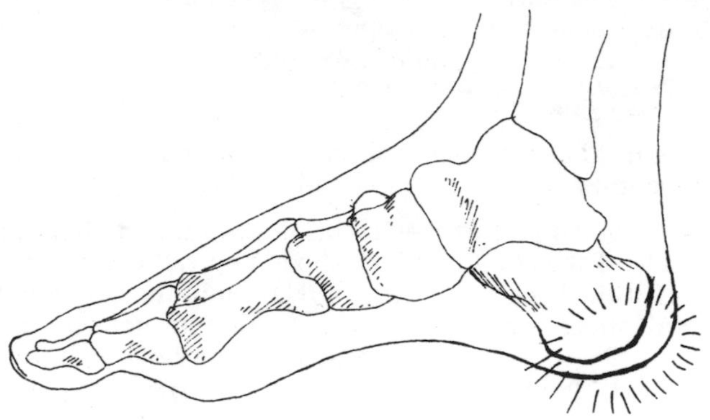

What is it?

A stone bruise is a sharply painful injury caused by direct impact of a hard object or surface against the foot. A stone bruise can be differentiated from other bottom-of-heel pain problems (see chapter 19) in that it occurs suddenly rather than gradually.

Things you will need for this treatment

see chapter 2 "Materials List" for brand names and substitutes

soap & water
antiseptic
ice bag
aspirin
adhesive felt or foam 1/8" and 1/4"
adhesive tape 1", 1½" or 2"
adhesive spray and skin protectant

Preparation for Treatment

► Make sure all materials and suggested medications are clean and up to date.

► Thoroughly scrub the entire foot with warm soapy water and a terry wash cloth. Pat dry with a soft clean towel.

► Read through all the instructions which follow, and make sure you understand them before beginning treatment.

Caution: *Do not proceed with this treatment until you have read the Guidelines to Treatment in Chapter 2*

Treatment

1. When you first have pain, apply ice to the bottom of the heel for 30 minutes.

2. Repeat the ice treatment at least two more times during the day, allowing 30 minutes for each application.

3. If swelling is present, elevate the leg (place the foot on two pillows above the level of the heart) as much as possible until the swelling diminishes. Plan on at least two days of rest from excessive standing, walking, and running once the swelling has disappeared. If you swell up again when you try to run, double the amount of rest.

4. Take two aspirin every four hours for two to seven days, depending on how long the pain continues.

5. Spray tincture of benzoin on the bottom of and back of the heel.

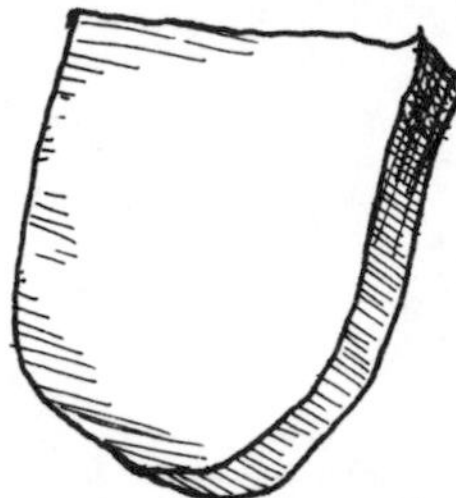

6. Cut 1/8'' adhesive foam to the shape of your heel. Place the pad on your heel.

7. Apply four 6'' strips of 1½''-2'' adhesive tape to the pad, as follows:

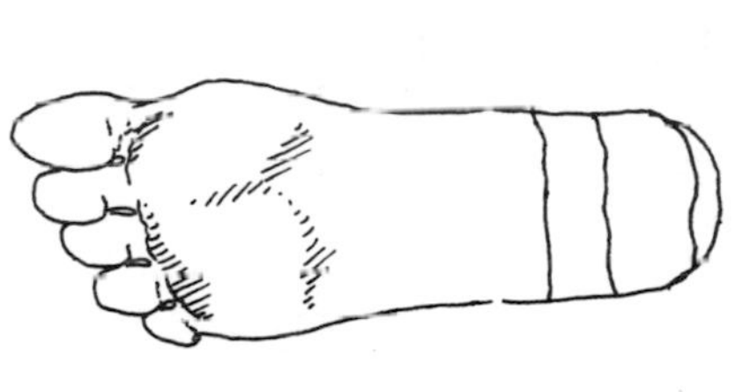

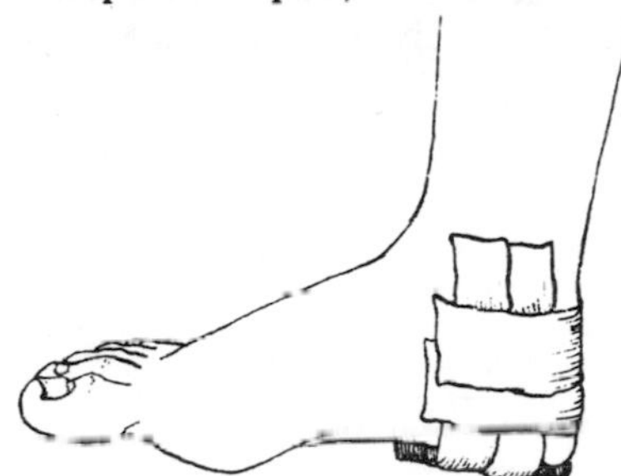

► Center one strip on the bottom of the heel pad and pull upward on both sides, attaching to the sides of the heel.
► Repeat with the second strip slightly behind the first, so that the bottom of the heel pad is covered.
► Center the third strip on the *back* of the heel (starting about one inch up from the bottom of the heel), pull around the heel and attach on the sides.
► Place the fourth strip so that it overlaps the third.

8. As an alternative (or an addition) to #7, place a properly fitted Spenco inlay in your shoes. If you wish, attach the cushion described in #6 to the bottom of the Spenco so that it can be moved easily from one shoe to another.

9. Additional relief can be obtained by using a heel cup padded with moleskin or 1/8'' foam (see illustration in chapter 20, treatment #6).

10-13. Follow treatment steps 7-10 in chapter 19.

When to Call the Doctor

If you have followed all of the recommendations above, and the pain and swelling persist, then seek professional evaluation from a podiatrist to determine whether you have sustained a stress fracture or any other condition requiring a doctor's attention.

Practical Pointers for Prevention

1. Make sure your shoes do not have excessive sole wear, especially in the heel. If they do, have the soles repaired or replaced.

2. When resuming athletic activity, make sure you have shoes with good rearfoot shock absorption and a flexible sole.

23. Cuts and Bruises

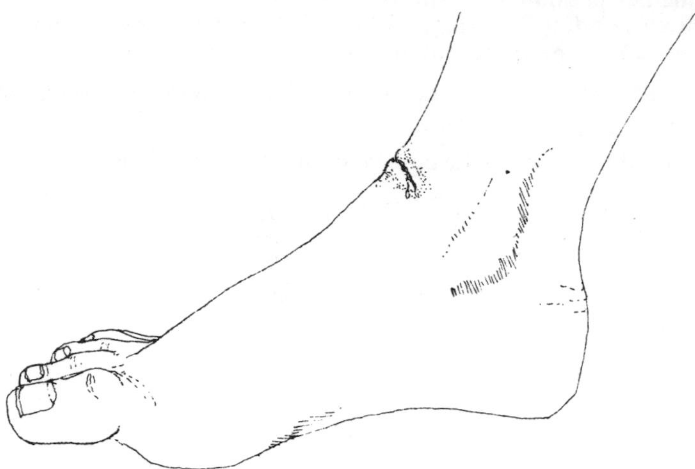

If a cut or bruised area is bleeding, but the bleeding can be controlled within a short period of time, it is likely that stitches are not necessary and that the injury can be treated at home.

Things you will need for this treatment

see chapter 2 "Materials List" for brand names and substitutes

soap & water
2"x2" gauze pad sterile
ice bag
ace bandage
pillows, 2
bandaids ("butterfly")

Preparation for Treatment

1. Make sure all the materials and medications you will be using are clean and fresh as discussed in chapter 2.

2. Read through all the instructions which follow, and make sure you understand them before beginning treatment.

3. Thoroughly scrub the entire foot with warm soapy water and a terry wash cloth. Pat dry with a soft clean towel.

Caution: *Do not proceed with this treatment until you have read the Guidelines to Treatment in Chapter 2*

Treatment

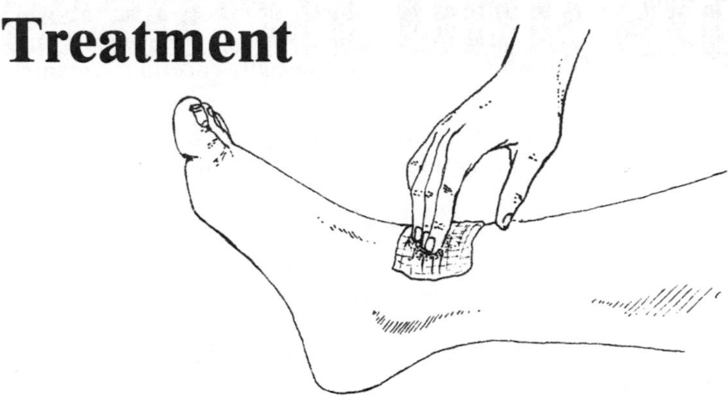

1. Cover the wound with a 2"x 2" sterile gauze pad and apply direct pressure on it for fifteen minutes. If the bleeding does not stop, re-apply pressure for another fifteen minutes.

2. Once the bleeding subsides, place an ice pack around the area for another fifteen minutes.

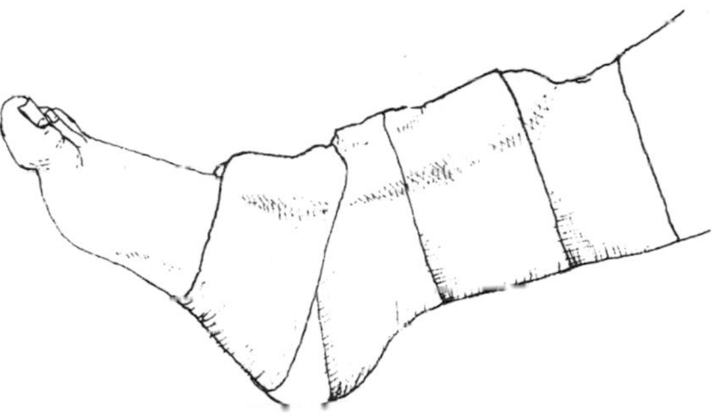

3. Cover the ice pack with an ace bandage and wrap around the area for compression. If mild bleeding continues, keep the foot elevated above the level of the heart (on two pillows) for several hours.

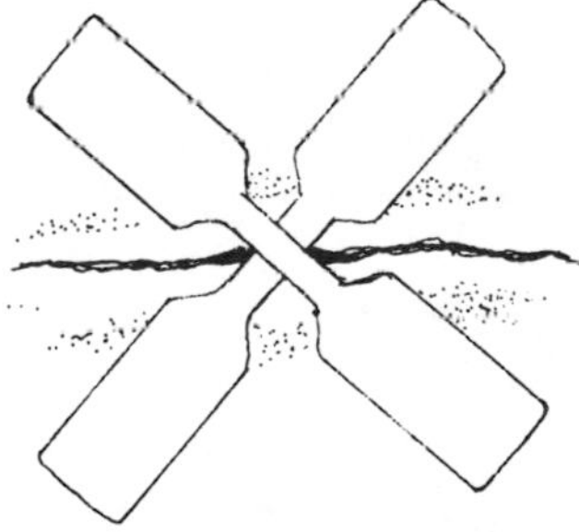

4. Once the problem is under control, apply bandaids in a criss-cross fashion to bring the wound edges together. So-called "Butterfly" bandages are specifically designed for this purpose and can be purchased at the drug store.

5. Ice can now be applied for the next 48 hours if necessary. Inspection of the area during the first couple of days may show some heat and swelling present, but this does not necessarily mean infection. It usually takes from 48 to 72 hours for an infection to occur.

When to Call the Doctor

If after two or three days the pain increases, the area feels hotter, and you see some oozing or pus, then you probably do have an infection. Another symptom of infection would be an increase in body temperature. If you think you have an infection, refer to chapter 15 or see a podiatrist. Don't use a tourniquet for a cut. It will only complicate the problem.

If the Injury Is a Puncture . . .

A puncture is a relatively deep hole in the flesh caused by a penetrating instrument such as a nail or knife. It usually bleeds less than an open cut, because the break in the skin is narrower. Use the same treatment for a puncture as you would for an open cut (above), but let it bleed for five to ten minutes because the wound is likely to be deeper and therefore more difficult to clean out. Make sure that you are especially careful in cleaning the area with soap and water.

If there is any dirt on the object which caused the puncture, you might need a tetanus shot and should see a podiatrist or a physician. Usually a tetanus booster is needed once every five years.

DON'TS

► Don't walk barefoot in city streets, alleys, empty lots, or other places where glass, nails, and trash are commonly found.

► Don't use a tourniquet for a cut. It will only complicate the problem.

24. Cramps

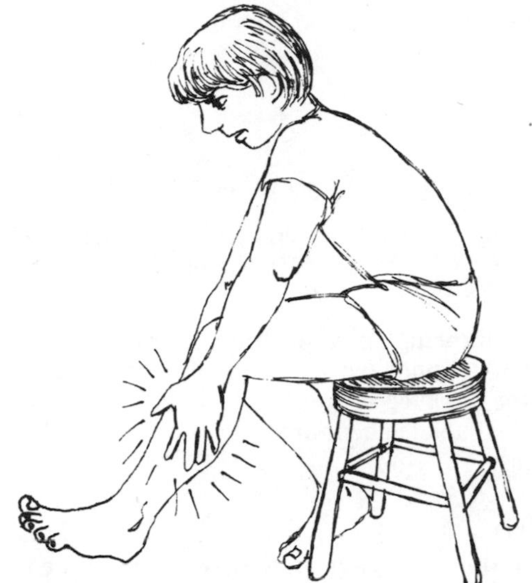

1. "Growing Pains" in Children

A muscle working at a mechanical disadvantage because of *faulty body mechanics,* whether in the back, foot, or elsewhere, is subject to abnormal fatigue. If the disadvantage is large enough, the muscle will become weaker rather than stronger.

Muscle cramps and "growing pains" may be caused by chronic muscle strain and fatigue. They commonly occur in the calves and in the muscles of the feet. They are most often associated with flat (pronated) feet and with foot strain caused by "tight heel cords" in which there is a continuous contraction of the calf muscle. Tight muscles in the back of the legs and thighs, including contracted hamstrings, are often present. Muscle cramps are probably initiated by over-use and over-stress, resulting in a lack of oxygen delivery to the tissues.

Treatment should be aimed at correcting the mechanical abnormality. For example, when cramps are caused by foot strain, the child's feet should be given more support under the arch, and the contracted calf and hamstring muscles should be stretched.

Things you will need for this treatment

see chapter 2 "Materials List" for brand names and substitutes

nitrogen-impregnated foam innersoles
non-adhesive felt ¼"
slant board
weights 2 pounds and 5 pounds
aspirin
baby oil
adhesive felt 1/8"
wet heat

Caution: *Do not proceed with this treatment until you have read the Guidelines to Treatment in Chapter 2*

Preparation for Treatment

► Make sure all materials and suggested medications are clean and up to date.

► Read through all the instructions which follow, and make sure you understand them before beginning treatment.

Treatment

1. Fit a pair of Spenco inlays into the child's shoes.

2. Make a varus wedge, long enough to extend from the back of the heel to the arch (see appendix on Shoe Inserts You Can Make). Fix the inserts to the Spencos, so they can be moved from shoe to shoe.

3. Have the child do the following exercises four times a week. For each exercise, each leg should be stretched for 30 seconds twice (see appendix on stretching).

- ► Wall pushes with the back leg straight
- ► Wall pushes with the back leg bent inward
- ► Hamstring stretches
- ► Toe touches
- ► Slantboard stretches

If your child is unable to do these exercises unassisted, then do the following.

- ► Have the child lie on his or her back, with legs extended straight. Grasp one of the child's feet, near the toes, and push it toward the knee for 30 seconds (if the child complains of pain, ease off until there is no pain). Release and then repeat.
- ► Repeat the above with the leg slightly bent at the knees, for 30 seconds, twice.
- ► With the child in the same position (flat on back) with one leg locked at the knee (straight), grasp the bottom of the foot and the back of the ankle and raise the entire straight leg up as far as possible (if the child complains of pain, pull back slightly). Hold this position for one or two seconds and slowly lower the leg. Repeat 20 times for each leg.
- ► Have the child sit on a table with legs hanging down. Hang two pounds of weight from the top of his foot (use an old pocketbook with a strap, or a paint can with a padded handle, and fill with rocks or other objects to the desired weight). Have the child pull his toes toward his face, without moving his leg. Repeat five times, holding for five seconds each time. Then do the same exercise with the foot turned inward.

Do all of the exercises above twice a day, four days per week.

4. Give aspirin (under age 12 use children's dose), two at bed time and two more as needed every 4-6 hours.

5. If the child walks on his toes or bounces conspicuously, make a heel raise of ¼'' felt, and thin down toward the front (see appendix on Shoe Inserts You Can Make).

DON'T

► Don't allow the child to walk barefooted.

► Don't allow the child to wear negative-heel shoes (shoes in which the heel is lower than the forefoot).

When to Call the Doctor

"Growing pains" should never be written off as something that will automatically go away as the child gets older. They are symptoms of problems that can be corrected at an early age but become irreversible in adulthood. If home treatment does not bring relief from this problem after one or two weeks, see a podiatrist.

2. Night Cramps in Adults

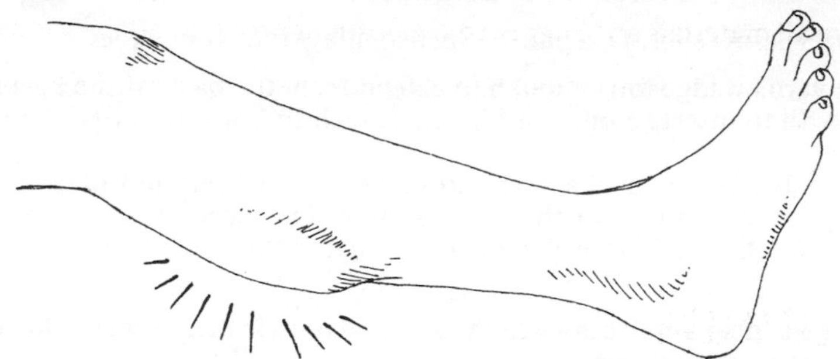

The cramps which occur in the muscles of the feet or legs at night—the so-called night cramps—are not symptoms of circulatory disorders of any kind. (Cramps occurring from poor circulation occur only as a result of exercise, and promptly disappear after a period of rest). Night cramps occur only during rest, and most often in bed. These muscle cramps are usually brought on by a sudden, exaggerated stretching of a muscle against little or no resistance from other muscles. They most commonly occur in the calf muscles (the strong muscle group in the back of the lower leg), but can also occur in the arch and toes.

Treatment

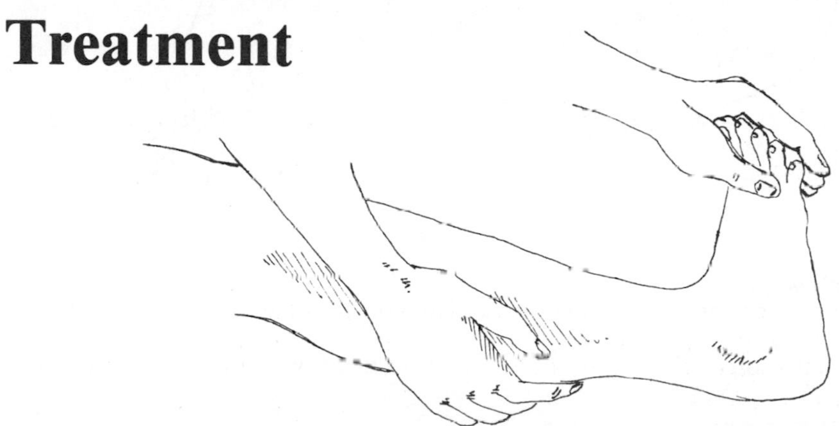

1. Immediate relief can be obtained by grasping the cramped limb with the hands and slowly but firmly helping it move in the opposite direction from the way the cramps have made it move.

► For calf muscle cramping (when the calf muscle knots up), grasp the foot with one hand and the calf with the other and slowly pull the foot upward (toward the leg). Hold this position until the calf muscle knot is released.

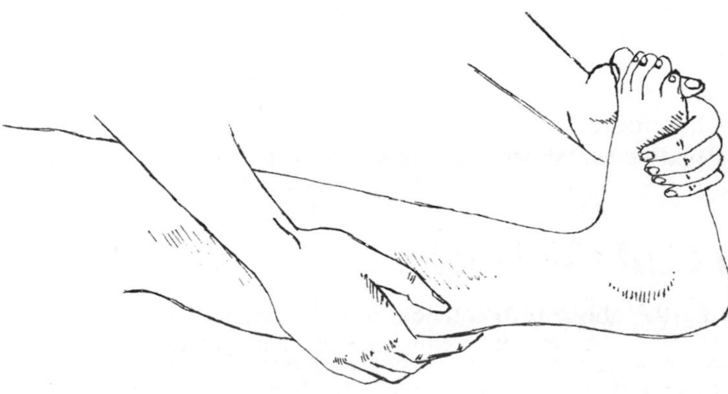

► For arch or toe cramping, hold the arch with one hand and toes with the other, and slowly pull the toes and the foot toward your face. Hold this position until the cramping sensation disappears.

2. Take some baby oil, apply liberally to the cramped area and gently massage the calf, arch, and/or toes for five to ten minutes with a back and forth motion.

3. Take two aspirin immediately and two more after four hours.

4. For longer term relief, fit a pair of Spenco inlays into your shoes.

5. Make a varus wedge long enough to extend from the back of the heel to the arch (see appendix on Shoe Inserts You Can Make). Attach to bottom of Spenco inlays in proper position:

► For calf cramps, add a heel pad made of 1/8" felt and place on top the varus wedging on the bottom of the Spenco inlay. This heel pad is made by cutting 1/8" felt into the shape of the heel, and attaching it to the bottom of the varus wedge at the heel.

6. Apply moist heat applications to the affected muscle three times a day until there is no trace of cramping (see chapter 2).

7. Do the following exercises four to seven days a week. For each exercise, each leg should be stretched for 30 seconds twice (see appendix on stretching).

► Wall pushes with the back leg straight
► Wall pushes with the back leg knee bent inward.
► Hamstring stretches
► Toe Touches

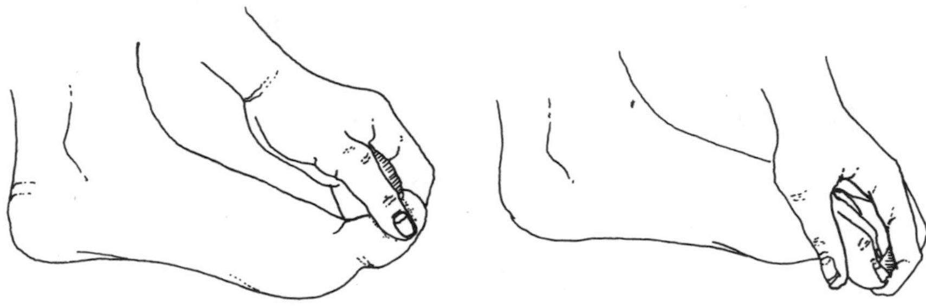

For Arch and/or Toe Cramps Only:

► With your weight off your feet (sitting or lying on your back), move your toes up and down as far as possible ten times in each direction.

► From a flat-footed standing position, move up and down on your toes 10 to 20 times.

For Calf Cramps Only:

► Sit on a table with legs hanging down. Hang five pounds of weight from the top of your foot (use an old pocketbook with a strap or a paint can with a padded handle, and fill with rocks or other objects to the desired weight (see appendix on Stretching).

► Pull your forefoot toward your face, without moving your leg. Repeat five times, holding for five seconds each time.

► Repeat the same exercise with the foot turned inward.

► Do these exercises twice a day, four days per week.

DON'T

► Don't walk barefooted.

► Don't use negative-heel shoes (shoes in which the heel is lower than the forefoot).

When to Call the Doctor

If after following the above recommendations, no relief is obtained within one or two weeks, see a podiatrist. If heat or swelling are present and/or if you have a fever, see a podiatrist.

Part 2
Problems Common to Athletes

25. Why Athletic Injuries Happen

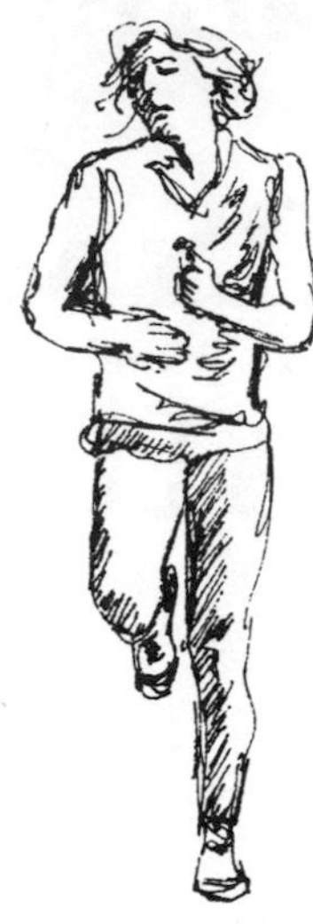

There are now some 30 million Americans who run or jog regularly. Millions more participate in such sports as football, baseball, softball, basketball, and soccer—all of which involve extensive running. Since running is the principal activity in which injuries are sustained in the majority of active sports, the guidelines outlined here are described mainly in terms of running injuries. But keep in mind that they are generally applicable to all athletes.

There are generally five basic reasons why injuries occur with running:

1. The athlete trains too hard or too long, causing the body more stress than it can recover from with normal rest.

2. Muscles become too tight, due to imbalances in muscle strength or lack of flexibility training (stretching).

3. The body is improperly aligned.

4. Improper running form puts excessive stress on certain muscles or joints.

5. Improperly designed athletic shoes do not provide sufficient shock absorption or "motion control" to protect the feet, legs, hips, and back.

Most running injuries are not traumatic or "accidental." That is, they do not occur suddenly. They are usually caused by a gradual—often predictable—overstressing of a susceptible part of the body. Podiatrists refer to such injuries as "overuse" injuries.

The purpose of any exercise program, whether it is swimming, cycling, aerobic dancing, jumping rope, or running, is to increase cardiovascular efficiency. To accomplish this, it is necessary to stress the body slightly beyond its current capability so that it will grow stronger. To be successful at such a program, the athlete must be able to handle stress *consistently*. Many athletes do too much too soon, thereby putting too much strain on their bodies and leaving themselves ripe for injury.

A typical example of "overuse" would be a runner who increases from three miles a day to five miles a day without a gradual buildup. Such an increase means a sudden transition from 21 miles to 35 miles per week—a transition most bodies are not prepared to make without breaking down. Another example would be a tennis player who suddenly increases from two times a week for an hour during the winter to three or four hours a day during his summer vacation. Stress may then accumulate over a period of days or weeks, until a point is reached where one extra day of training, one extra mile, or one more race becomes the breaking point. To prevent such overuse injuries from catching up with you, we recommend the following basic rules of training:

1. *Train, Don't Strain!*
For a distance runner, the key to staying injury-free is to run at a comfortable, relaxed pace at least 75%-95% of the time. If you are running so fast (in most of your workouts) that you can't carry on a comfortable conversation as you run, you are probably accumulating too much stress and heading for eventual breakdown.

If you are not feeling up to par on a particular day, slow down or cut the workout shorter than you had planned. Don't feel guilty about taking a day off if you don't feel well. Doing hard exercise when your body isn't ready for it will do you more harm than good.

Get into the habit of taking your pulse each morning before getting out of bed. If your pulse on a given morning is six to ten more beats-per-minute higher than your average, this may be a warning to take it easy on the exercise that day.

If you have been accumulating a lot of mileage, watch out for the symptoms of over-training: fatigue, declining enthusiasm for athletic activity, inability to relax, insomnia, loss of appetite, frequent headaches, and sore throat.

Overtraining occurs not only when the *amount* of exercise is excessive; it can also occur when the *pattern* of exercise does not permit sufficient recovery. The ideal pattern is one in which each "hard" workout is followed the next day by an "easy" day. If you run hard for two days in a row, you are asking for trouble.

2. *Warm-up*
Before starting to run, do ten minutes of slow static stretching (see appendix on stretching). Start off the run at a *slower* pace than your average training pace. This allows the muscles and body to become loose and warmed up. Run at this slower pace for five minutes, or until you begin to perspire. Then you are ready to increase your pace. Likewise, end your run with a few minutes of "cooling down" at a slower pace. Finish up with a few minutes of walking. *Never* stop suddenly and sit down after a hard run, no matter how tired you feel!

3. *Don't Rush*
When you go out for your daily run, try to pick a time when you do not have to rush. Otherwise you will not be relaxed enough and may be tempted to skip some of your stretching or warmup. A rushed workout will not be as enjoyable and positive an experience as it could be, and will therefore be more conducive to injury. If you run early in the morning, it may be a good idea to warm up with a little easy jogging before you do your stretching, because the muscles are tighter earlier in the morning. Later in the day, you can do your stretching first and then start to run.

4. *Listen to Your Body*
Most of the stresses which lead to injury can be felt, and experienced athletes often learn to recognize the signs of impending injuries *before* they happen. If you feel unusually run down or achy, reduce your mileage for the day or cut your run short and go home. If you have a chronic injury and the area of that injury starts to ache or get tight, this also may be a warning to stop or take time off.

5. *Beware of Training Conditions that Often Lead to Injury*
In addition to inadequate warmup and excessive strain, the following situations are frequent causes of injuries.
Sudden changing from flat to hill running.
Running downhill with too long a stride in order to break yourself from falling.
Increasing your distance too quickly or decreasing your time in minutes per mile too suddenly.
Rapidly changing the type of surface that you train on, especially from soft surfaces to hard ones.
Getting involved with racing before you have had enough background in training.
Always running on the left side of the road, causing the slant (crown) of the pavement to distort your running form. To remedy, reverse directions every other day. For similar reasons, if you run on a track, run counter-clockwise one day and clockwise the next. If you have weak ankles, avoid rough, uneven terrain. The best surface to run on is an even dirt path or grassy field.

6. *Be Aware of Other Factors Than the Training Itself*
Athletic injuries are not always caused by the stress of physical activity alone. Contributing factors may include insufficient sleep, eating habits, excessive emotional strain, and excessive stress at work.

7. *Cultivate Good Running Form*
Run with your body relaxed and erect (*not* leaning forward). The normal style is to land on the heel (*not* the toes), rolling from the outside corner of the heel towards the outside border of the front of the foot and evenly across the ball of the foot to the big toe. When your weight has been transferred from the heel to the ball, the toes "push off" forcefully to propel you forward. Running on the balls of your feet for long distances may eventually lead to injury.

If landing on your heels is difficult, then try to run flat-footed rather than land on the ball of the foot. Your stride should be comfortable. Most people think that a longer stride will increase their speed or improve their performance, but in fact it will only lead to straining and often to injury—particularly in the knees. Your arms should be held comfortably at your sides, with your forearms at right angles to your body.

8. *Check for Faulty Body Alignment*
Improper body alignment can lead to injury. See the appendix on foot structure and function.

9. *Body Type*
The "ideal" distance runner usually has a body type for which two times the height in inches equals the weight in pounds. If your body type does not resemble the ideal, that doesn't mean you can't enjoy distance running or even become successful in competition, but it does mean you should be conscious of your limitations and recognize that it may take a longer period of time to achieve your goals than it might take someone with a different body type. To rush yourself in an effort to match someone else's rate of progress is to court injury.

10. *Other Sports*
Participation on a regular basis in more than one sport can often lead to overload or overstress. Pace yourself carefully, make sure you follow training principles carefully, and limit yourself to no more than three hard workouts a week *in all your sports combined.*

11. *Coming Back Too Soon*
Many athletes, in their eagerness to get back to activity after an injury, push too hard too soon and are quickly reinjured. For every day lost, you lose approximately three days of conditioning no matter what kind of shape you were in. Thus, a two to three week layoff cannot be reversed overnight. To give yourself maximum protection against reinjury, recondition yourself very gradually (see chapter 27).

12. Women who wear high-heeled shoes are more likely to sustain certain injuries. If you *must* wear high heels, try to alternate different heights while bringing them progressively lower (but don't change your accustomed height too suddenly). If you are an athlete, use training shoes with the thickest heels you can get, to minimize the contrast between your dress shoes and training shoes. It may also help to use a quarter inch heel-raise in your training shoes (see the running shoe section in the appendix on shoes).

26. General Rules for Self-Treatment

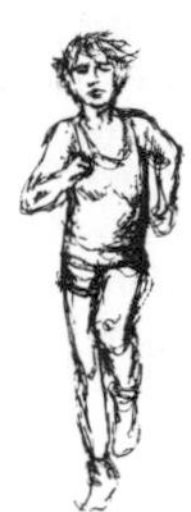

Pain should never be ignored, despite what many coaches tell their athletes. Pain is always a sign that something is wrong, and only by paying close heed to it, can you determine whether it is something you can risk overriding or not. There are four basic types of pain associated with running injuries.

1. First Degree - The pain is present at the beginning of the run, usually goes away as the run continues, and sometimes returns afterwards. It does not interfere with your running form at all.

2. Second Degree - The pain is present at the beginning and may gradually increase, but never gets much worse. It may linger on afterward for several hours. It does not interfere with your running form.

3. Third Degree - The pain is present at the beginning, gets worse as the run progresses (especially with hard workouts), and definitely interferes with running form. The pain lingers on after running and is usually present throughout the day. On easy days, the pain will be present but is usually milder.

4. Fourth Degree - You are not able to run at all. Even walking produces severe pain, and often results in a limp.

General Steps

1. Stretch carefully, both before and after running (see appendix on stretching).

2. Warm up. For the first three to five minutes, run at a slower pace in order to increase your body temperature and get your muscles heated up. At the end of the run, diminish your speed for the last three to five minutes before stretching again.

3. Do not increase your training distance, speed, or intensity until the pain has receded.

4. As long as you feel pain, avoid all of the following:
   - Speed or sprint interval workouts
   - Racing
   - Racing shoes
   - Hills and uneven terrain
   - Any increase in distance
   - Anything you are not used to

5. Wear a good pair of training shoes. Make sure they fit well. Make sure there is no excessive sole wear, especially in the heel area, and that the uppers are not sagging or caving in. If the shoes are new, make sure you break them in carefully by walking in them for a few days before running and then using them for shorter runs initially. Make sure the shoes have good shock absorption and motion control characteristics (see appendix on running shoes).

6. Rest and treat the injury with ice for the first 24 to 48 hours. If swelling occurs, use elevation and compression as much as possible (see chapter 2).

7. After 24 to 48 hours, begin an ice therapy regimen. Ice therapy is an alternation of exercise and the application of ice. First put an ice pack on the injured part for six to twelve minutes or until it gets numb, and then carefully stretch out and flex the part. Repeat the sequence as follows: *ice,* exercise, *ice,* exercise, *ice* (see chapter 2).

8. Take two aspirin every four hours for two days initially, and then every six hours for up to two weeks (see chapter 2).

9. Continue to do general stretching exercises on non-running days. If the injured area of the body is irritated by a particular stretch, reduce the amount of stretching or eliminate that stretch entirely.

10. If swelling persists, recurs with running, or is present after a few days' rest, seek professional care.

11. It is advisable to seek professional care when any injury accompanied by a severe pain does not resolve itself within a few days. Any injury that has not healed in two to five weeks should be seen by a podiatrist even if it started as a minor ache.

12. Any infection where there is pus, heat, persistent swelling and/or redness should be checked by a podiatrist.

13. If for *any* reason you feel that you would like to have something checked out by a doctor, you should definitely have it done. NOTE: If you think that your injury is around a joint, then have it checked within a few days.

14. In addition to the general recommendations above, the following recommendations apply (depending on the severity of the injury) as indicated:

Degrees of Pain

First Degree

Start by holding your weekly training mileage at its present level. If you are no better after a few days, diminish the total mileage by 25% the first week and 50% the second week, etc. If necessary, cut your training to every other day. Do not increase your distance at all until the pain has diminished. Apply ice massage to the injured part for five to ten minutes after running.

Second Degree

Cut your weekly training distances by 25%, immediately. Consider running every other day, and walking briskly on the alternate days. Or quit running completely until the pain has disappeared or diminished to a first degree level. Cut your running pace substantially. For example, if you normally run seven minute miles, slow down to nine or ten minute miles. Apply ice massage to the injured part for five to ten minutes after the run and again at another time of the day.

Third Degree

Start running at a very easy pace. As soon as the pain increases its intensity, *STOP* and easily stretch the muscle groups around the injured area. Then walk fifty steps and start the easy run again. If the pain is present after the run or gets progressively worse during the run, take two to seven days off. Ice for fifteen minutes after the run and one or two more times at another time of the day. Begin to run again only when you can *walk* without any pain. Also try bicycling or swimming.

Fourth Degree

Take at least one week off. Use aspirin to reduce inflammation. After one week, if the pain is gone, resume running every other day, doing 50% of your usual mileage. If the layoff is prolonged, read the chapter on "Coming Back from Injury" (chapter 27).

When to Run Again—General Rule After Layoff

When you can walk with no pain you are ready to jog (nine to ten minutes per mile). If you can jog without pain for at least one week, you are ready to run.

27. Coming Back from Injury

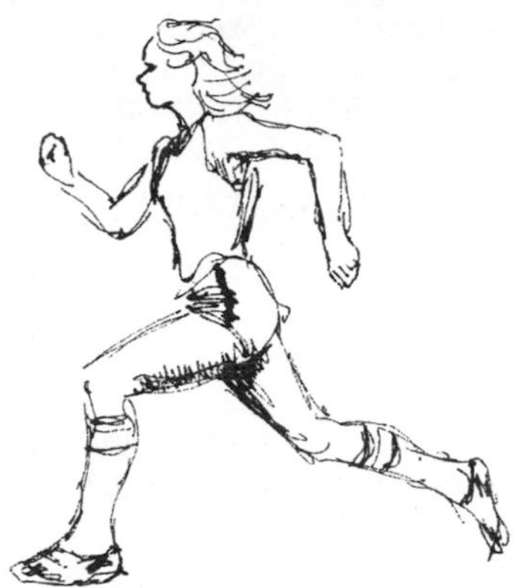

No matter what kind of shape your are in, if you are forced into a prolonged layoff due to an injury, it will take just two to four weeks to lose most of your conditioning. When the injury has healed, therefore, it is necessary to resume training quite gradually in order to prevent re-injury.

General Rules

1. Warm up and go through a full set of general stretching exercises before each workout or run (see appendix on stretching).

2. Wear athletic shoes that fit well, do not have excessive sole wear, and do not have uppers that are sagging or stretched out of shape. If the shoes are new, make sure they are broken in properly. If you are a runner, make sure the shoes have good shock absorption and motion control characteristics (see appendix on shoes).

3. Run on as smooth and level a surface as you can find. Even if the surface is hard, it is better than uneven terrain.

4. Until you are fully recovered, avoid (or go easy on) all of the following:

- Hills
- Speed
- Wearing racing shoes
- Racing
- Uneven terrain
- Excessive distances
- Anything at all that you are not used to

5. During a prolonged layoff, try to find an alternative exercise program to help maintain some of your cardiovascular fitness. This will make the layoff easier on you mentally, and will enable you to get back to your regular activity more quickly after you heal. Here are some good alternatives to running:

► Four to five miles of *biking* generally equals one mile of running.

► One quarter mile of *swimming* equals about one mile of running.

► *Running in a swimming pool* gives the body exercise while keeping weight off the feet.

► Two and a half miles of vigorous *walking* equals about a mile of running.

► *Walking on an inclined treadmill* can help to maintain fitness with a minimum of stress on the feet.

6. As you ease back into running, try alternating one day of running with another day of swimming, biking, or weight lifting—or even a day off.

7. Gradually increase your running days and decrease your alternate days over a two to four week period until you are back in the groove.

8. If you have been off for two to seven days, you can come back at about the same mileage as when you got hurt. If you have been off for two to three weeks, you should start back at about 50% of your previous weekly mileage.

► Plan on no "hard" days (long distance or high speed) for about one month.

► Run at a very slow pace at first.

► Gradually increase your total mileage, by ten percent or so each week, depending upon how you feel. This ten percent can be added to one day or divided among several. But the total increase should not be more than ten percent.

► Avoid racing and speedwork (and don't wear racing shoes) until you have been back at your previous fitness level for a good four to six weeks. Also avoid running on hills during this period.

9. If you have been off for three to six weeks (or longer, depending upon what other fitness activities you are doing and how you feel), you should:

► Start back at no more than 25% of your previous weekly mileage.

► Increase weekly mileage by no more than 10% per week.

10. Increase your distance first, and *then* work on your speed.

11. Review a training log if you have kept one in the past and try to determine whether your injury occurred at a time when you were over-trained, had not been stretching properly, or had not been warming up. You may have noticed some kind of unusual achiness or warning several weeks or days before the injury occurred. Try to determine whether there was any tell-tale pattern which might explain your injury and help you to prevent its recurrence. If you do not keep a training log, it would be a good idea to start one (see chapter 28).

28. Prevention of Recurrence

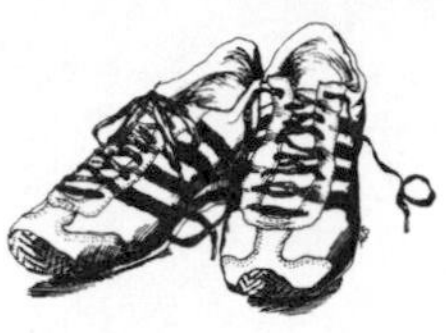

Athletes who are healthy often become careless about the need to protect against injury—which is one reason why many athletes injure themselves over and over again. Because injury most often results from overuse, the harder an athlete strives to excel, the more he flirts with striving *too* hard and going over the fine line that separates superb physical conditioning from physical collapse. When you have recovered from injury, the temptation is to want to forget all about it—and along with it the tedious stretching exercises you had to do so carefully while recovering. To grow careless, however, is to invite almost certain reinjury. For maximum protection against repeated breakdown, follow these rules:

1. Get into the habit of doing good stretching exercises *before and after* running (see appendix on stretching). If you are extremely tight, repeat the exercises at another time of the day. If you run in the morning, be especially careful and thorough with the stretching because your muscles will be tighter and more brittle at that time of day. You may find that your body responds better if you begin by jogging easily for a few minutes before doing your stretching, and *then* start your regular run. It is also a good idea to stretch out at night before going to bed, if you are going to run early in the morning.

2. "Warm into" your run. For the first three to five minutes, go slower than your average pace. This will loosen up your muscles, increase your body temperature, and lessen your chance of injury. It is especially important to warm up gradually when the weather is cold.

3. Wear athletic shoes that fit well, do not have excessive sole wear, and do not have uppers that are sagging or stretched out of shape. If the shoes are new, make sure they are broken in properly. If you are a runner, make sure your training shoes have good shock absorption and motion control characteristics (see appendix on running shoes).

4. If you feel your legs or back tightening up during a long run, stop and stretch. Do wall pushes (also known as tree pushes or telephone pole pushes) toe touches, hamstring stretches, and side stretches (see appendix on stretching).

5. Any major changes in your training routine (increasing your distance, increasing your training pace, moving from flat to hilly country or from soft to hard surfaces, etc.) should be made as gradually as possible.

6. Alternate between hard and easy days of training. Don't do hard workouts more than three times a week, and don't ever do them two days in a row.

7. Don't go for a long or hard run if you are feeling tired or achy from the previous day's workout. Run at a very easy pace, if at all.

8. Don't underestimate your body's needs for good nutrition and rest. Athletes who ignore these needs *always* pay the price eventually. One of the body's ways of collecting on overdue debts is to get injured—thereby forcing the athlete to provide rest which he (or she) would not provide voluntarily: remember that as your mileage increases, your need for sleep and energy increases also.

NOTE: When returning from an injury to a normal running schedule, reflect on past performance to make sure you were not overtraining initially. If you were, adjust your training goals accordingly.

If you have not kept a record of your training program in a log before now, this is a good time to start. Record the following data each day:

- Miles run
- Pace
- Total time spent
- Weather conditions
- Surfaces run on
- Shoes used
- Unusual aches or pains
- Unusual tightness or tiredness
- Any changes in normal routine

29. Toe Jamming

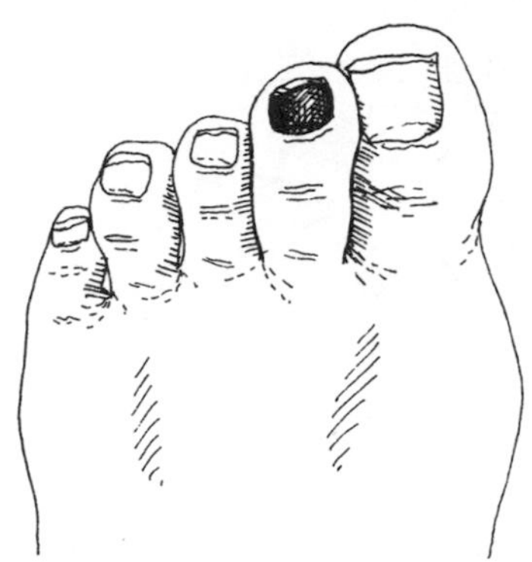

What is it?

Toe jamming occurs when a toenail gets sandwiched between the shoe and the underlying nail bed. The toenail cuts into the soft nail bed, causing it to bleed. A blood blister or blood clot (hematoma) then forms under the nail plate, causing additional pressure and pain. The clot often dries up leaving a blackened, thickened toenail which in many cases will fall off. If left untreated, however, redness, swelling and infection may occur.

CAUTION: If you are diabetic or have an unsteady hand, circulatory problems, a severe infection, or if you are just plain chicken, you had better see a podiatrist immediately rather than attempt to do anything yourself.

Things you will need for this treatment

see chapter 2 "Materials List" for brand names and substitutes

soap & water
paper clip
match
antiseptic
bandaids
2"x2" gauze pads-sterile
lamb's wool
ice bag
adhesive tape
soaking solution
antibiotic cream (if you have any)
petroleum jelly
lamb's wool

Preparation for Treatment

► Make sure any instruments you use are clean. Wash them in soap and water and rinse off with alcohol or some other recognized antiseptic.

► Make sure all materials and suggested medications are clean and up to date.

► Thoroughly scrub the entire foot with warm soapy water and a terry wash cloth. Pat dry with a soft clean towel.

► Read through all the instructions which follow, and make sure you understand them before beginning treatment.

Caution: *Do not proceed with this treatment until you have read the Guidelines to Treatment in Chapter 2*

Treatment

The only way to solve this problem is to relieve the pressure and drain the blood from underneath the nail.

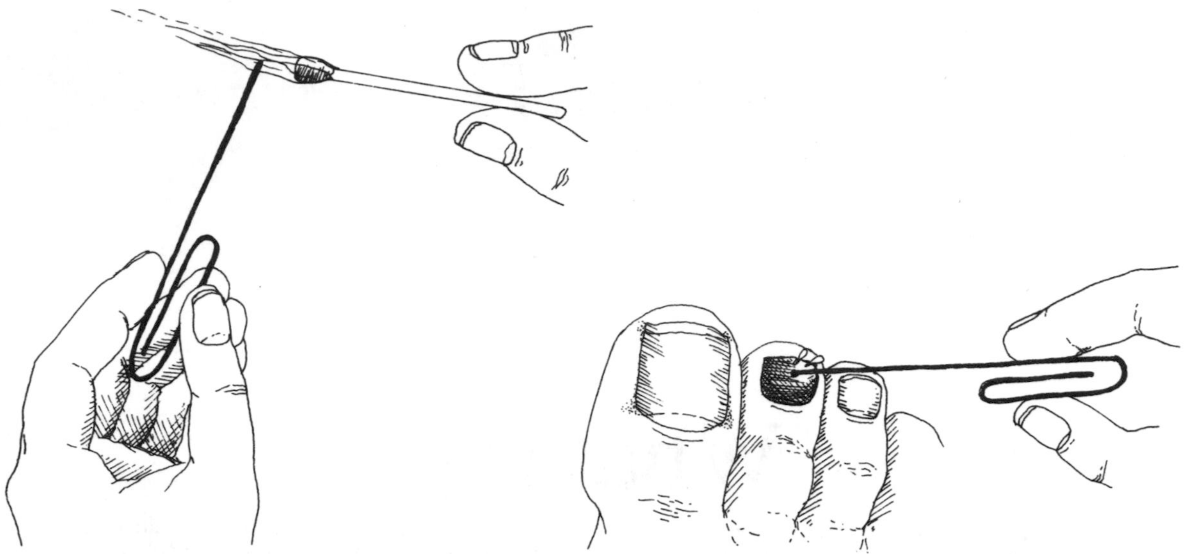

1. *Draining the blood clot...*
   Take a paper clip and heat it by placing it to a match or flame. Then place the hot clip directly on top of the nail plate (the plate has a gelatin-like consistancy and will melt). With your thumbs, apply downward pressure on either side of the nail. The fluid underneath will shoot out through the hole created. It is sometimes necessary to use more than one hole.

2. *After you have drained the blood clot...*
   ► Wipe off the area on the toe gently with soap and water on a gauze pad.
   ► If you have cut the nail bed and there is some bleeding, elevate the foot and apply an ice pack for ten minutes with light compresssion.
   ► Apply an antiseptic solution and place a clean bandage over the toe. You can do this by putting a piece of gauze over the nail plate and wrapping around with some tape, or by using bandaids with the gauze part placed over the nail.

3. *During the next few days...*

The toe may be tender to the touch. If so, treat as follows:

► Soak for 20 minutes in a solution of two Domeboro tablets dissolved in one gallon of warm water, or two tablespoons of epsom salts in a gallon of warm water, or two tablespoons of a mild detergent in a gallon of warm water. Do this twice a day.

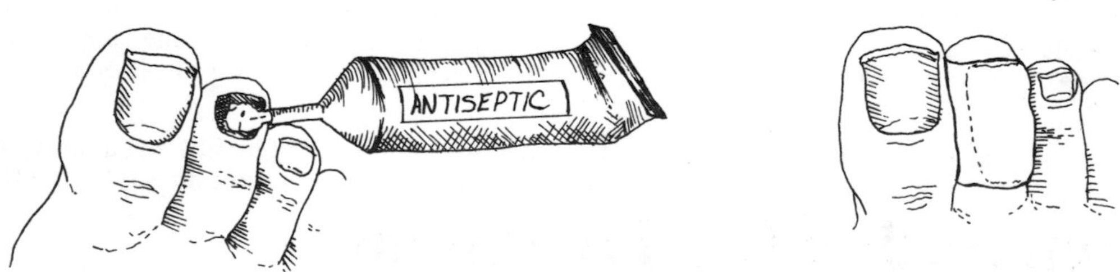

► After you soak, apply Merthiolate (which will act as a drying agent), bandaid and antibiotic cream such as Neosporin (if you have any). If you are going to run later that day or the next day, place Vaseline on top of the nail and around the tip of the involved toe. Cover with some lamb's wool and tape down, using half-inch adhesive tape or some bandaids in a criss-cross fashion with the gauze part over the lamb's wool or the nail plate. After running, clean the nail and toe area with warm soapy water on a gauze pad. Repeat the entire process if fluid or blood blistering has recurred.

► To eliminate the original source of pressure on the toe, slit the fabric of the toe box directly over the toe, or increase the toe box depth (see running shoe section in the appendix on shoes).

When to Call the Doctor

If you think you have an infection, see a podiatrist immediately. If do-it-yourself treatment provides only temporary comfort and the problem soon returns, the nail may have to be permanently removed by a podiatrist through a minor procedure that can be done under local anesthetic with very little pain and almost no disability.

Practical Pointers for Prevention

► Check to see if the toe box of your shoe is too narrow, and if necessary buy shoes with a wider toe box (see running shoe section in the appendix on shoes).

► Check to see if your shoe is the proper length. You should have a thumb's width from the end of the longest toe to the end of the running shoe, and you should be able to wiggle your toes freely.

► Check to see if there are any seams in front of the shoe which may be irritating the toe or the toenail.

► Make sure that the nails are cut, but also be sure not to cut the toenails too short, leaving the skin underneath the nail exposed.

► If you have running shoes or athletic shoes with leather uppers that are stiff and cracked, you may need to replace the shoes.

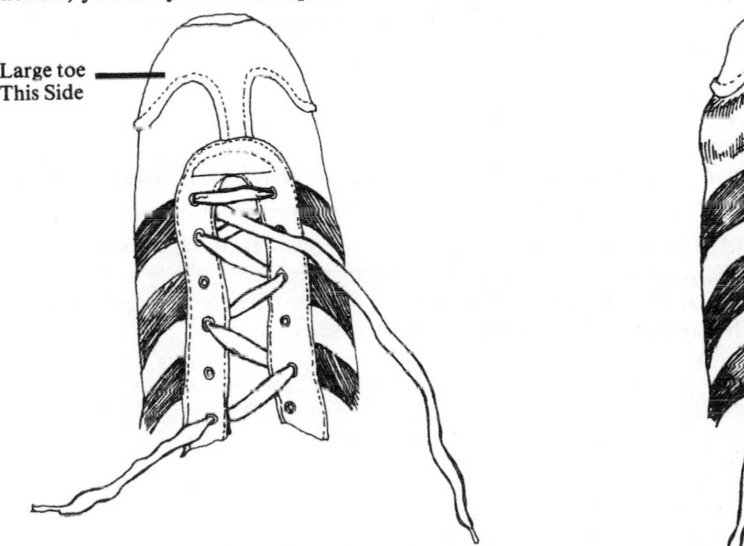

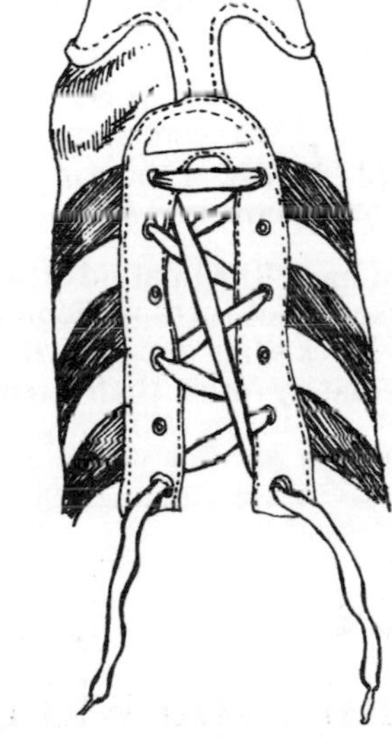

► There is a special way to lace the shoes to increase the space in the toe box area, especially for the first and second and sometimes the third toes. First, one lace is placed normally in the shoe. Then the second lace is inserted into the bottom-most loop and laced directly diagonal to the top loop on the other side.

► You may be able to increase the toe box area of a running shoe by stuffing a sand-filled sock into the front of the shoe. Leave this in the shoe for two to three days (see chapter 17, Practical Pointer #1).

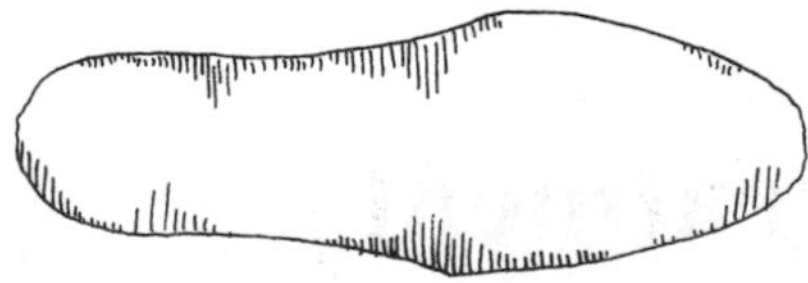

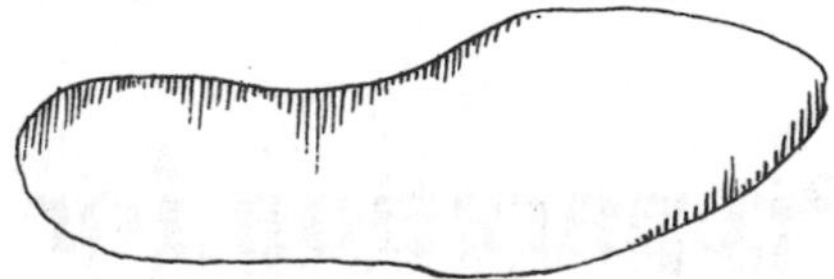

► Try wearing a *straight-last* running shoe instead of a *curved last* shoe. The straight last shoe will provide more space in the toe box.

30. Toe Tendonitis

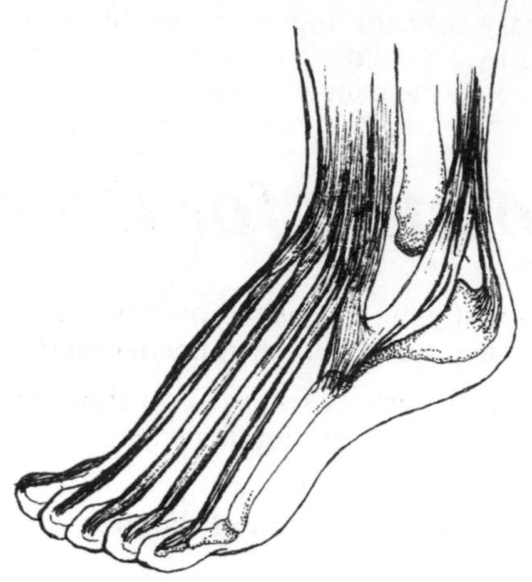

What is it?

Pain which is felt when the toes move, especially when toeing off (pushing off or propulsion in walking and running) may be due to an inflammation of the tendons that connect the muscles which move the toes.

Caution: *Do not proceed with this treatment until you have read the Guidelines to Treatment in Chapter 2*

If you have Rheumatoid arthritis,Raynaud's phenomenon, or allergic reaction to cold, do not use the ice therapy recommended. If severe swelling or excessive pain is present in any of the toes after one or two days of treatment with ice and rest, then see your podiatrist immediately rather than attempt to do anything more yourself.

Things you will need for this treatment

see chapter 2 "Materials List" for brand names and substitutes

soap & water
ice bag
adhesive spray and skin protectant
adhesive foam or felt 1/8"
adhesive tape ½"
lamb's wool
soft polyurethane foam
nitrogen-inpregnated foam innersoles
aspirin

Preparation for Treatment

1. Make sure all the materials and medications you will be using arc clean and fresh as discussed in chapter 2.

2. Read through all the instructions which follow, and make sure you understand them before beginning treatment.

Treatment

1. Apply ice and compression (on thirty minutes, off thirty minutes) as much as possible for the first 24 to 48 hours over the affected toe or toes.

2. Take two aspirin every four hours for two days, then two aspirin every six hours for up to seven days.

3. Immobilize the affected toe by taping it to the adjacent toe or toes as shown.

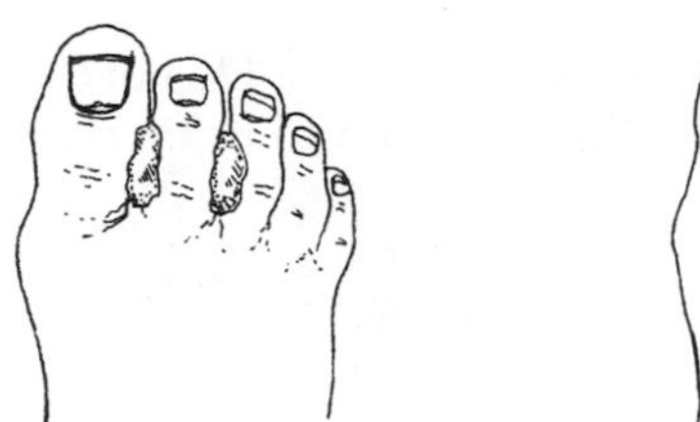
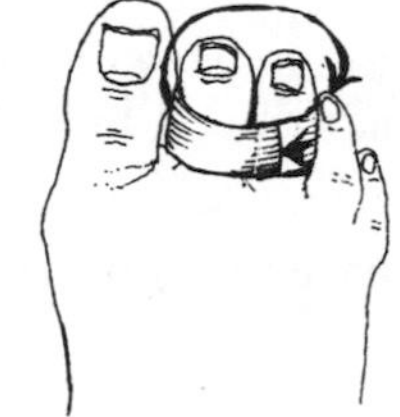

2nd Toe

Place lamb's wool between the first and second and second and third toes, to prevent irritation. Wrap a strip of half-inch tape around the second and third toes, starting on top of the third toe.

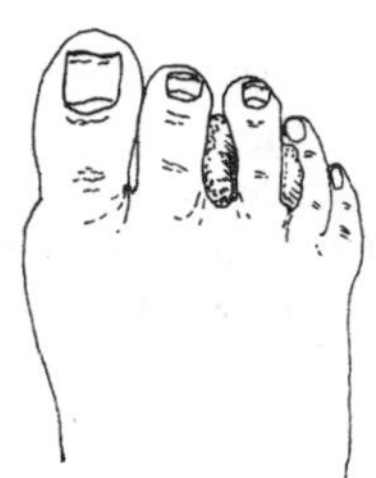
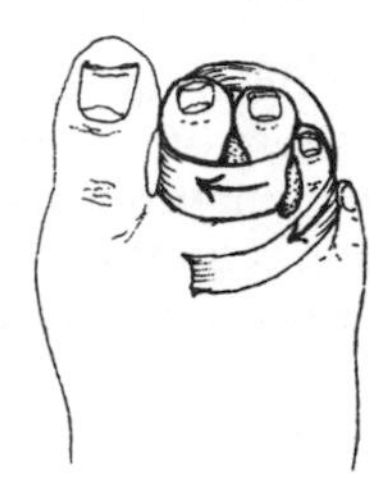
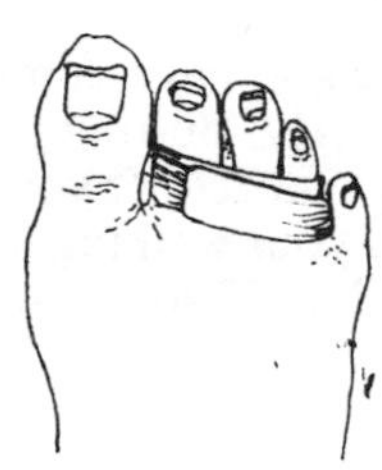

3rd Toe

Place lamb's wool between the second and third and third and fourth toes. Wrap a strip of half-inch tape around the three middle toes, starting on the top of the third toe.

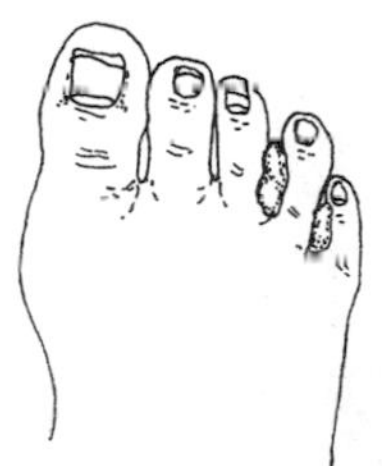
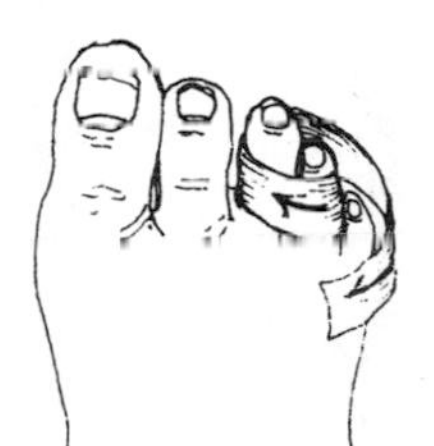
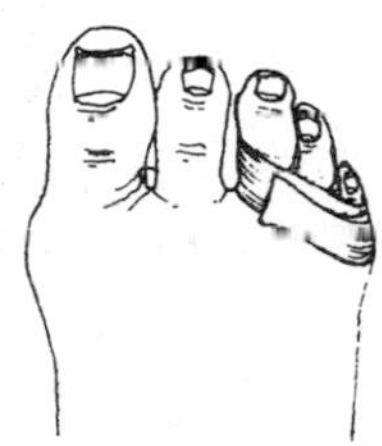

4th Toe

Place lamb's wool between the third and fourth and fourth and fifth toes. Wrap a strip of half-inch tape around the third, fourth, and fifth toes, starting on the top of the fourth toe.

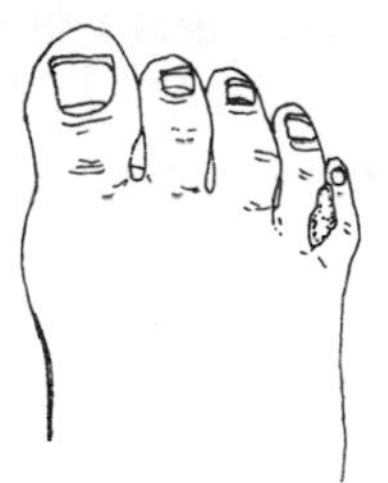
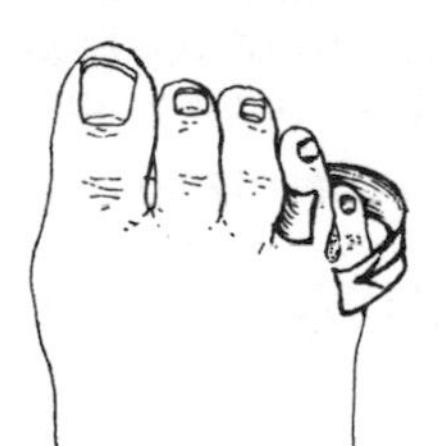
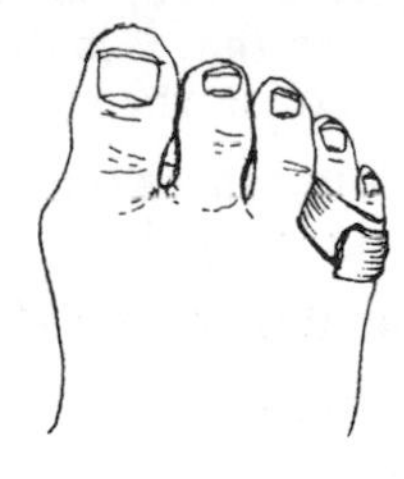

5th Toe

Place lamb's wool between the fourth and fifth toes. Wrap a strip of half-inch tape around the fourth and fifth toes, starting at the top of the fourth toe.

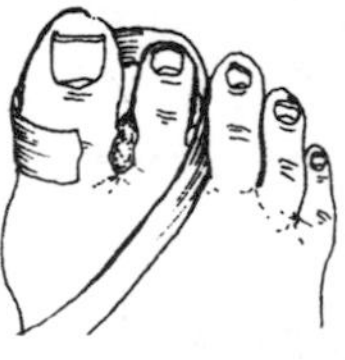
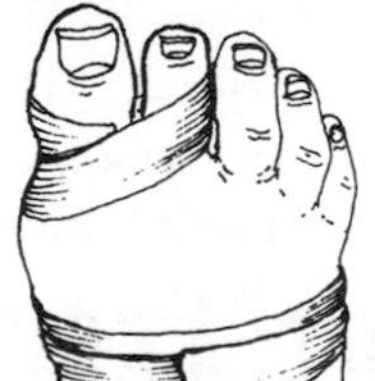
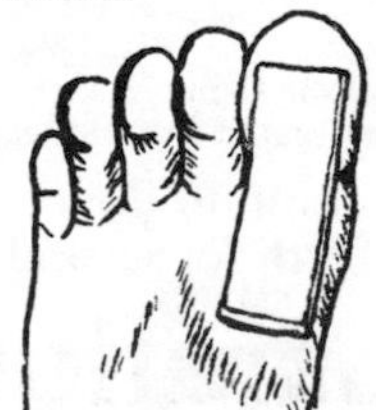

Big Toe

Place lamb's wool between the big toe and second toe. Also place a piece of 1/8" foam under the big toe. This will serve both as a cushion and as a splint to curtail movement. Wrap a strip of half-inch tape around the big and second toes by starting on top of the big toe, going around the second toe, then around the big toe, and finally around the whole foot once or twice to help stabilize the big toe.

4. After 24 to 48 hours of improvement, begin applying *heat* to the area two times daily (see chapter 2).

5. When you are ready to run again or walk vigorously, diminish toe movement by . . .
   ► Using extra socks
   ► Taping the affected toe to adjacent toe or toes as previously described
   ► Adding polyurethane foam to the toe box area

   OR

   Using a Spenco innersole or Scholl's sponge foam innersole to bunch the toes together more.

6. When you start to run, stay on soft level surfaces. Do not land on the ball or the front of the foot, and do not run on hills. (If you prefer to or do run on the ball, see practical pointers #1).

7. Run at a slower pace than normal.

Practical Pointers for Prevention

1. Some people have congenitally tight calf muscles, with a tendency to get off their heels too quickly, putting a lot of stress on the front of their feet. Have someone watch you walk. If you get off your heels prematurely and put excessive stress on your toes (that is, if most of your walking or running is on the front of the foot), this may be the cause of your tendonitis. If so, your shoes may have excessive sole wear in the forefoot (ball of

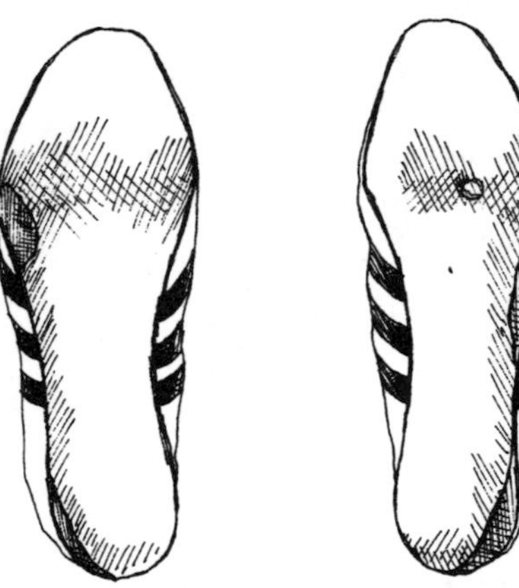

foot) area. If either the front-of-foot walking style or the front-of-foot sole wear is particularly pronounced, put a heel raise in your shoes. Make this raise out of felt or foam, and skive it so that it is thinner toward the front. Raising your heel will help you to put more weight on it when you walk or run (see appendix on Shoe Inserts You Can Make).

2. Do not use shoes that are too narrow in the toe area, and do not use so much padding in the toe area that blistering and friction occur.

3. Get running shoes with good shock absorption, flexibility and toe box depth.

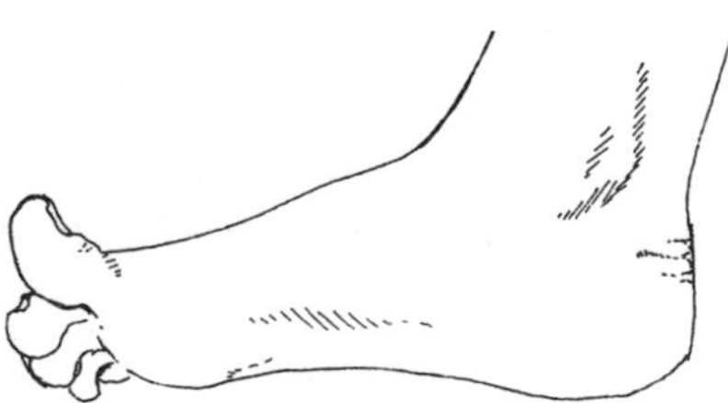

4. In addition to doing your regular stretching routine, stretch the toes or wiggle them back and forth for several minutes before running.

DON'TS

► Do not wear high-heeled shoes.

► Do not use exercise sandals or loafers, because they make the toes work too hard to grip the shoes and keep them on.

31. Blisters

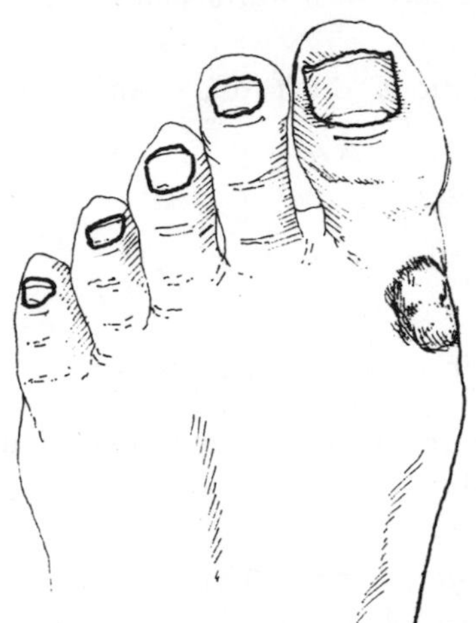

What Are They?

A blister is an accumulation of fluid under the superficial skin surface, usually caused by excessive friction and pressure. The area around the blister is very sensitive to pressure, and continued irritation may cause redness, swelling, and eventual infection.

Things you will need for this treatment

see chapter 2 "Materials Lists" for brand names and sub-

soap and water
antiseptic
ice bag
match
pin or needle
2"x2" gauze pads
adhesive felt or adhesive foam 1/8"
moleskin
adhesive tape ½" and 1" or 1½"
bandaids
adhesive spray and skin protectant
antibiotic cream (if you have any)
antiseptic cream
petroleum jelly
lamb's wool

Caution: *Do not proceed with this treatment until you have read the Guidelines to Treatment in Chapter 2*

Preparation for Treatment

► Make sure any instruments you use are clean. Wash them in soap and water and rinse off with alcohol or some other recognized antiseptic.

► Make sure all materials and suggested medications are clean and up to date.

► Thoroughly scrub the entire foot with warm soapy water and a terry wash cloth. Pat dry with a soft clean towel.

► Read through all the instructions which follow, and make sure you understand them before beginning treatment.

Treatment

If the blister is less than one inch in diameter and you are in no pain, leave it alone. Otherwise proceed as follows:

1. Apply an ice pack to the blistered area (for up to five minutes). This will provide some numbness and alleviate the pain.

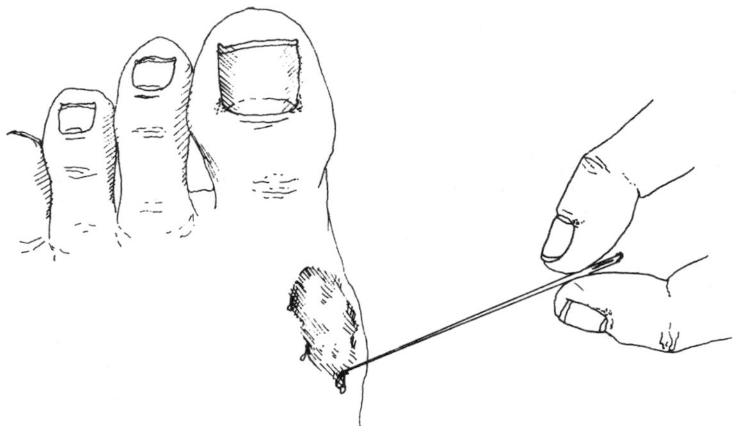

2. To drain the blister, puncture it in several places around its outer edges with a sterile pin or the tip of a scissor. (to sterilize the pin or scissor tip, either place a lighted match to it or dip it in alcohol.)

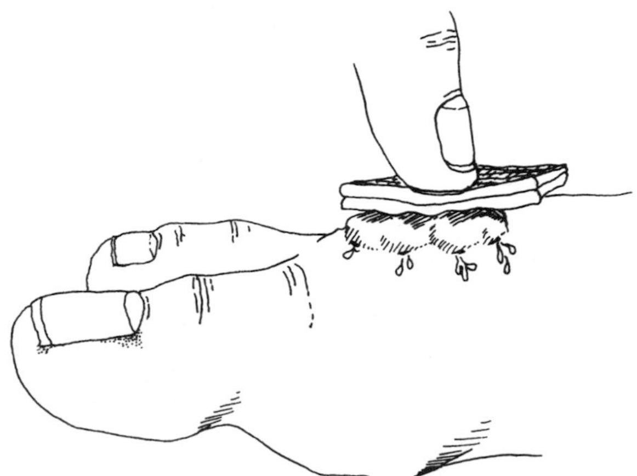

3. Squeeze the fluid out of the sides by applying gentle pressure to the top of the blister with your finger.

4. Leave the roof intact, and after several hours (or when the blister has filled with fluid again), repeat step #2. Continue to repeat once a day as required.

5. If the blister occurs under a callous, use the same procedure as described in step 2.
   - ► Penetrate your puncture needle through the callous itself.
   - ► Keep the callous filed down and under control after the blister has cleared up.
   - ► See chapters 8 and 9.

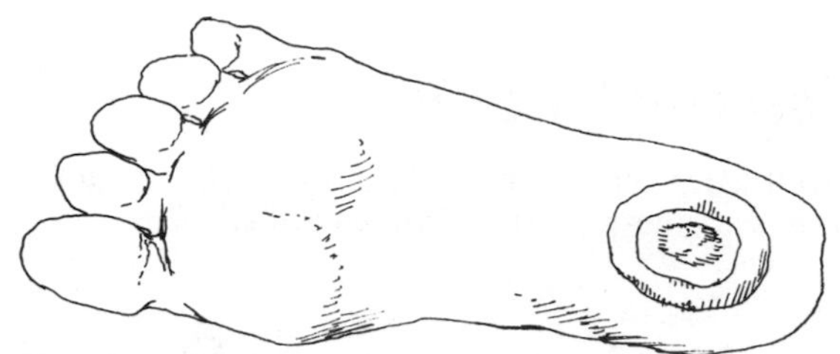

6. For blisters on the bottom of the feet (see chapters 8 and 9 for padding procedure):
   ► Using 1/8'' adhesive felt or foam, cut a hole slightly larger than the blister.
   ► The remaining circle of padding (outer diameter minus inner diameter) should be between ¼ and ½ inch in width.

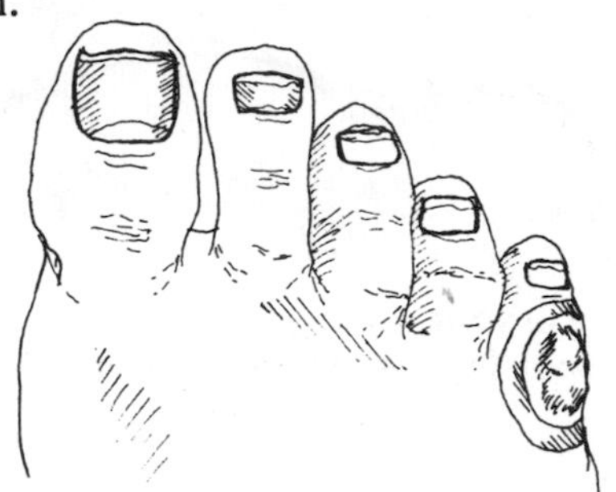

   ► Place pad on skin surrounding the blister.

7. For toe blisters:
   ► Cut a hole in a piece of moleskin slightly larger than the blister.
   ► The remaining circle of padding should be between ¼ and ½ inch in width (outer diameter minus inner diameter).
   ► Place pad on skin surrounding the blister.

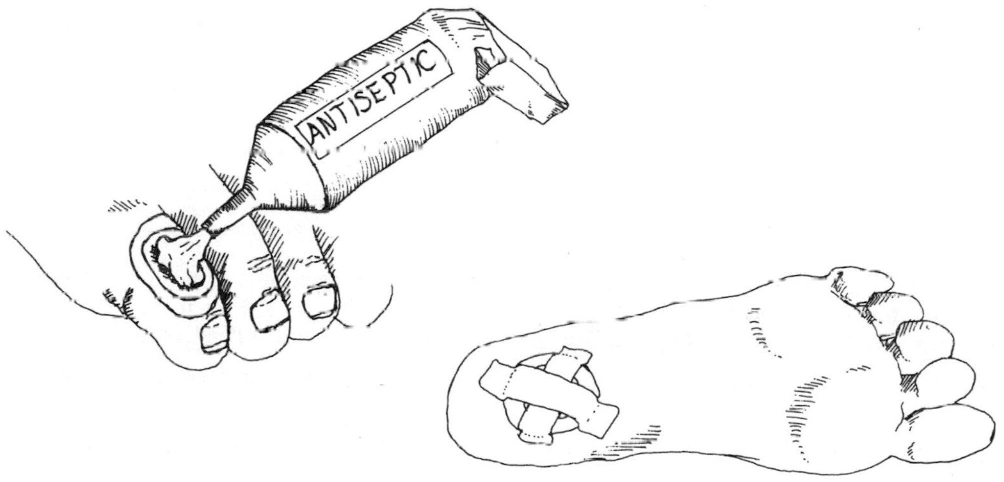

8. Put a liberal amount of antiseptic cream in the opening. Cover with sterile gauze and tape down.
   ► For the bottom of the foot, use 1'' or 1½'' tape in criss-cross fashion.
   ► For the toes, use bandaids and half-inch tape.
   ► For the tip of the toe, one piece of tape or bandaid goes from the bottom of the toe around the tip and onto the top; a second piece of tape or bandaid is placed around the first piece to hold it in place.

9. To help the tape adhere better, spray the skin first with tincture of Benzoin.

10. If you want to continue running until the blister is healed, apply a liberal amount of vaseline over the blistered area.
   ► For the toes: After the vaseline, cover the toes with lamb's wool or criss-crossed bandaids with the gauze pads over the nail plates.
   ► For the bottom of the feet: Pad around the blister as described earlier in the treatment and tape it down (see chapters 8 and 9).

When to Call the Doctor

If pain is not reduced after one to three days, or if you see any signs of heat, redness, swelling, or infection, see your podiatrist immediately.

Practical Pointers for Prevention

1. For toe blisters, see the running shoe section of the the appendix on shoes, for information on how to increase the forefoot and toe space of running shoes and to alleviate the pressure of the shoes on the toes.

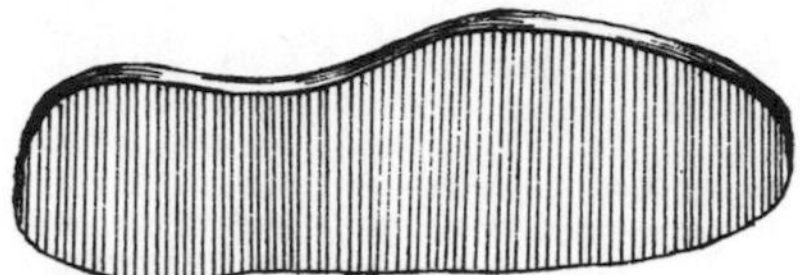

2. Place a Spenco inlay in your running shoes. These friction-resistant inlays can be purchased in your size in a sporting goods store or drug store.

3. Check your shoes for any rough seams or spots which could be causing blistering on the inside of the uppers.

4. If you have been having problems with blistering and are not using socks in your running shoes, start using them now.

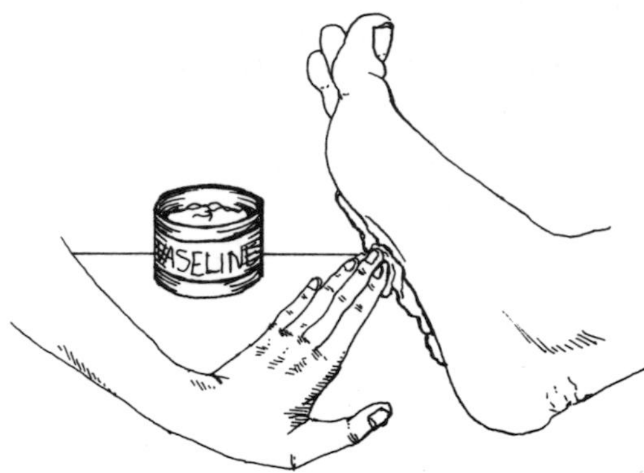

5. Before a long run or a race, especially in hot or inclement weather, apply a handful of vaseline to the entire bottom of the foot. Put a ped or running sock over it, and you will have a good friction-resistant surface. The use of powder can also be effective here.

6. Always wear clean white socks. The best kind is 100% cotton or a cotton and wool blend.

7. If you wear inlays, orthotics, heel cups, etc., be sure that they are properly placed in the shoes.

8. If you are wearing new running shoes, be sure that they have been broken in properly. Walk around with them for several days before attempting to run in them, and then use them initially only on shorter runs (see running shoe section of appendix on shoes).

DON'TS

- ► Don't remove the roof of the blister. Always leave the roof on.
- ► Don't use crinkled, soiled, or damp socks.
- ► Don't use tube socks that fit several sizes.
- ► Don't start runs in shoes that are wet from a previous run.

32. Pain in Ball of Foot

(Dancer's Foot)

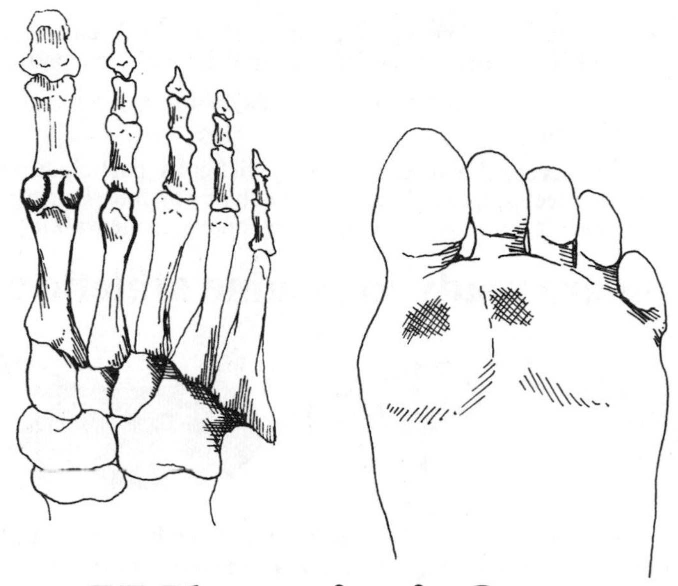

What is it?

"Dancer's Foot" is the name given to localized pain in any one of several areas on the ball of the foot corresponding to the heads of the metatarsal bones. The most common locations are under the head of the second metatarsal bone behind the second toe area, and under the first metatarsal head (sesamoid or accessory bone area) just behind the big toe.

Things you will need for this treatment

see chapter 2 "Materials List" for brand names and substitutes

soap & water
ice bag
adhesive spray and skin protectant
adhesive foam or felt 1/8" and ¼"
adhesive tape ½"
nitrogen-impregnated foam innersoles
aspirin

Caution: *Do not proceed with this treatment until you have read the Guidelines to Treatment in Chapter 2*

Treatment

1. Apply ice for five to ten minutes at the end of the day or after athletic activity. Repeat icing two to three times a day during the acute stage.

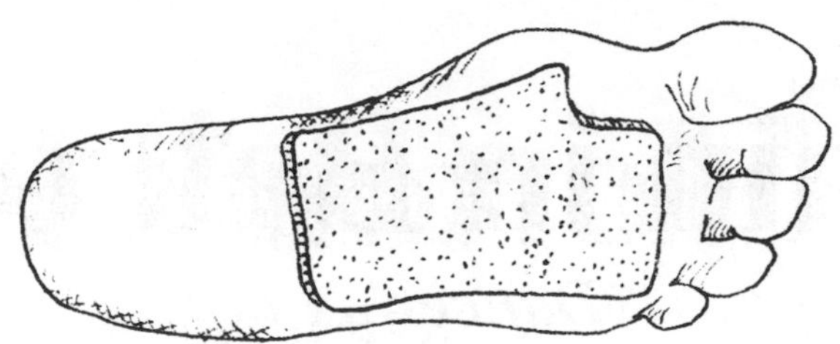

2. During the acute stage, make a pad out of 1/8" or 1/4" felt to remove the pressure from the painful spot. For more detailed instructions on making a pad, see chapter 8.

3. Take two aspirin every four hours for two days, and two aspirin every six hours for up to seven days after that.

4. If the pain is so severe that you are having difficulty participating in sports or even walking, get off your feet and rest the area as much as possible. During this time, keep the area padded to protect it from the pressure of any unavoidable walking.

After you are ready to resume athletic activities...

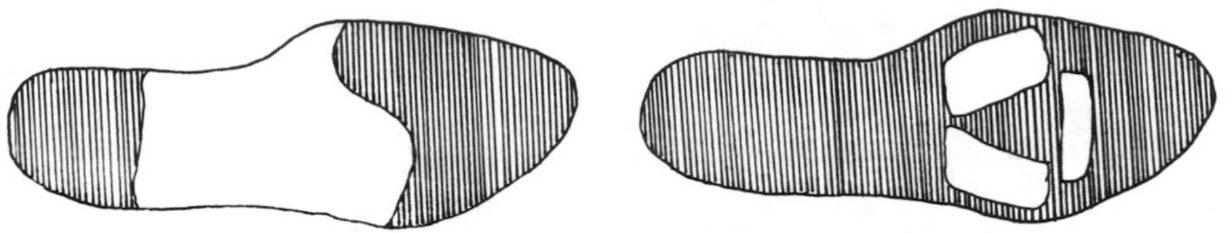

1. Place the padding on a Spenco inlay instead of directly on your foot, so that you can have extra protection while running that you may not need at other times.

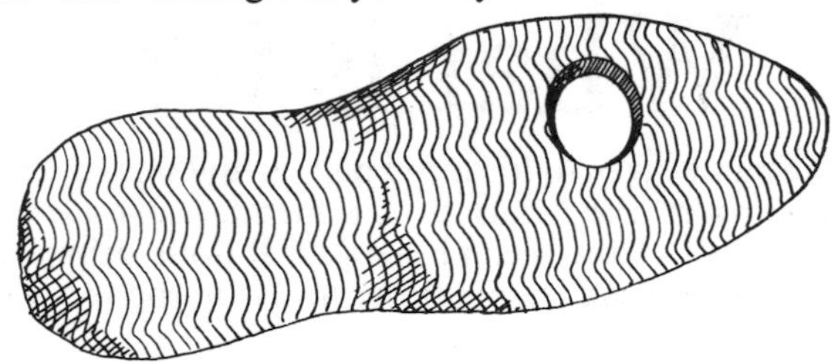

2. Make sure your athletic shoes have good forefoot shock absorption and flexibility. If you are a runner and your ball-of-foot pain is chronic, cut a portion of the sole out of your running shoe to create a depression that will keep the weight off the painful area. This can also be done to most walking shoes. The best type of shoe to use for this condition is a ripple sole.

3. If you are a runner, avoid speed workouts, racing or running on your toes or the balls of your feet. If you prefer to run on the balls of your feet, then add a heel raise made out of ¼" felt thinned down toward the front. The heel raise can be either inserted directly in your running shoes or attached to the bottom of a Spenco inlay (see appendix on Shoe Inserts You Can Make).

4. Do not wear racing shoes until the pain has disappeared.

5. If you are a dancer or gymnast and cannot or prefer not to use inserts, use a dancer's pad taped directly to your foot (see chapter 8).

When to Call the Doctor

If severe swelling or excessive pain is present in any of the injured areas after four days of treatment as described above, then see your podiatrist.

DON'TS

- Don't wear high-heeled shoes.
- Don't wear exercise sandals.
- Don't walk barefoot.

33. Morton's Foot

(Short first metatarsal bone)

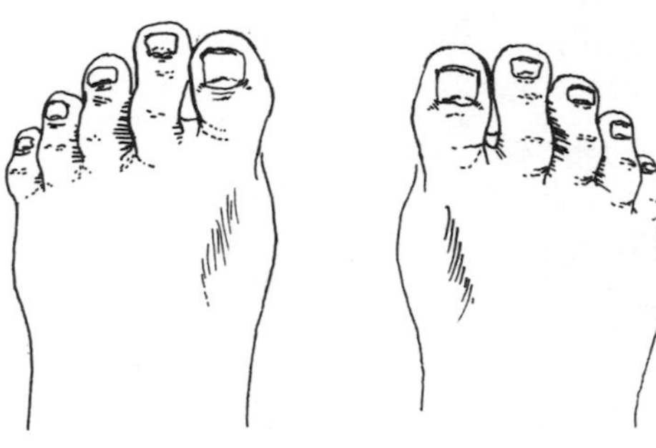

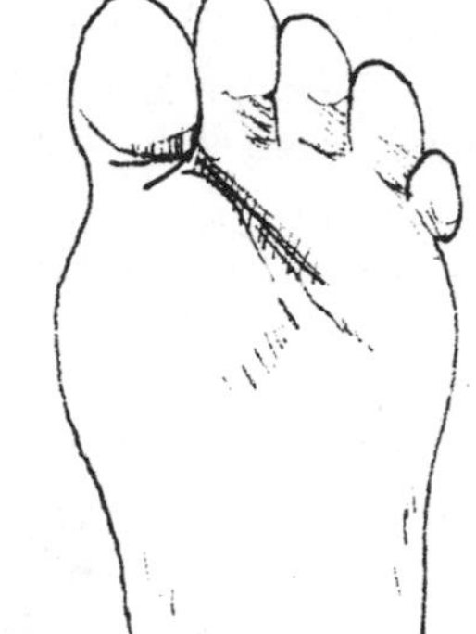

What is it?

Morton's foot is an inherited foot type, a mechanical weakness which is usually characterized by a second toe which is excessively longer than the first (big) toe. In a normal foot, the skin folds behind the big toe are perpendicular to the axis of the foot; but in Morton's Foot they may run at a different angle. There may also be a callous or thickened build-up of skin under the second and third metatarsal heads. In running sports, this type of foot tends to roll in (pronate) at the ankle, lowering the arch and increasing the susceptibility to injury.

Note that Morton's Foot is a foot type, *not* a disease. If you do have a Morton's foot and you want to accomodate it in order to reduce your chances of injury, we recommend the following:

Things you will need for this treatment

See chapter 2 "Materials List" for brand names and substitutes

Nitrogen-impregnated foam innersoles
1/4" or 1/8" adhesive foam or felt

Treatment

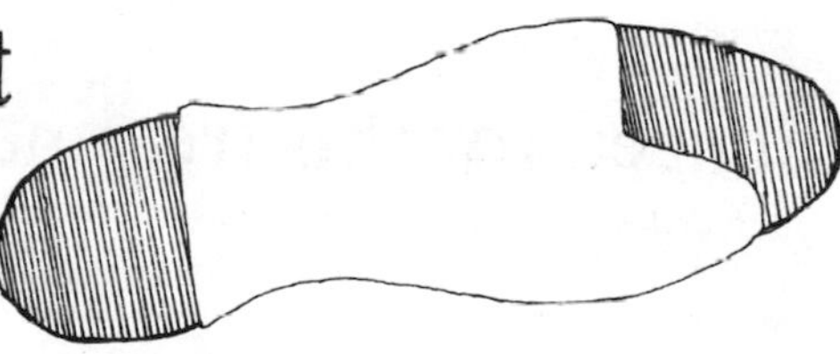

1. Take a Spenco inlay, fit it to your shoe size, and put it up against your foot with the bottom facing the floor. Then place 1/8" foam or ¼" foam or felt on the inlay, filling in the arch and extending it up to the big toe.

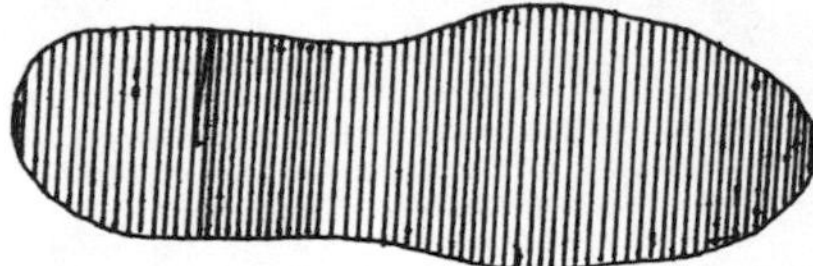

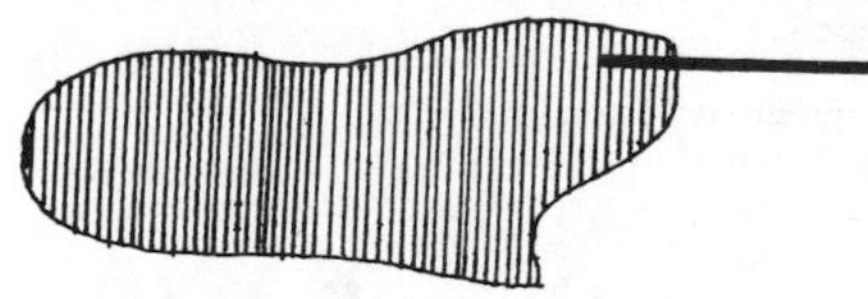

2. An alternative technique is to cut away the part of the Spenco inlay behind and beneath the second, third, fourth and fifth toes.

NOTE: If you have heavy callouses under the second and third metatarsal heads, you can pad around the callouses to alleviate the pressure on them (see chapter 8).

3. If you have Morton's Foot, you probably also roll your feet inward (pronate) excessively and can therefore reduce this abnormal motion by adding a varus wedge to your Spenco inlay. Make this wedge long enough to extend from the heel all the way to the arch. For instructions, see the appendix on Shoe Inserts You Can Make.

34. Bump on Top of Foot

(Dorsal exostosis)

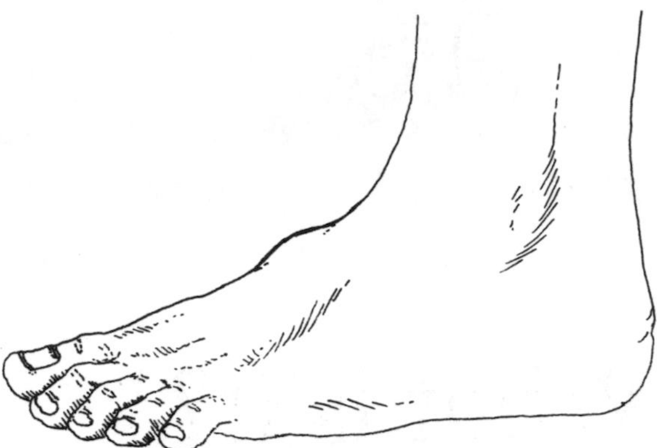

What is it?

A dorsal exostosis is a bony enlargement on top of the foot which can often become irritated and painful.

Caution: *Do not proceed with this treatment until you have read the Guidelines to Treatment in Chapter 2*

Things you will need for this treatment

see chapter 2 "Materials List" for brand names and substitutes

soap & water
ice bag
aspirin
moleskin
adhesive foam 1/8"
petroleum jelly
2"x2" gauze pads
adhesive tape 1½"
adhesive felt ¼"
nitrogen-impregnated foam innersoles
adhesive spray and skin protectant

Preparation for Treatment

1. Make sure all the materials and medications you will be using are clean and fresh as discussed in chapter 2.

2. Read through all the instructions which follow, and make sure you understand them before beginning treatment.

3. Thoroughly scrub the entire foot with warm soapy water and a terry wash cloth. Pat dry with a soft clean towel.

Treatment

1. Place an ice pack directly over the painful area for up to 30 minutes. Continue the application of ice (up to 30 minutes on, 30 minutes off) for as much of the first 24 hours as you can. If the area is swollen, elevate the foot on two pillows while applying the ice pack.

2. After 24 hours, begin ice therapy by applying ice on the bumpy area for six to twelve minutes or until numbness ensues. Then actively exercise the foot by moving it up and down or walking for a few minutes until the pain returns. Then repeat the icing for six to twelve minutes or until the area is numb, and exercise again. Repeat this entire process as follows (that is, *ice*-exercise; *ice*-exercise; *ice*).

3. Aspirin can be useful for anti-inflammatory purposes. Take two every four hours for two days, then two every six hours for up to a week (see precautions in chapter 2). Stop using aspirin once the pain has disappeared.

4. When there is no pain or swelling during walking, you are ready to resume your athletic activities.

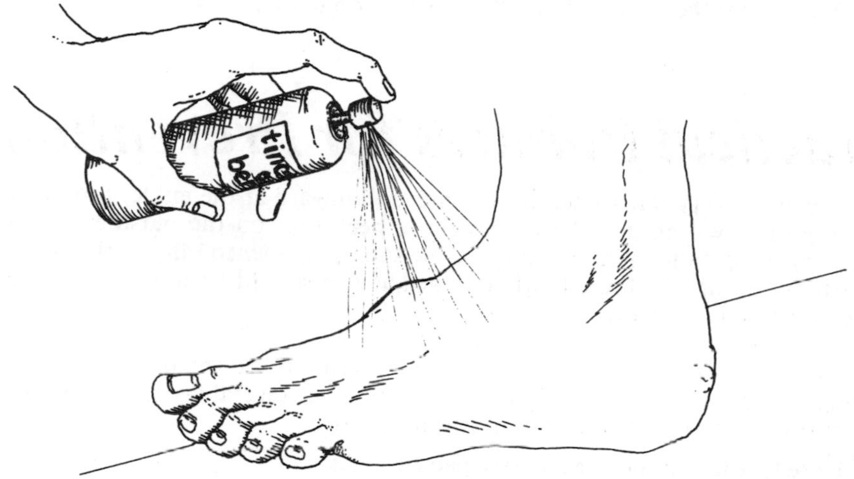

5. To protect the area from further irritation, spray tincture of Benzoin on the area to be taped.

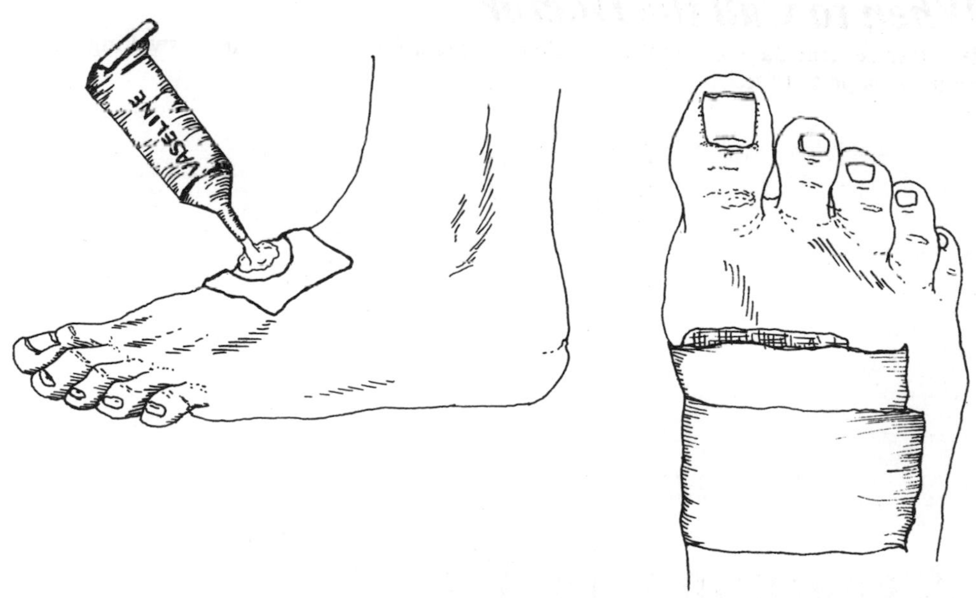

6. Cut a hole in a piece of moleskin or 1/8" foam and place it around the bump. Remember to make the hole slightly larger than the bump itself. The remaining circle of padding should be between ¼" and ½" in width around the bump. Put vaseline on the bump and tape a 2x2 gauze pad over the circle.

7. If pain or swelling returns after a day or two, repeat the ice treatment and rest the foot from athletic activity for a day.

8. If the pain actually makes you limp or interferes with your running form, or if severe swelling occurs, then take two to seven days off with ice therapy daily and aspirin. Pad as above to relieve the pressure on walking and pad the back of the tongue on all of your shoes. Take 1/8" foam or several layers of moleskin and adhere to the inside of the tongue of the shoe (see chapter 21, treatment#10.

DON'TS

1. Don't lace your shoes too tightly.
2. Don't put tape on too tightly.
3. Don't run if there is severe swelling, pain, or limping.

Practical Pointers for Prevention

1. If you are very flat-footed or pronate (roll inward at the ankle) too much, or if you are severely bow-legged and have excessive heel wear on the outsides of your running shoes, try using either a varus wedge in the shoe or a Spenco inlay with a varus wedge attached. If you are flatfooted, an arch wedge also should be used. See the appendix on Shoe Inserts You Can Make.

2. The lacing of the shoe may be a cause of irritation to the bump on top of the foot, leading to excessive pressure. If so, use 1/8" foam or several layers of moleskin on the inside of the tongue of the shoe. See illustration above.

3. To reduce irritation, use an extra pair of socks.

When to Call the Doctor

If, after several days of treatment, there is persistent heat, redness, swelling, or severe pain, see a podiatrist.

35. Achilles Tendonitis

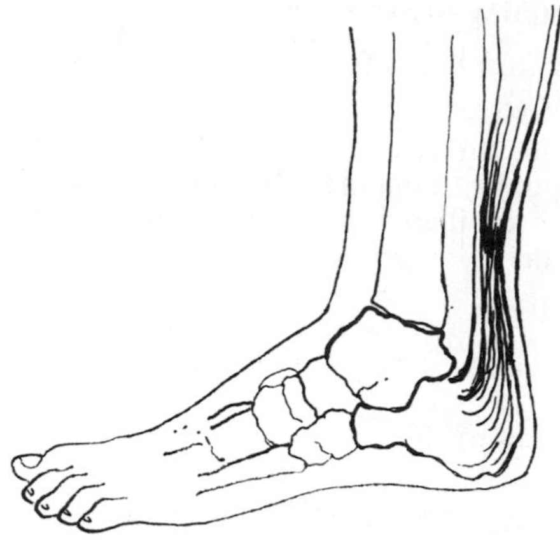

What is it?

Strictly speaking, Achilles Tendonitis is an inflammation of the large tendon in the back of the lower leg. The term is also used as a catchall phrase for several other tendon problems for which the recommended treatment is the same. (The only achilles problem requiring a different treatment is a strain at the junction of the calf muscle and the achilles tendon, identifiable by pain in the *middle* of the calf—in which case, use the treatment for calf strain described in chapter 38.)
NOTE: Proper attention to detail is important because achilles tendon injuries can become chronic if not initially treated properly.

Things you will need for this treatment

see chapter 2 "Materials List" for brand names and substitutes

soap & water
ice bag
aspirin
piece of rope or towel
adhesive spray and skin protectant
non-adhesive felt ¼"
adhesive tape 1½"
nitrogen-impregnated foam innersoles

Caution: *Do not proceed with this treatment until you have read the Guidelines to Treatment in Chapter 2*

Preparation for Treatment

1. Make sure all the materials and medications you will be using are clean and fresh as discussed in chapter 2.

3. Read through all the instructions which follow, and make sure you understand them before beginning treatment.

3. Thoroughly scrub the entire foot with warm soapy water and a terry wash cloth. Pat dry with a soft clean towel.

Treatment

1. Apply ice to the affected area four or five times a day, for 20-30 minutes each time. Keep the leg elevated and rested while applying the ice.

2. If the achilles area is severely swollen, elevate the leg above the level of the heart by propping it on two pillows. Do not run until at least two days after the swelling goes down. If you swell up when you start running again, stop immediately. This time, double the number of days off before attempting to run again.

3. Take two aspirin every four hours for the first two days, then every six hours for the rest of the week (see chapter 2).

4. After 24 to 48 hours, ice the affected area for six to twelve minutes or until numb, then actively exercise the foot by doing the following exercises until the pain returns, then repeat the ice treatment for another six to twelve minutes until the area is numb again, and exercise again. Repeat the entire process as follows: *ice,* exercise; *ice,* exercise; *ice.*

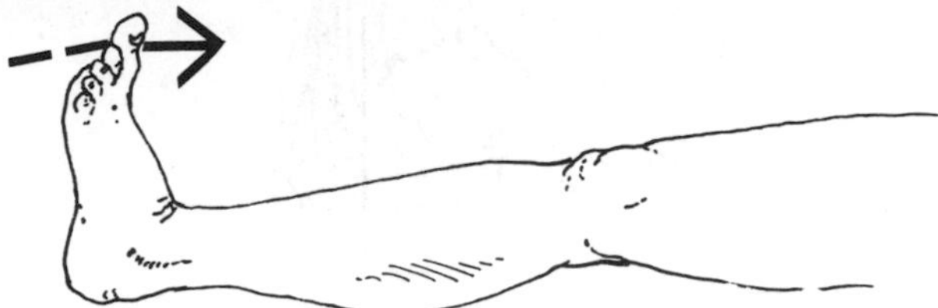

► While sitting on the floor with legs extended straight out in front of you, bend the foot at the ankle so that the top of the foot moves toward your face as far as possible; then hold this bent position for ten seconds. Repeat five to ten times.

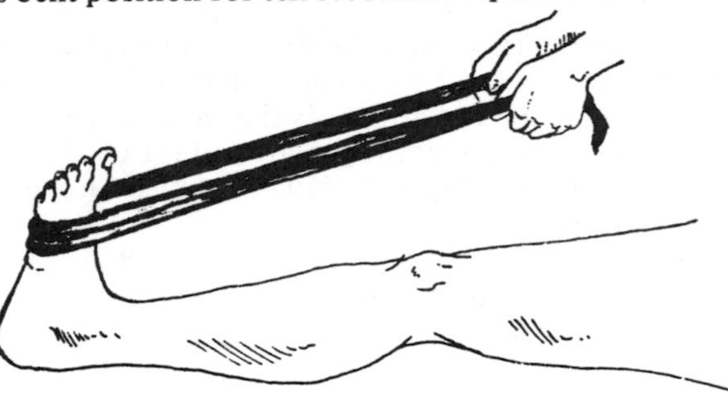

► Repeat this exercise using a rope or towel to pull the top of the foot toward you a bit further, thereby extending the range of the stretch. Hold for ten seconds. Repeat five to ten times.

When Ready to Resume Running

1. To test your readiness to start running again . . .

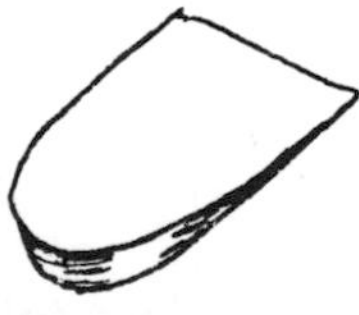

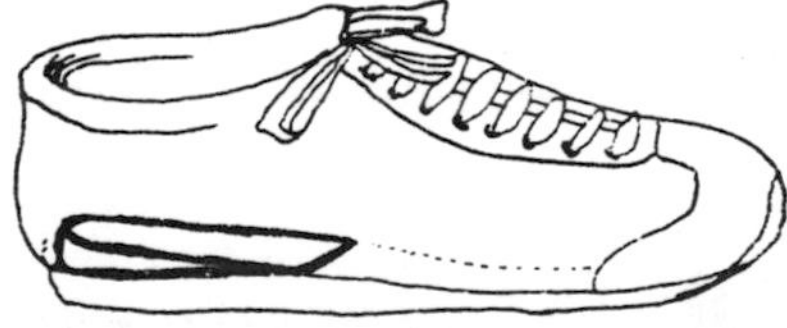

► Cut a ¼" piece of felt to the shape of the heel, scive it down so that the front end is thinner than the back, and place it in the heel of your shoe.
► Place identical raises in both shoes, unless one of your legs is shorter than the other.
► Add more thickness to the lift as required to eliminate pain in walking—but only as long as your foot doesn't slip out of the shoe! If added thickness does not alleviate the pain, take two to four weeks off.
► If you can walk without pain, try to run. If pain is present in running, add more of a raise if you can do so without slipping out of the shoe. If you cannot run without pain, you need at least one to two weeks of rest.

► If you have to stop running, try swimming or bicycling to maintain cardiovascular fitness during the layoff. Also continue general stretching exercises to maintain flexibility, giving special emphasis to achilles tendon stretching with ice therapy (see Treatment #4).

2. Do the following stretching exercises three times daily (before and after running and before bed).

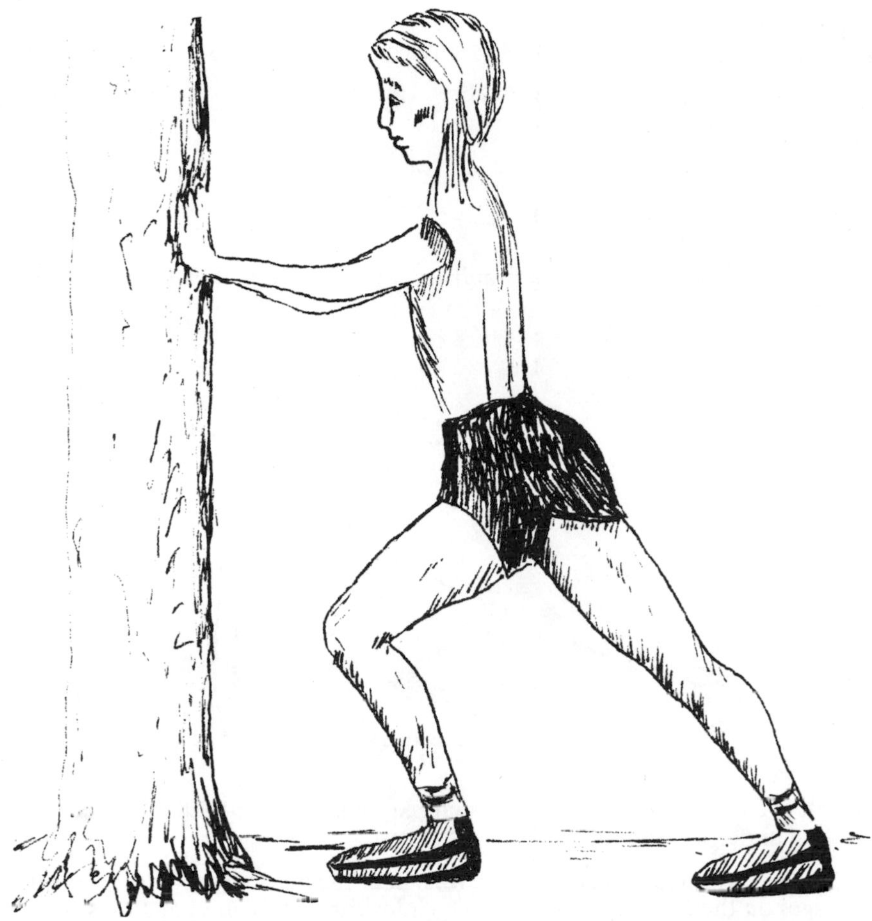

► Wall pushes (with each leg stretched separately), two times for 30 seconds each time—one set with back leg straight, and one set with back leg bent inward at the knee.
► Stair stretches, two times for 30 seconds each time (see appendix on Stretching).

3. Heat the achilles area before running by applying hot towels for two to four minutes, or hot towels and liniment, or, if in a hurry, at least liniment.

4. There is a special way to tape the achilles tendon to take the stress off of it, called an equinus taping. This is useful for acute problems or during the first days back after a layoff.
► Clean the area with soap and water and rinse with alcohol.
► Spray tincture of Benzoin on the area to allow the tape to adhere better.
► If using a heel pad also (#1 above), put the pad on the bottom of the heel first.

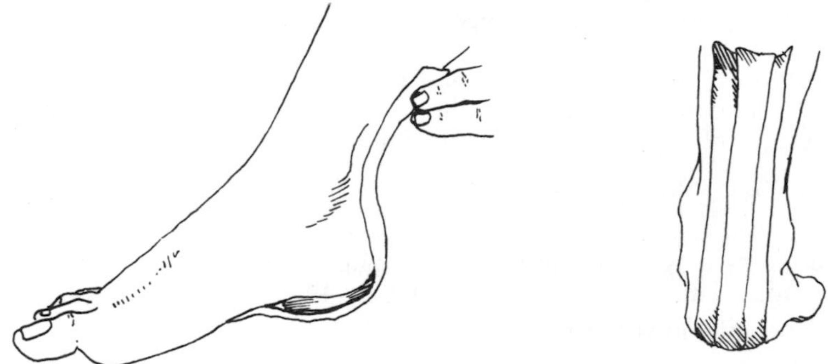

► Cut three strips of 1½"-2" wide tape about 8-12" long (depending on the size of the foot and leg). Take the first strip and place it over the center of the heel just in front of the heel and heel pad.
► Make sure the foot is relaxed with the toes pointing in a downward direction.
► Pull the tape upwards.
► Repeat with strips two and three, covering the entire bottom of the heel or heel pad.

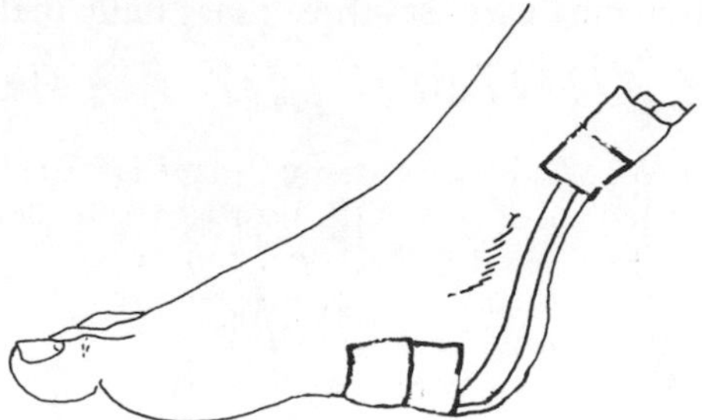

► Anchor these strips on the foot and leg with four four-inch strips of 1½-2'' tape as shown.

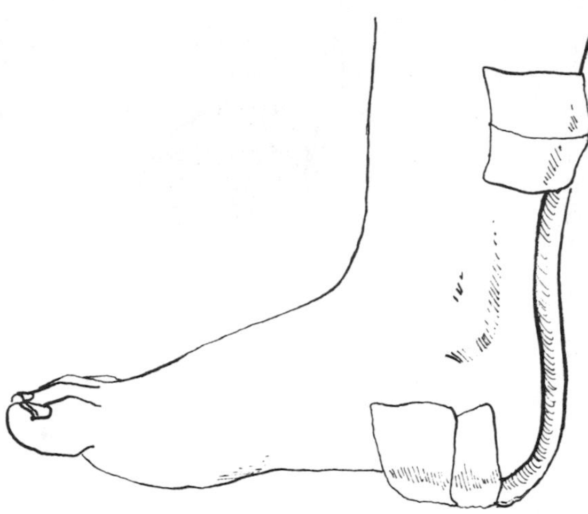

► You can incorporate an artificial external achilles tendon made out of rubber tubing under this taping.

5. If the arch flattens out severely or rolls in at the ankles (pronates) severely, put varus wedges on the bottoms of two Spenco inlays and place in your shoes (see appendix on Shoe Inserts You Can Make).

   NOTE: Whatever you put in one shoe must also be put in the other, unless you are compensating for a leg length discrepancy.

6. Do not run until at least two days after the swelling goes down. If you swell up when you start running again, stop immediately. This time, double the number of days off before attempting to run again.

7. If you feel pain during running, apply ice to the area for six to twelve minutes within half an hour after you finish.

8. If you are resuming running after a rest, start at a slow, easy pace.
   ► Run on level, even, soft surfaces only. The ideal surface is a soft dirt track, an artificial track, or a level grass field.
   ► Do absolutely no hill running, speed training, or racing until the condition is improved.
   ► When running, try to land on the heel first (though it may be risky to make sudden, radical changes in your normal running form). Landing on your toes or forefoot will almost certainly aggravate the achilles tendonitis.

9. If you are a ''toe runner,'' use heel raises (see #2 under ''Pointers for Prevention'' below).

10. Do not attempt to increase mileage until you have recovered fully. If anything, *decrease* your training miles for two to six weeks. If you prefer, run every other day initially, or two days on and one off.

When to Call the Doctor

If you have followed the foregoing instructions faithfully, but if you cannot move your foot downward (toes toward the floor) or put weight on your foot, see your podiatrist immediately.

Practical Pointers for Prevention

1. Use good training shoes, *not* discount-store "jogging" or "sport" shoes.
► Do not use racing flats or spikes until the injury is healed.
► Select a training shoe with a strong heel counter and good rearfoot motion control. Be sure the shoes have a heel elevation at least half an inch higher than the forefoot (see appendix on running shoes).
► Make sure that the heels of the running shoes are kept up and not allowed to become worn down. If they are, have them repaired or get new shoes.
► Make sure the shoe is flexible enough at the forefoot (where the shoe bends) so that it will bend easily.

2. Use a heel raise in your running shoes.
► Cut a ¼" piece of felt to the shape of the heel, skive it down so that the front end is lower than the back, and put it in the shoe under the heel.
► Place identical raises in both shoes, unless you have a shorter leg on one side.

3. As an alternative to putting a heel raise in your shoe, tape a pad directly to the bottom of your heel. Tape the pad on with four 6" retention straps (see chapter 22), or with Equinus taping as described in this chapter under Treatment #4.

4. Another alternative is to attach a heel raise to the bottoms of a pair of Spenco inlays (see appendix on shoe inserts you can make).

36. Sprained Ankle

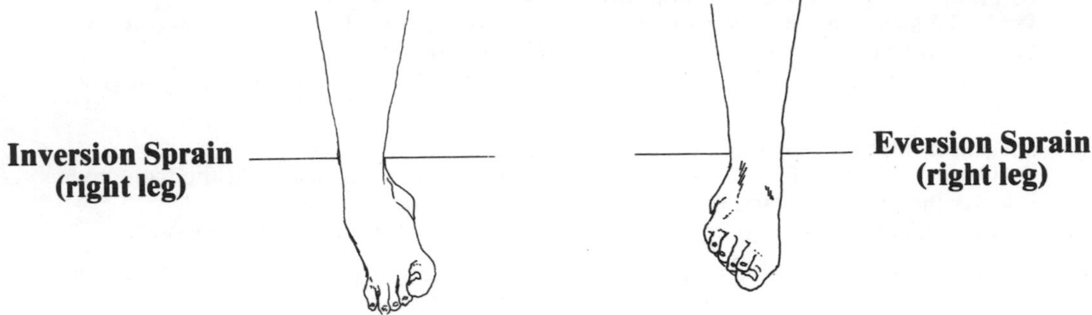

What is it?

An ankle sprain is an injury to the ligaments around the ankle. Ligaments are bands of non-elastic soft tissue which attach bone to bone (tendons attach muscles to bone). In an ankle sprain, these ligaments are stretched or partially torn. The most common kind of ankle sprain is an "inversion" sprain, in which the foot lands and rolls to the outside (ankle turns out). The injury occurs just below the ankle joint and on the outside of the foot. Often the entire foot and ankle will become rapidly swollen and discolored (black-and-blue). In an "eversion sprain" (much less common), the ankle is turned in.

> **NOTE:** Proper attention to detail is important, because even moderate sprains can cause more trouble than fractures.

When to Call the Doctor

If you sprain your ankle and cannot "walk it off" in five minutes, go home. In a case like this, a professional opinion should be obtained. An ankle sprain is one of the most neglected of common injuries, and a lack of proper initial treatment can lead to a lifetime of chronic instability or other ankle problems.

Things you will need for this treatment

see chapter 2 "Materials List" for brand names and substitutes

soap & water
ace bandage
adhesive spray and skin protectant
adhesive tape 1½"
ankle brace or support
aspirin
petroleum jelly
2"x2" gauze pads
ice bag

Preparation for Treatment

1. Make sure all the materials and medications you will be using are clean and fresh as discussed in chapter 2.

2. Read through all the instructions which follow, and make sure you understand them before beginning treatment.

3. Thoroughly scrub the entire foot with warm soapy water and a terry wash cloth. Pat dry with a soft clean towel.

Caution: *Do not proceed with this treatment until you have read the Guidelines to Treatment in Chapter 2*

Treatment

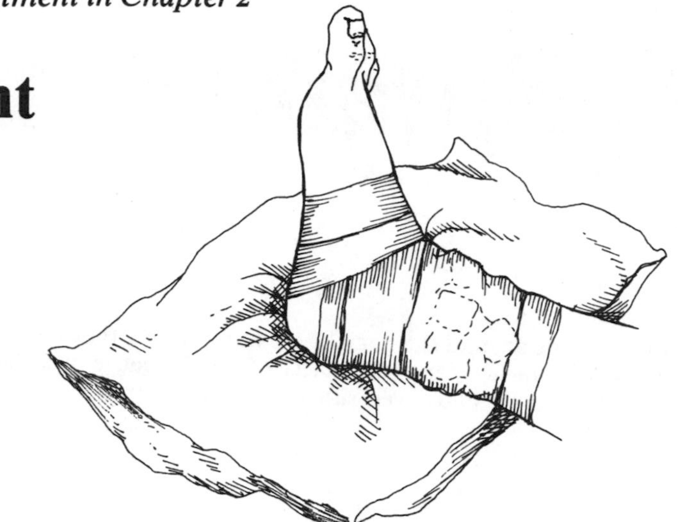

1. Apply ice, 30 minutes on and 30 minutes off for several hours (see chapter 2 for specific techniques of preparing an ice pack), elevate the foot on two pillows, and wrap with an ace bandage for compression. Keep the bandage on for the first 24 hours.

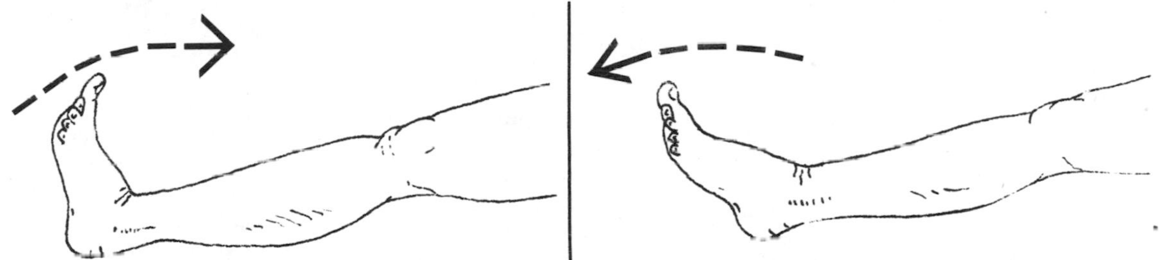

2. After the first 24 hours, start passive dorsi-flexion and plantar-flexion exercises as shown, ten times for ten seconds each, two to three times a day. For *dorsi-flexion*, move the feet towards the face as far as possible. For *plantar-flexion*, stretch the feet away from the face as far as possible.

3. Re-wrap the ace bandage several times the first few days as the swelling diminishes.

4. Take two aspirin every four hours for two days.

5. On the second day, add these exercises:

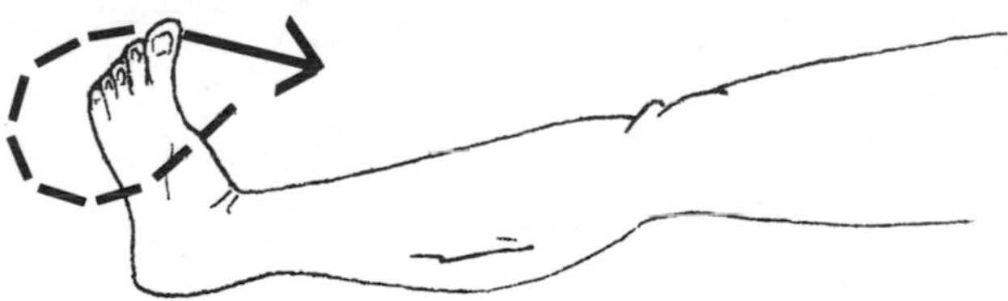

► Holding the foot perpendicular to the leg, turn the foot *inward* as far as possible (on the *left* foot, the *right* border of the foot turns upward toward the knee, etc.). Repeat ten times for ten seconds each time.

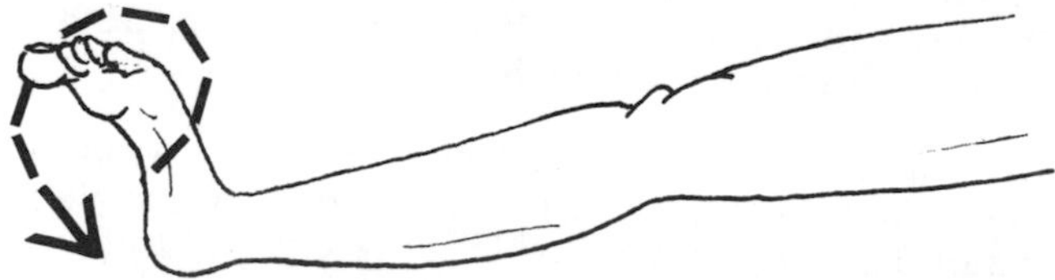

► Repeat the same exercise turning the foot *outward* as far as possible.

6. If the sprain is severe, strap the ankle. For an inversion sprain, try the following strap:

► Wash the entire foot and lower leg with soap and water.
► Shave all hair away from the area.
► Apply tincture of Benzoin to the entire area to be taped.

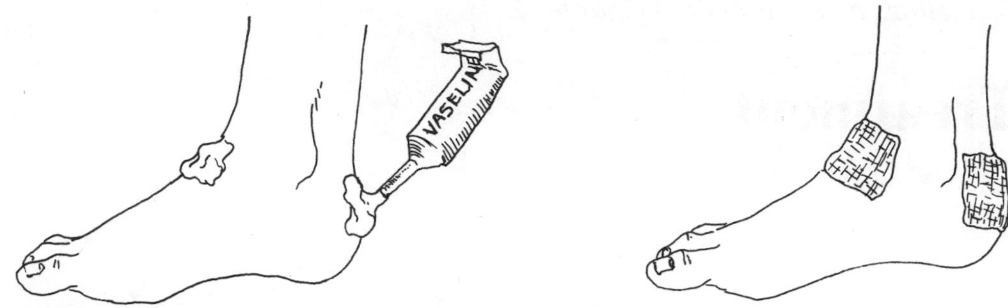

7. ► Put vaseline around the back of the bump where the achilles tendon is inserted into the back of the heel, and put a piece of 2"x 2" gauze over that. Put a lot of vaseline in front of the ankle, and cover with a 2"x 2" gauze pad.

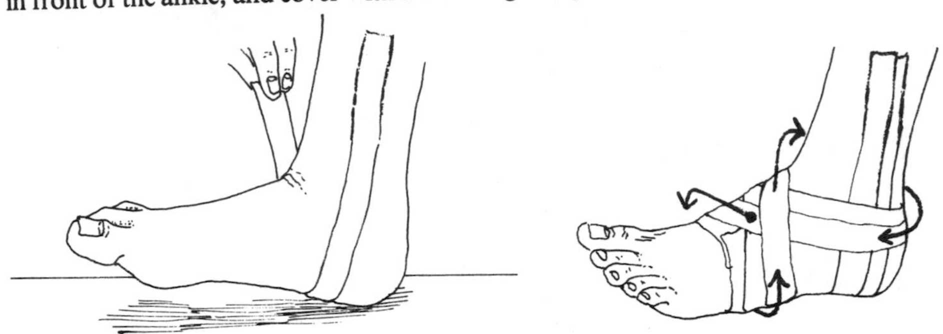

► Take a piece of 1½" adhesive tape approximately twelve inches long, start it about four inches above the inside part of the ankle, run it down the lower leg, around the bottom of the heel, and about four inches up the outside of the ankle. Remember to keep your foot at right angles, and perhaps even twist the outside of your foot a little towards your face to take the pressure off the outside of the ankle. Repeat another retention strap as described above. (For an eversion sprain, twist the inside of your foot a little bit toward your face).

► Take a roll of tape and, starting at the top of the foot above the arch, wrap it alternately around the foot and the ankle to form a figure-eight.

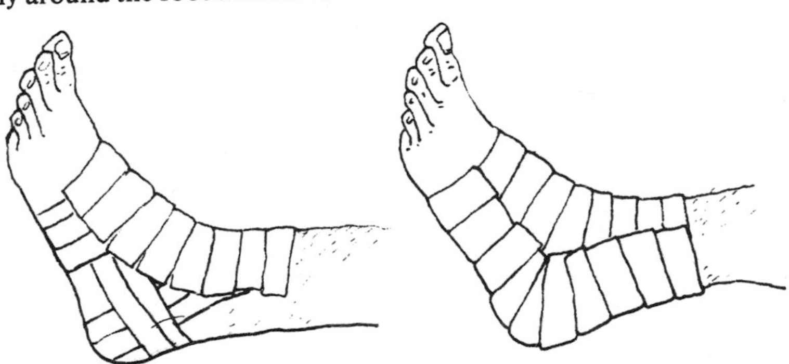

8. Cut about a dozen four-inch strips of 1½" tape (you may need more, depending on your foot size). Starting near the toes, wrap one strip across the top of the foot. Then wrap a second strip slightly overlapping the first. Continue until the whole top of the foot, front of the ankle, and front of the lower leg are covered. Then repeat this process for the bottom of the foot and back of the ankle and lower leg, again starting at the front near the toes.. Try to avoid putting wrinkles in the tape.

9. As an alternative to strapping for a less severe sprain, wrap the ankle with an ace bandage and tape. While wrapping, keep the foot at a right angle to the leg, perhaps even twisting the outside of the foot a little bit toward your face to take the pressure off the outside of your ankle. Start the wrap at the top of the foot, go around the inner arch, and come around the outside of the foot to anchor the bandage. Then wrap around the inside of the ankle, the back of the ankle and lower leg, and around the inside of the foot again, to form a "figure 8." Repeat the "8" one or two more times, going higher around the ankle each time. Clip the ace bandage down. Do not clip the end of the bandage on the bottom of the foot or directly in front of the ankle. An alternative is to anchor the bandage with tape.

10. On the third day, begin ice therapy. Apply ice for six to twelve minutes, enough to numb the ankle area. Then stretch the ankle and walk on it until you feel discomfort or pain. Repeat the icing for six to twelve minutes. Then stretch and walk again until the pain comes on, repeating the ice treatment a third time. Follow this routine every day until you can walk painlessly without taping. The sequence for this treatment is: *ice*-exercise-*ice*-exercise-*ice.*

11. When the swelling is completely diminished and pain is no longer present in normal walking, resume normal activities.

After You Have Recovered . . .

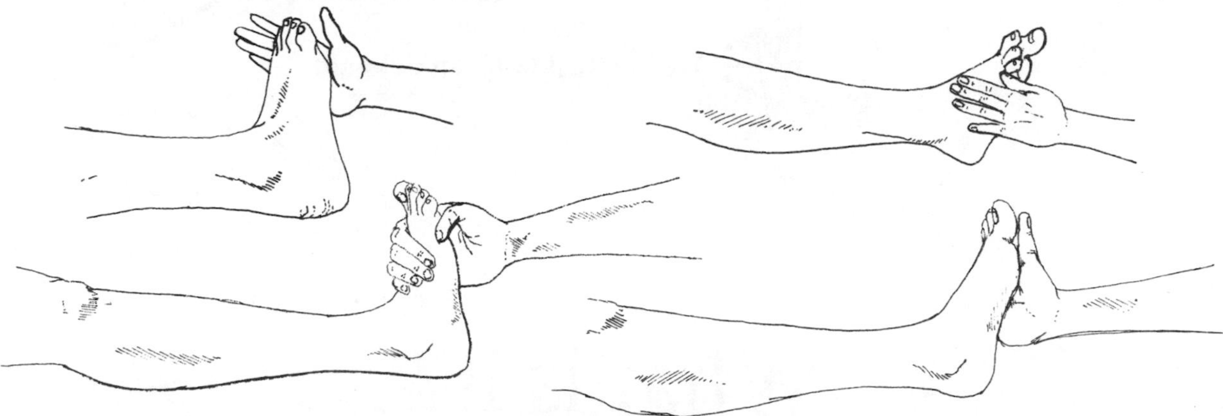

1. Once the ankle is well, it is important to begin strengthening it. At this time, change your exercise program from ankle stretching to ankle resistance. Push the foot in each direction (inward, outward, upward, downward) five times for a steady ten seconds each time. You can push against a wall for the inward, outward, and downward resistance. For upward resistance, put your foot under a piece of furniture and press upward as though to lift the furniture. As an alternative, you can have someone assist you by providing resistance with the hand, as shown. Do these exercises two or three times a day for at least a month after the ankle feels well.

2. If you are involved in activities that require running, strap the ankle before the activity for at least two weeks after the initial pain is gone (see Treatment steps 1–8). If the sprain was mild, use an ace bandage (Treatment step 9).

3. Run or play on smooth, even terrain, with no gravel and no potholed surfaces. Avoid racing, and avoid runs that require a lot of turning. Be especially careful in racquet sports which require quick starts and stops.

4. If athletic activity produces swelling without pain, use ice for 30 minutes after each practice or competition. Use ice a second time at another time of day, along with resistance exercises.

5. If there is any noticeable discomfort from the previous day's activities, take a day off and try again.

6. Stretch the ankle and do resistance exercises even on no-sport days, using ice for 30 minutes after stretching.

7. Never use excessively worn athletic shoes when trying to come back from an injury, especially an ankle injury. The outside sole of the heel is the most important area to look at. If you have chronic ankle problems, always make sure the soles are kept in good repair.

8. Athletic shoes with wide soles at the heel provide better ankle stability. For sports requiring the use of cleats, use shoes with as many cleats under the heel as possible for maximum stability. For basketball, use only high-top shoes.

9. To know how strong the injured ankle is, compare the strength of that ankle to your other ankle and you will know when to stop your rehabilitative ankle strength program. Once they are equal in strength you can stop the resistance exercises and just use basic stretching.

10. A good way to strengthen the ankles while you are running is to run in figure eight patterns (or run up and down the white lines of a parking lot) for a few minutes two to three times a week.

37. General Ankle Pain

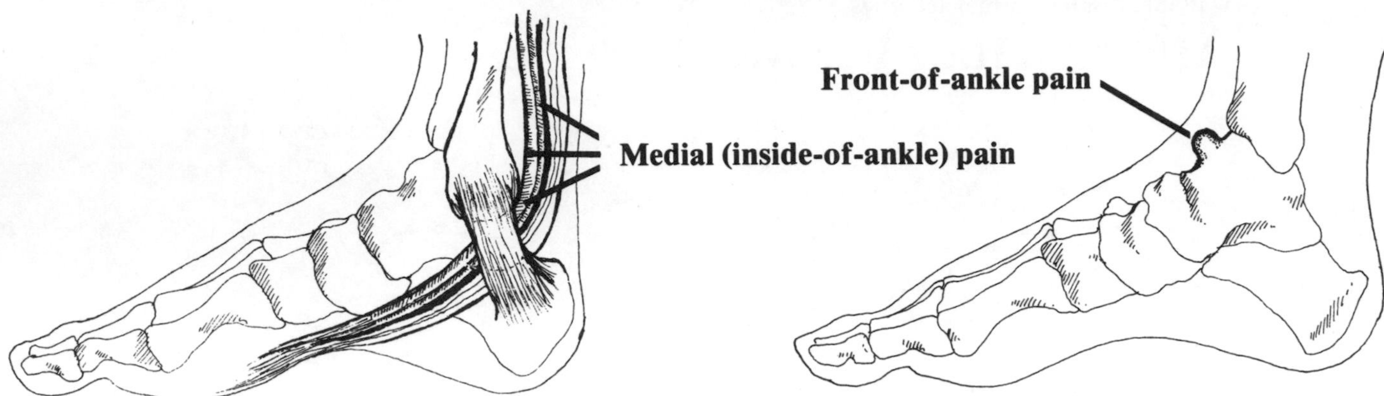

What is it?

Pain in the front of the ankle, when there is no history of injury, is usually due to a spur on top of the talus, the bone which connects the foot to the leg. The pain is usually more noticeable in uphill running, or in running at faster speeds, when there is a greater tendency to dorsiflex (move the toes toward the leg), therefore diminishing the space in the ankle joint. If there is a spur present on the top of the talus bone as illustrated, the tendon and nerves running from the area get pinched and the pain occurs.

For pain on the inside of the ankle, see the section of ''Medial Ankle Pain'' in this chapter.

Things you will need for this treatment

see chapter 2 ''Materials List'' for brand names and substitutes

soap & water
ice bag
aspirin
non-adhesive felt ¼''
nitrogen-impregnated foam innersoles
adhesive tape 1½'' to 2''
alcohol
adhesive spray and skin protectant

Preparation for Treatment

► Make sure all materials and suggested medications are clean and up to date.

► Thoroughly scrub the entire foot with warm soapy water and a terry wash cloth. Pat dry with a soft clean towel.

► Read through all the instructions which follow, and make sure you understand them before beginning treatment.

Treatment

1. Rest for two days, applying ice to the ankle for 15-30 minutes, twice a day.

2. Take two aspirin every four hours for two days, then two aspirin every six hours for up to one week.

3. When there is no more pain on walking, then you are ready to try and run.

4. Apply ice for six to ten minutes before athletic activity (discontinue once you are free of pain).

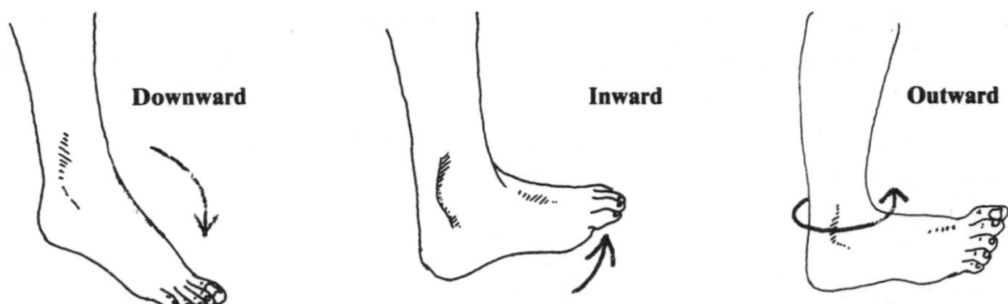

5. Before and after running, stretch the ankle in three directions—downward, inward, and outward. Hold the ankle stretched for five seconds and do five repetitions in each direction. These additional exercises may be discontinued once you have been free of pain for at least one month.

6. Use heel raises made out of ¼'' felt, thinned downward toward the toes. Use raises in both heels to avoid causing imbalance between the legs, except when one leg is shorter (see chapter 44).

7. If you are a runner, stay on level, smooth surfaces. Avoid speedwork. Do not race (or wear racing shoes) until the pain is completely gone.

8. If there is still some discomfort after athletic activity, ice the ankle for six to ten minutes before and after your workouts (discontinue once you are free of pain).

9. If you are bow-legged, if you have severe wear on the outside corner of your heel, or if your feet roll in (pronate) excessively, you should use varus wedges either directly in the shoes or underneath the Spenco inlays fitted to your foot (see appendix on Shoe Inserts You Can Make).

10. Make sure the soles of your shoes, particularly the heels, are kept in good repair at all times (see appendix on shoes).

11. Use athletic shoes with good rearfoot shock absorption and strong heel counters for good rearfoot "motion control" (stability). For sports requiring cleats, the more cleats you have, the better the control.

DON'T

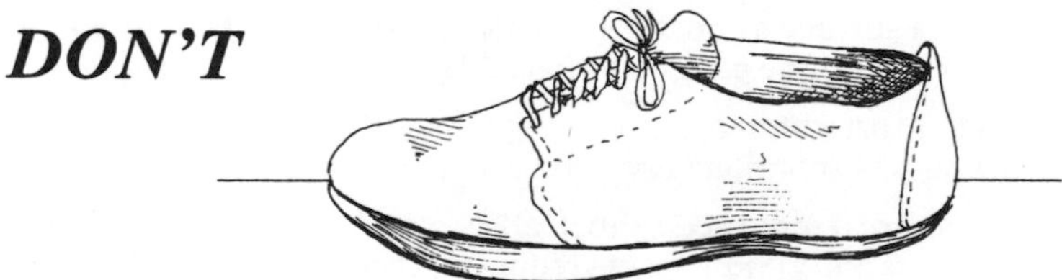

12. Do not wear negative-heel shoes, as they will force the feet to dorsiflex (move the toes toward the leg) too much and add excessive stress, actually tending to worsen the original injury.

When to Call the Doctor

If after following all the above directions, the pain remains the same or worsens, take a week or two off from athletic activity. If the problem persists, see a podiatrist. If swelling persists after four days of ice, rest and elevation, see a podiatrist.

Medial Ankle Pain

Pain occuring on the *inside* of the ankle is usually caused by a strained ligament, tendonitis, or a nerve impingement. In any of these cases, the following treatment may be helpful.

Treatment

1. Rest for two days, applying ice to the ankle for 15-30 minutes, twice a day.

2. Take two aspirin every four hours for two days, then two aspirin every six hours for up to one week.

3. When there is no more pain on walking, then you are ready to try and run.

4. Apply ice for six to ten minutes before athletic activity (discontinue once you are free of pain).

5. If the problem is acute, wash each foot with soap and water, pat dry with a terry towel, and wipe off with rubbing alcohol. Apply tincture of benzoin to the arch, heel and ankle.

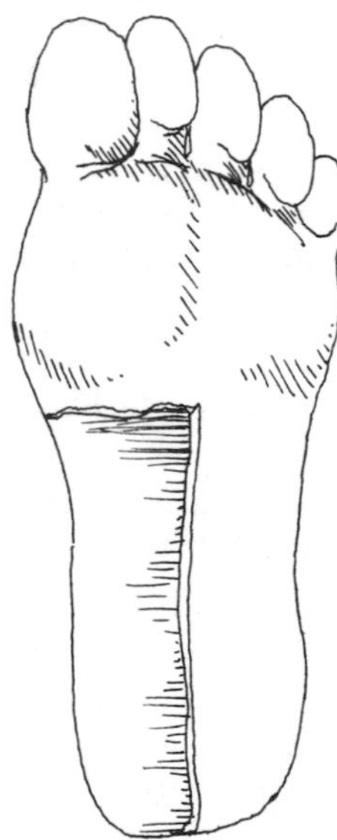

6. Apply the following padding and taping to the feet. Using ¼'' felt, cut out a varus pad for your heel and extend it into your arch.

NOTE: See chapter 18, treatment #4 and #5 for taping instructions.

7. Once the acute stage is over and the symptoms have subsided, duplicate the padding you used in #6 above and glue onto the bottom of a Spenco inlay (see appendix on Shoe Inserts You Can Make).

8. Run on as level and smooth a surface as possible. Avoid speed workouts of any kind. Do not race (or wear racing shoes) until the pain is completely gone.

9. If there is still some discomfort after athletic activity, ice the area for six to ten minutes before and after workouts (discontinue once you are free of pain).

10. Use athletic shoes with good rearfoot (heel) shock absorption and strong heel counters for good ''motion control'' (stability). For sports requiring cleats, the more cleats you have, the better the control .

11. Make sure the soles of your shoes, particularly the heels, are kept in good repair at all times (see running shoe section in the appendix on shoes).

38. Calf Strain

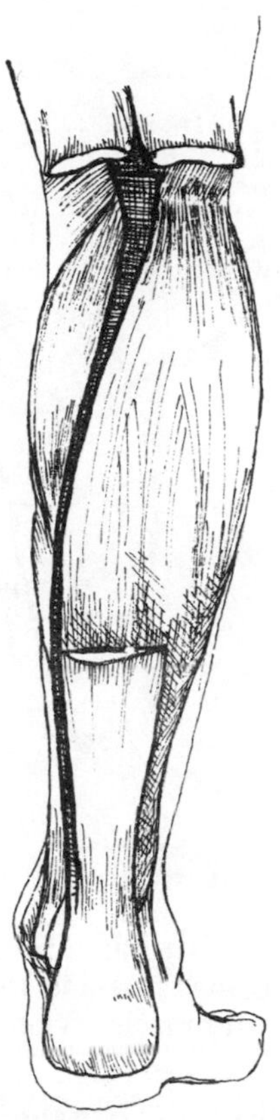

What is it?

A calf strain is an injury to the muscle group in the back of the lower leg. The muscle fibers become over-stretched, partially torn, or occasionally even ruptured. Calf strain is characterized by a sudden localized pain, swelling and sometimes a black-and-blue discoloration.

You can also experience pain in the mid-calf area due to an inflammation of the achilles tendon as it joins up with the calf muscle group from above. There will usually be no swelling or black and blue discoloration, but the treatment will be the same as for calf strain.

Things you will need for this treatment

soap & water
ice bag
ace bandage
non-adhesive ¼'' felt
rope or towel
aspirin

Caution: *Do not proceed with this treatment until you have read the Guidelines to Treatment in Chapter 2*

Preparation for Treatment

► Make sure all materials and suggested medications are clean and up to date.

► Thoroughly scrub the entire foot with warm soapy water and a terry wash cloth. Pat dry with a soft clean towel.

► Read through all the instructions which follow, and make sure you understand them before beginning treatment.

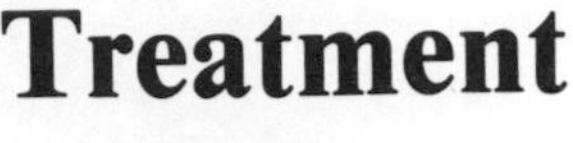

Treatment

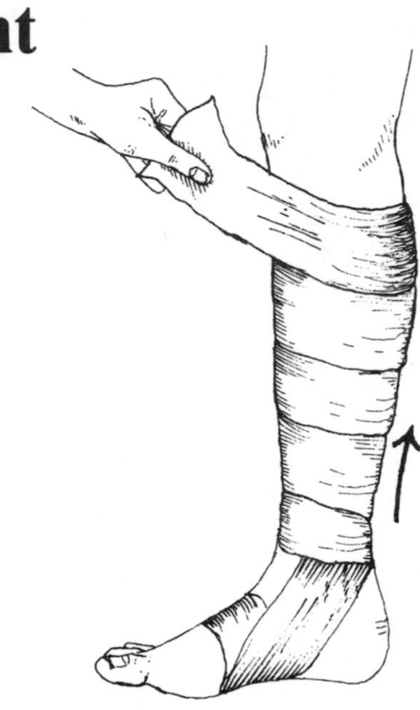

1. Apply an ice pack directly to the injured area for 10 to 20 minutes, twice a day. Use an ace bandage for compression, anchoring it around the foot and wrapping it in an upward spiral so that it supports the whole calf muscle. When you are off your feet, elevate the injured leg on two pillows.

2. Take two aspirin every four hours for two to three days, then every six hours for up to one week.

3. After 48 hours start adding passive stretching exercises with ice therapy, as follows:
► Apply an ice pack for six to twelve minutes or until the calf is numb.
► Sit on the floor with your legs stretched out straight, and pull the tops of your feet back towards your face (bending the foot at the ankle) two times, holding the stretch for 30 seconds each time.
► Repeat this stretch with a rope or towel wrapped around the foot and pulled backwards for a little extra extension (see chapter 19).
► This ice therapy should be done as follows: *ice*-exercise-*ice*-exercise-*ice*. Repeat once or twice a day for up to one week after symptoms have subsided.

4. If you have pain when walking, wear an ace bandage all day, applied as described in #1 above.

5. A heel raise in your shoe will help to take stress off the muscle. Cut a piece of ¼" felt to fit in the heel of the shoe, and skive down so that the front is thinner than the back. Put identical pieces in both shoes, unless the injured leg is shorter than the other leg (see chapter 44). If you need more support, use the equinus taping explained in chapter 35.

6. Do not run until you can walk without pain (though you may need the help of an ace bandage and heel raise).

When Returning to Action...

1. Wear athletic shoes in which the heel is raised well above the ball of the foot. If you are a runner, make sure that your shoes are flexible enough to bend easily, and that the heels are not allowed to wear down badly (see the running shoe section, appendix on shoes).

2. For the first few days back, wear the ace bandage and the heel raise, and heat the calf with a heat-producing ointment before running and ice for 6 to 12 minutes afterward (discontinue once you are free of pain).

3. Do wall pushes with the knees straight two times for 30 seconds each, and with the knees bent two times for 30 seconds each, both before and after running and at least one other time during the day.

> **Wall push:** Stand flat-footed about three feet from the wall. Bring one foot forward and lean toward the wall (keeping the rear foot flat on the floor) until you feel a good stretch in the calf of the rear leg. Relax and hold this position for a minute. Then repeat the same exercise but bend the back knee in order to stretch the lower part of the calf muscles (see appendix on stretching).

4. Begin anterior and posterior tibial strengthening exercises to reduce the muscle imbalance which is probably one of the causes of the injury (see appendix on stretching).

Practical Pointers for Prevention

1. If you are resuming sports activity after a long layoff, start at a slow, easy pace (see chapters 27 and 28).

2. Run on a level, even, soft surface. The ideal surface is a soft dirt track, an artificial track, or a flat grassy field. Do no hill running, speed training, or racing until the calf has completely recovered.

3. When running, try to land on the heel first (though any sudden change of form may be risky). Toe or forefoot running is almost certain to aggravate this problem. If you are a toe runner, use a ¼'' heel raise cut out of felt as described in Treatment #5 above.

DON'TS

1. Don't attempt to increase mileage until you have recovered. If anything, *decrease* your mileage for a week or two. If you prefer, run every other day, or two days on and one off.

2. Do not go barefoot.

3. Do not wear negative-heel shoes for everyday use. Wear shoes with heel heights of about 1½ inches. If you like wearing flat shoes, add heel raises made of ¼'' felt.

4. For further suggestions, see chapter 35 (under Practical Pointers).

When to Call the Doctor

If after following all the above instructions, the pain remains the same or worsens, take a week or two off from athletic activity. If the problem persists, see a podiatrist.

If swelling persists after four days of ice, rest and elevation, *or* if the injured calf is warmer to the touch than your other calf, and/or you have a low-grade temperature, *or* if you can't move your foot downward (away from your face) when your weight is not on it . . . see a podiatrist.

39. Shin Splints

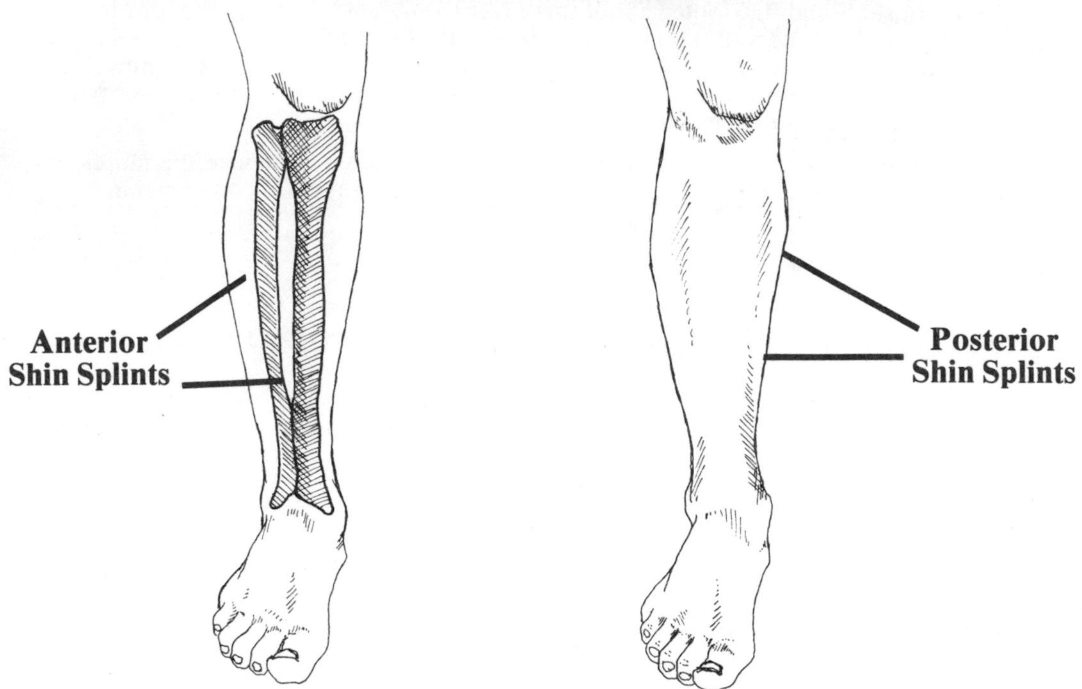

What is it?

"Shin splints" is a catch-all term used to describe various causes of pain in the lower leg brought on by athletic activity. The most common problems are inflammations of the muscle (myositis), tendons (tendonitis) or bone covering of the lower leg (periostitis), where the muscle attaches to the bone. There are also some more serious problems for which shin splints are sometimes mistaken, such as stress fractures of the lower leg bones, or compartment syndromes (a compartment syndrome is caused by abnormal pressure in one or more of the muscular compartments of the lower leg and is considered a medical emergency).

There are two common types of shin splints:

Anterior Tibial shin splints are characterized by pain in the lower front of the leg and radiating down the outside of the leg.

Posterior Tibial shin splints are characterized by pain along the inside of the lower leg and ankle.

Things you will need for this treatment

see chapter 2 "Materials List" for brand names and substitutes

soap & water
ice bag
aspirin
nitrogen-impregnated foam innersoles
adhesive felt 1/8"
non-adhesive felt ¼"
baby oil
adhesive spray and skin protectant
tennis elbow brace
ankle brace
weights, 5 pounds
adhesive tape 1½" or 2"
soft polyurethane foam

Caution: *Do not proceed with this treatment until you have read the Guidelines to Treatment in Chapter 2*

Preparation for Treatment

► Make sure all materials and suggested medications are clean and up to date.

► Thoroughly scrub the entire foot with warm soapy water and a terry wash cloth. Pat dry with a soft clean towel.

► Read through all the instructions which follow, and make sure you understand them before beginning treatment.

Treatment

The recommendations below are intended for both of the shin splint problems described above. Specific recommendations for the anterior and posterior types of shin splints respectively will follow.

Shin splints can often be "run through."

► If you have pain in walking, you should not attempt to run.

► If you can walk without pain, with or without an elbow brace, you can try to jog.

► If you can jog with or without an elbow brace with minimal discomfort, and the discomfort you have does *not* increase as the workout goes on, you can begin to run.

► You can race after you can run four to six weeks without pain.

1. Rest (keep off your feet as much as possible) for 24-48 hours.

2. Apply ice to the involved part of the lower leg for 15-30 minutes two to three times a day, and elevate the involved leg above the level of the heart (on two pillows) as much as possible for the first 48 hours.

3. Take two aspirin every four hours for the first two days and then two every six hours for up to seven days.

4. After two days, start ice therapy and active exercises once or preferably twice a day, until ready to resume running. Place the ice on the skin for 6-12 minutes, or until the area feels numb. Move the ice in an up-and-down (massaging) motion. (See chapter 2). The ice therapy regimen should follow this pattern: *ice,* exercise, *ice,* exercise, *ice.* Do the following exercises from a sitting position:

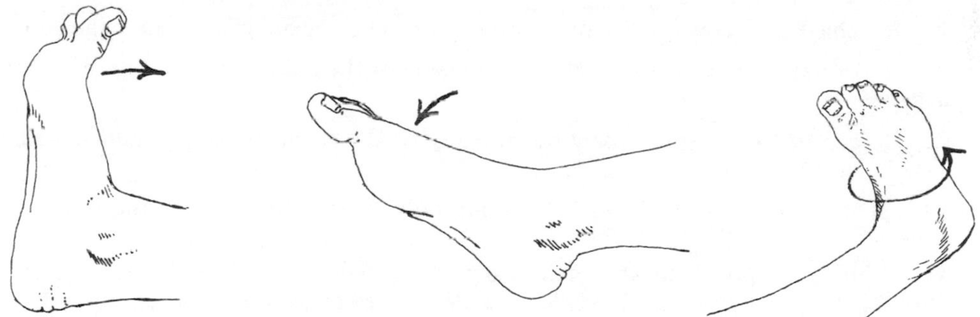

► Move the foot toward the front of the leg (without lifting the leg) as far as possible, and hold for five seconds. Repeat five times.

► While sitting in the same position, move the foot *away* from the front of the leg as far as you can stretch it, and hold for five seconds. Repeat five times.

► Turn the foot inward, then move it upward toward the front of the leg as far as possible and hold for five seconds. Repeat five times.

5. Before bedtime apply baby oil liberally to the involved shin. Massage the front of the leg in an up and down motion for ten minutes. Use as much pressure as you can, using pain as your guide as to how much to use.

6. Shin splints are often related to excessive pronation (rolling inward of the ankles with or without feet flattening out) and poor shock absorption. To compensate for excessive pronation and aid in shock absorption, fit a pair of Spenco inlays into your shoes.

7. Make a varus wedge long enough to extend from the back of the heel to the arch (see appendix on Shoe Inserts You Can Make). Attach to the bottom of the Spenco inlay in the proper position.

When ready to resume training...

1. Wear training shoes with good rearfoot shock absorption and motion control. Make sure the heel fit is snug and the width of the sole on the bottom of the heel is about three inches. Also make sure the heel sole wear of the shoes is not excessive (see running shoe section in the appendix on shoes).

2. Avoid hard and uneven surfaces, racing, racing shoes, or slanted (crowned) road surfaces until you have been able to run free of pain for two to six weeks (depending upon how long a layoff you have had).

3. If you can, run initially on soft surfaces such as grass or dirt.

4. Cut back on your training schedule in proportion to the length of time you were off (see chapters 27 and 28).

5. Make sure you take time to warm up before running, and to stretch well before and after your workout. Pre-running stretches should include wall pushes with knees locked (30 seconds each leg, twice), wall pushes with knees bent (30 seconds each leg, twice) and stair stretches (30 seconds each leg, twice). See appendix on Stretching.

6. Ice the leg or legs for 6-10 minutes before and after running (do the icing before the warmup).

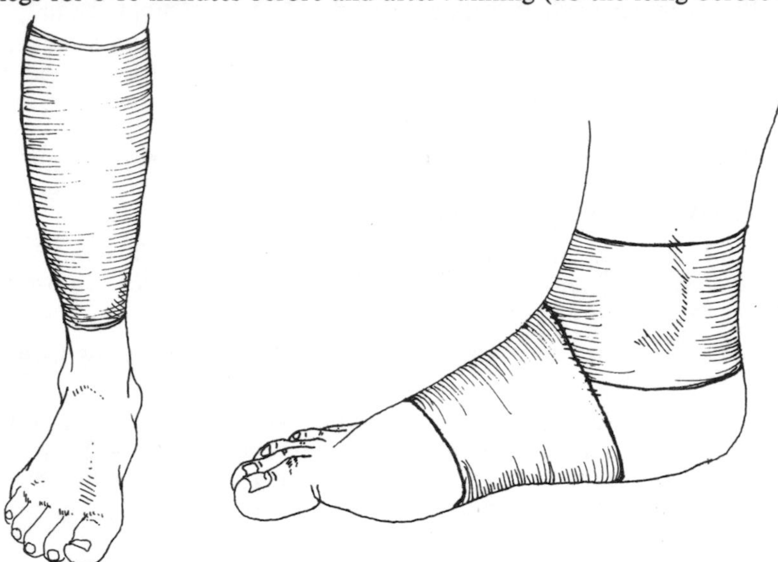

7. Purchase an elbow brace from a drug store and place on the leg where the pain is.

8. If your shin splint pain is behind the inside of the ankle, an ankle brace can be used instead.

9. Before bedtime, apply baby oil liberally to the front of the leg and massage as in Treatment #5.

10. It may be helpful to plan on running only every other day for the first few weeks back.

11. Shin splint problems are often associated with lower leg imbalances. Therefore, it is important to strengthen the lower leg muscles as well as to stretch the calf muscles (see appendix on stretching, section on strength training).

For Anterior Tibial Shin Splints...

1. Use criss-cross taping, with or without the elbow brace. Prepare the skin by shaving the front of the leg and spraying it with tincture of Benzoin. Take a 1½ or 2" adhesive tape, cut in strips six inches long. Start taping from one inch below the area of pain on the front of the leg, and criss-cross each strip all the way up the leg to an inch above the point where the pain initially began. Leave no spaces between the pieces of tape. Do not tape around the entire leg, just the front half. As you place each strip, anchor the lower end tightly down, then pull very strongly in an upward direction before applying the rest of the strip to the leg.

2. Make a heel raise out of 1/8" adhesive felt and add it to the Spenco inlay you have already fabricated. If you need a thicker heel raise, add 1/8" layers one at a time, over a period of several weeks.

For Posterior Tibial Shin Splints...

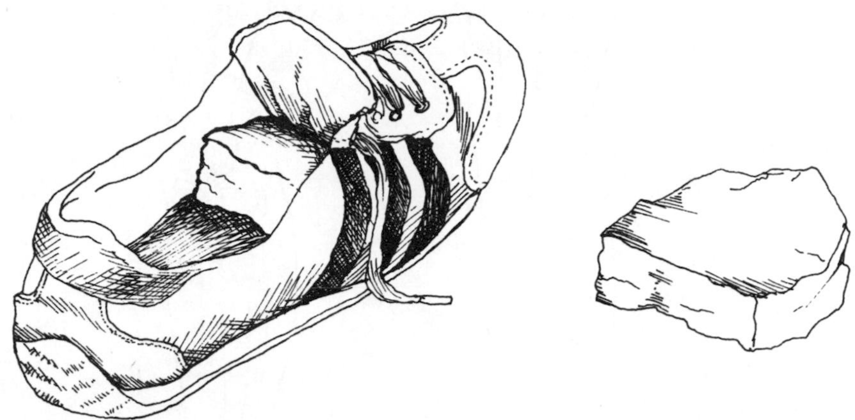

1. Diminish toe movement by placing a piece of ½" to 1" polyurethane foam directly into the bottom front of the running shoe (between the Spenco inlay and the innersole of the shoe). Alternately, try wearing an extra pair of socks. (see appendix on stretching)

2. Run with your body erect (not leaning forward) and your stride at a comfortable length. Try to concentrate on landing gently, if you do not do so already.

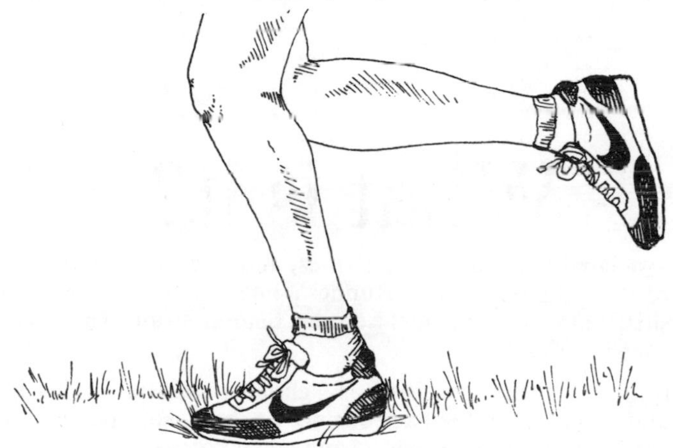

3. Try not to land directly on your toes. If you prefer to or naturally do so, use heel raises made out of ¼" adhesive felt, thinned toward the front. Attach to your Spenco inlays (see appendix on Shoe Inserts You Can Make).

When to Call the Doctor

1. If severe swelling, pain, and/or discoloration occur and persist after four days of treatment, see a podiatrist.

2. If you feel numbness and/or interference with lower leg coordination when walking after a run, see a podiatrist.

Note: Stress fractures and other serious conditions often start out as shin splints. The symptoms are initially the same. If the pain increases in spite of all your efforts to help yourself, or if a localized hard area develops or bump occurs on the leg, stop running and consult a sports medicine podiatrist. There is a good chance at this point that you have a stress fracture, and that a layoff (as well as professional treatment) will be necessary.

40. Knee Pain

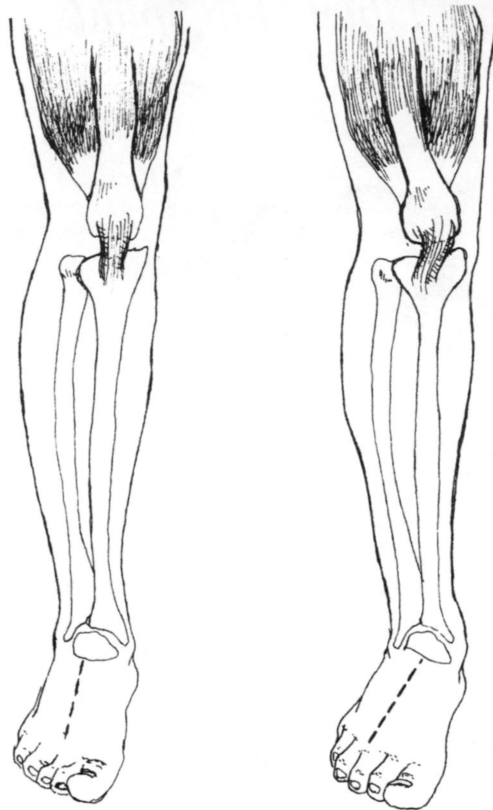

What is it?

Knee problems associated with running activities, and due to overuse or "overtraining," can include any of several conditions. "Runner's knee" is a catch-all term for disorders that include bursitis, tendonitis, ligament strain, tendon strain, cartilage irritation, and sometimes even bone injuries.

Knee pain in a runner is often identified as "chondromalasia." This is an actual softening, erosion, and cracking on the back surface of the knee cap itself. It is not as common a problem as recent literature suggests, and when it does actually occur it is likely to require a much longer recovery time than most of the non-traumatic overuse or running-related knee injuries that we will be dealing with in this chapter.

CAUTION: A knee injury caused by a direct blow or trauma, where there is swelling, locking, loss of motion, black and blue discoloration, or collapsing of the knee joint, should be seen immediately by an orthopedist.

Things you will need for this treatment

soap & water
ice bag
pillows, 2
aspirin
ace bandage
nitrogen-impregnated foam innersoles
adhesive felt ¼"
non-adhesive felt ¼"
moleskin
adhesive tape 1½"
knee brace
petroleum jelly
weights 5 to 10 pounds

Caution: *Do not proceed with this treatment until you have read the Guidelines to Treatment in Chapter 2*

Preparation for Treatment

1. Make sure all the materials you will be using are clean and fresh as discussed in chapter 2.

2. Read through all the instructions which follow, and make sure you understand them before beginning treatment.

Treatment

The following recommendations are to be followed for general knee pain. Additional recommendations, related to specific types of pain, will follow.

> **NOTE:** Pay careful attention when dealing with knee pains. If the knee is properly treated and rested during the first few days, you can often avoid more serious problems which would lead to more prolonged layoffs.

1. Rest (keep off your feet as much as possible) for 24-48 hours.

2. Apply ice to the knee, at least 15-30 minutes, two to three times a day, and elevate the involved leg above the level of the heart (on two pillows) as much as possible for the first 48 hours.

3. Take two aspirin every four hours for the first two days and then two again every six hours for up to seven days.

4. After two days, start ice therapy and active exercises. Ice the knee for six to 12 minutes or until numb. Then do the ice therapy regimen described below, using the following sequence: *ice,* exercise; *ice,* exercise; *ice.*

► Sit on the floor with the legs extending straight out in front of you. Tighten the thigh muscles, lock the knee, and lift the leg slightly off the floor. With the entire leg rigid, hold for 15 seconds, then lower slowly and relax. Repeat 15 times.

► Repeat the exercise above with the foot turned inward. Repeat 15 times.

► Do 20 to 40 leg lifts with each leg, as follows: Lying on your back, raise a straightened leg slowly until it is as close to vertical as possible (as seen in chapter 41, treatment #4). Hold for two seconds, and lower slowly.

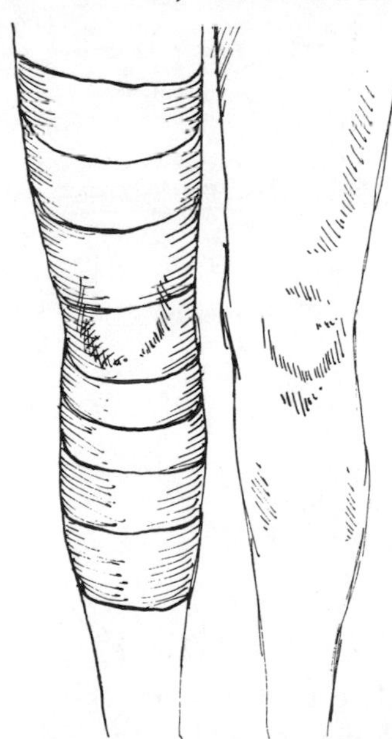

► If the knee feels sensitive during these exercises, then try wrapping it with an ace bandage for extra support. If it is still too sensitive, then you must rest a few more days before trying these exercises again.

To wrap an ace bandage, start just *below* the knee and wind behind the knee just below the skin creases. Wrap several times around the leg, overlapping each wrap and moving towards the hip. The wrapping should be laid on firmly, but not tightly, and should cover the lower half of the upper thigh and upper half of the lower leg.

5. Most knee injuries are related to excessive pronation and bow-legged structure (see appendix on foot structure and function). If you are bow-legged or pronate excessively, fit a pair of Spenco inlays into your shoes.

6. Make a varus wedge long enough to extend from the back of the heel to the arch (see appendix on Shoe Inserts You Can Make). Attach to the bottoms of the Spenco inlays in the proper position.

7. Limb length discrepancies can also lead to knee problems. If you think you may have one leg longer than the other, see chapter 44 and make appropriate adjustments to your inserts.

When ready to resume running...

You may resume *jogging* when you can walk on level surfaces without pain (you may still experience some pain up and down stairs). If necessary, use a knee brace or an elastic bandage to stay free of pain. You are ready to resume running when you can jog comfortably.

1. Wear training shoes with good rearfoot shock absorption and motion control. Make sure the heels of the shoes are not worn down too much (see shoe appendix).

2. Avoid hill training, racing, racing shoes, slanted (crowned) road surfaces or a lot of curves, until you have been able to run painfree for two to six weeks, depending upon how long a layoff you had (See chapters 27 and 28). Also, make sure you run with a short stride.

3. Cut back on your training schedule accordingly. Make sure you warm up properly before running and concentrate on hamstring and quadricep stretches (see stretching appendix).

Special Considerations According to Location of Knee Pain

1. For pain on either side of the knee cap itself:
   A tight elastic bandage or an ace bandage wrapped as described in Treatment section #4.
   NOTE: Running long distances with an elastic knee brace can cause a skin irritation, so apply a liberal amount of Vaseline around the knee area before using the brace.

2. Pain along the outside of the lower thigh and next to the outside of knee joint:
   An elastic bandage snugly wrapped around the knee as described in Treatment #4 is useful. Stretching is also helpful. Do the following exercises:

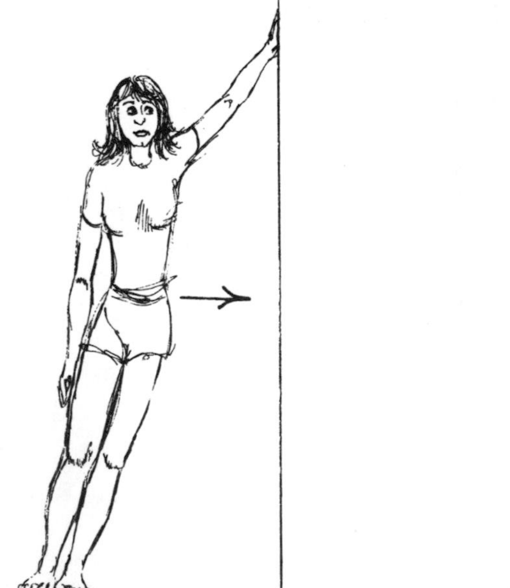

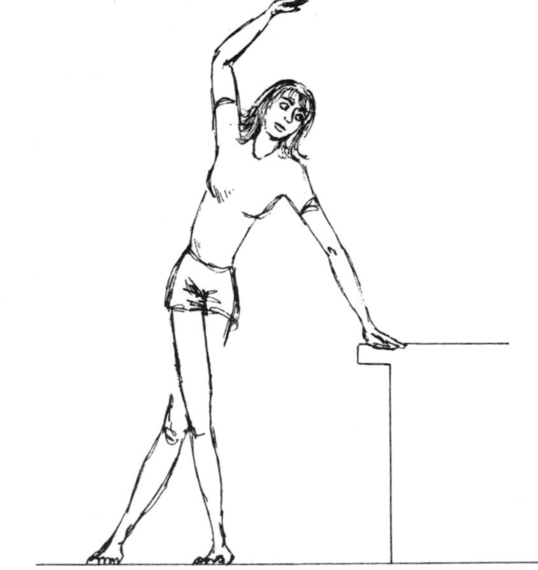

► To stretch the left side place a stiff left arm against a wall and lean your left side into the wall two times; hold for 30 seconds each time.
► Stand erect, balance yourself with your left arm against a table, and lift your right arm over your head. Tilt your body over to the left as far as possible. Repeat two times, holding for 30 seconds each time.

3. For pain *directly under the knee cap,* cut a horseshoe shaped piece of ¼" felt (non-adhesive, so it will not stick to the hair on your leg) and place around the knee cap with the bottom of the horseshoe around the bottom of the knee cap. Wrap and hold in place with an ace bandage as described in Treatment section #4. If only adhesive-backed ¼" felt is available, cover the sticky side with tape or moleskin.

The relative-strength ratio of the hamstring (back of thigh) and quadriceps (front of thigh) often can be a factor in a knee injury. The ratio should be quadriceps/hamstrings = 3/2. To test this ratio:

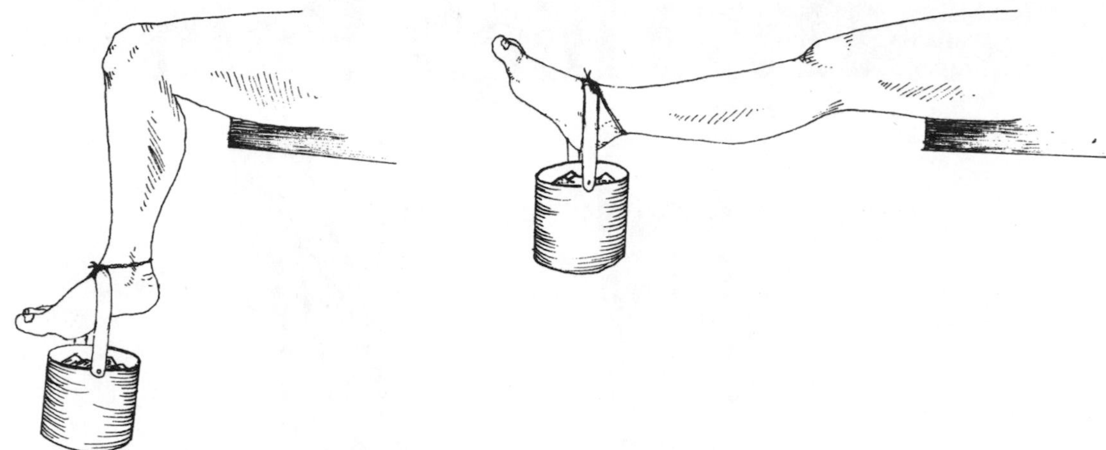

► Take 10 pounds of weight (either fill a pocketbook with 10 lb. of rocks, or go to a local gym and use a universal machine).
► While sitting on a counter top or table, with legs dangling, hang the weight from one foot. Lift the leg until it is straight out in front of you, then lower. Count how many times you can lift the leg.

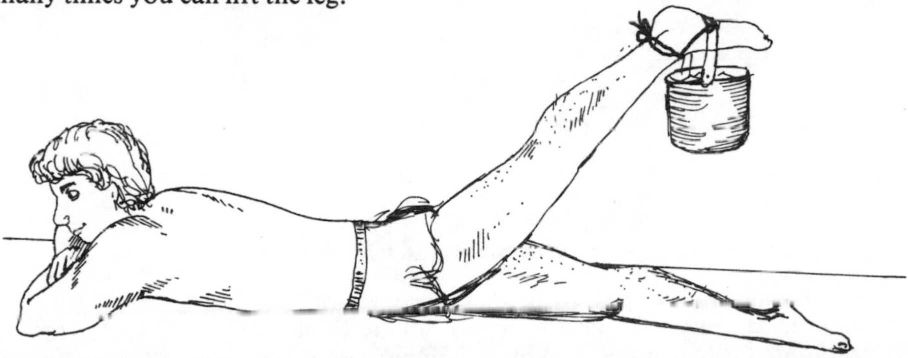

► Now lie flat on your stomach, attach the weight to the ankle, and see how many times you can lift your leg to perpendicular.

The results should be quadriceps/hamstrings = 3/2. If your ratio is significantly different, you should build the weaker muscle group accordingly.

To strengthen either group do the same exercises as in the test—but for the quadricep exercise use the exercise position described in Treatment #4 (knee partially bent, but *not* at a 90° angle), and start with 5 lb. Do three sets of twelve repetitions, three times a week, and hold the leg in the extended position for 10 seconds each time.

When three sets of twelve repetitions becomes easy, increase the weight by 5 lb. and cut back to six repetitions, then work back up to 12 over a period of several weeks.
► Repeat the test every month until you are balanced.
► If you wish to continue lifting after you are balanced, do so for all muscle groups.

When to Call the Doctor

If severe swelling, pain, and discoloration persist after four days of treatment, see a doctor. If after a few days of rest your knee joint gives way or locks, see a doctor. If, after a prolonged layoff, the symptoms return shortly after you begin running again, see a podiatrist.

DON'TS

► Don't do any weight training with knees bent at 90°.
► Don't do any knee squatting exercises.

41. Thigh Pain

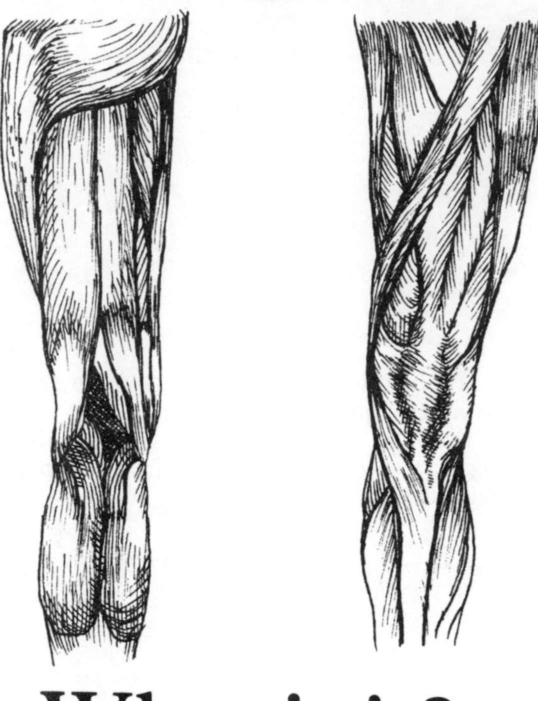

What is it?

A thigh strain occurs when the muscle fibers become overstretched, partially torn, and occasionally even ruptured. Hamstring (back of the thigh) and quadricep (front of the thigh) strains are both characterized by occasionally gradual but usually sudden localized pain and swelling and sometimes black and blue discoloration.

CAUTION: For further information on thigh injury, see chapter 42.

Things you will need for this treatment

see chapter 2 "Materials List" for brand names and substitutes

soap & water
ice bag
ace bandage
non-adhesive felt ¼"
rope or towel
pillows, 2
aspirin

Preparation for Treatment

► Make sure all materials and suggested medications are clean and up to date.

► Read through all the instructions which follow, and make sure you understand them before beginning treatment.

Caution: *Do not proceed with this treatment until you have read the Guidelines to Treatment in Chapter 2*

Treatment

1. Apply an ice pack directly over the injured area for 10 to 20 minutes, twice a day.

2. Use an ace bandage for compression, anchoring it just below the knee cap and wrapping it in an upward spiral all the way to the groin so that it supports the entire hamstring muscle group. When at rest, elevate the injured leg by putting two pillows underneath your knee (see illustration in chapter 42, treatment #1).

3. Take two aspirin every four hours for two to three days, then two every 6 hours for up to one week.

4. After 48 hours, start passive stretching exercises with ice therapy, as follows:
► Apply an ice pack for six to twelve minutes or until the injured area is numb.

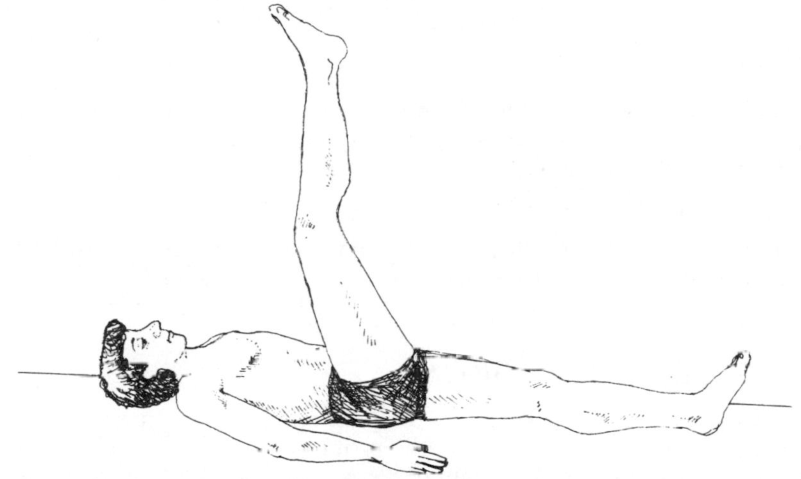

► Lie on the floor with your legs stretched out straight. Raise the injured leg off the floor, keeping the knee straight (straight leg raise). Hold for up to 30 seconds, lower and repeat twice.

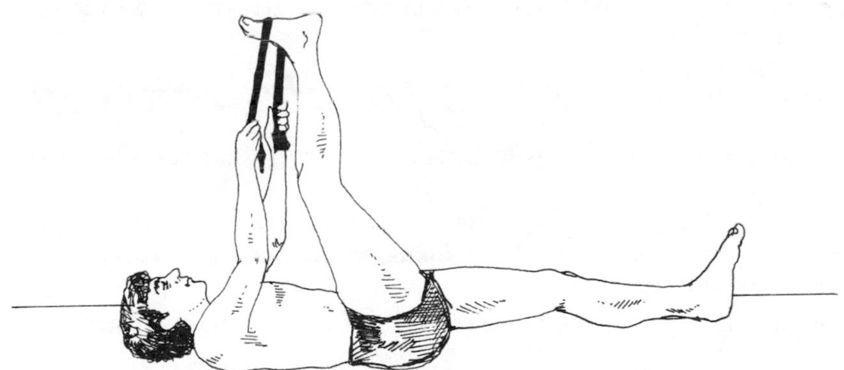

► Repeat this stretch with a rope placed around the foot for additional leverage. Pull back on the rope as you do this exercise.
► The ice therapy should follow this pattern: *ice,* exercise; *ice,* exercise; *ice.* Repeat once or twice a day for up to one week after symptoms have subsided.
► Do the quadricep stretch as described in chapter 42.

5. If you have pain when walking, wear an ace bandage all day, applied as described in #2 above.

6. A heel raise in your shoe will help to take stress off the muscle (see appendix on Shoe Inserts You Can Make).

7. Do not jog until you can walk without pain (though you may continue to need the support of an ace bandage and heel raise). Do not run until you can jog for two to four weeks without pain.

When Returning to Action . . .

1. Wear athletic shoes in which the heel is raised well above the ball of the foot. If you are a runner, make sure that your shoes are flexible enough to bend easily, and that the heels are not allowed to wear down badly (see running shoe section, appendix on shoes).

2. For the first few days back, wear the ace bandage and heel raise, and ice the thigh for six to ten minutes before and after running (discontinue once your running is free of pain).

3. Do leg raises two times for 30 seconds each, both before and after running and at least one other time during the day.

4. Do toe touches two times for 30 seconds each, before and after running and one other time.

5. Do head-to-knee touches two times for 30 seconds each time, before and after running and one other time (see appendix on stretching).

6. Do the quadricep stretch (see appendix on stretching).

DON'TS

1. Don't attempt to increase mileage until you have recovered. If anything, *decrease* your mileage for a week or two. If you prefer, run every other day, or two days on and one day off (see chapter 27).

2. Do not go barefoot.

3. Do not wear negative-heel shoes for everyday use. Wear shoes with heel heights of about 1½ inches. If you like wearing flat shoes, add heel raises made of ¼'' felt.

When to Call the Doctor

If after following the above instructions, the pain remains the same or worsens, take a week or two off from athletic activity. If the problem persists, see a podiatrist or sports doctor. If swelling persists after four days of ice, rest and elevation, *or* if the injured thigh is warmer to the touch than your other one, and/or you have a low grade temperature *or* you can't bend your knee when your weight is on it, see a podiatrist or sports doctor.

> **NOTE:** If the thigh area becomes lumpy or severely black and blue, or if you cannot walk, or if you get severe, gripping pain in the thigh, see a sports doctor immediately.

Practical Pointers for Prevention

1. If you are resuming sports activity after a long layoff, start at a slow, easy pace (see chapters 27 and 28).

2. Run on level, even, soft surfaces. The ideal surface is a soft dirt track, an artificial track, or a flat grassy field. Avoid hill running, speed training, or racing until you have completely recovered.

3. When running, try to land on the heel first (though any sudden change of form may be risky).

4. Check your quadricep/hamstring ratio, and, if not correct, do the necessary weight work (see chapter 40 for testing and weight work).

42. Hip Pain

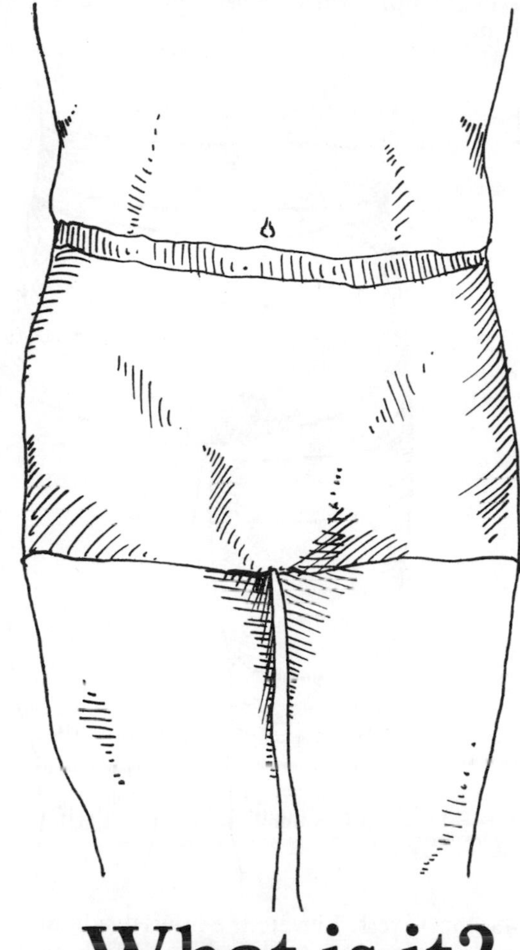

What is it?

Hip, groin, and buttock overuse injuries are most often a sign of muscle strain, tendon strain, or hip joint bursitis. These conditions are often associated with pain accompanied by a snapping sound at the hip joint, and sometimes by a feeling that the hip is ''going out of joint.''

CAUTION: A hip, groin, or buttock injury caused by a direct blow or trauma, where there is resulting swelling, locking, loss of motion, and/or black and blue discoloration should be seen immediately by an orthopedist.

Things you will need for this treatment

soap & water
ice bag
aspirin
baby oil
nitrogen-impregnated foam innersoles
non-adhesive felt ¼''
adhesive felt 1/8''
ace bandage (nylon stocking)
heat ointment
weights 5 to 10 pounds

Preparation for Treatment

► Make sure any instruments you use are clean. Wash them in soap and water and rinse off with alcohol or some other recognized antiseptic.

► Make sure all materials and suggested medications are clean and up to date.

► Read through all the instructions which follow, and make sure you understand them before beginning treatment.

Treatment

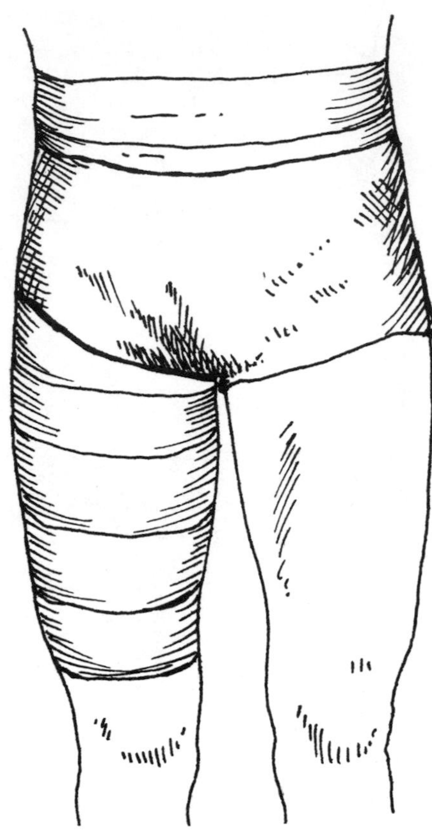

1. For the first 24 to 48 hours, rest. Elevate the injured side on two pillows above the level of the heart. Place an ice pack over the area, alternating 30 minutes on and 30 minutes off. Wrap an ace bandage around the area for support and compression. When wrapping an ace bandage around the hip joint area, it is wise to anchor it by wrapping it once or twice around the waist.

2. Take two aspirin every four hours for two days, then two every six hours for up to a week.

3. After two days, use ice therapy two or three times a day (see chapter 2). Use a paper cup filled with frozen water so you can gently massage the hip area in a circular motion as you are applying the ice.

4. Do the following stretching exercises, keeping your weight off your feet. If any of these exercises irritate the hip area too much, ease off of them or eliminate them from your program for the time being.

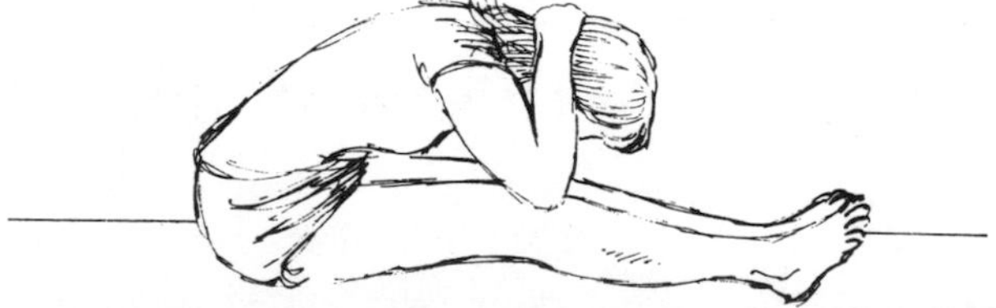

► To stretch the hamstring muscles (back of the thigh), sit on the floor with your head toward your knees as far as you can go. Hold for up to 30 seconds. Repeat twice.

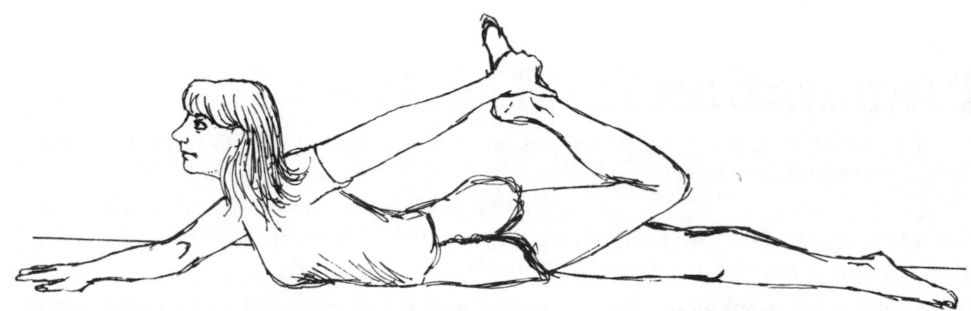

► For the left quadricep (front of the thigh), lie on your right side with your body straight. Grasp the top of your left foot with your left hand and pull it back toward your buttocks so that the heel is as close as you can g et it to the buttocks. Hold for 30 seconds. Repeat two times.

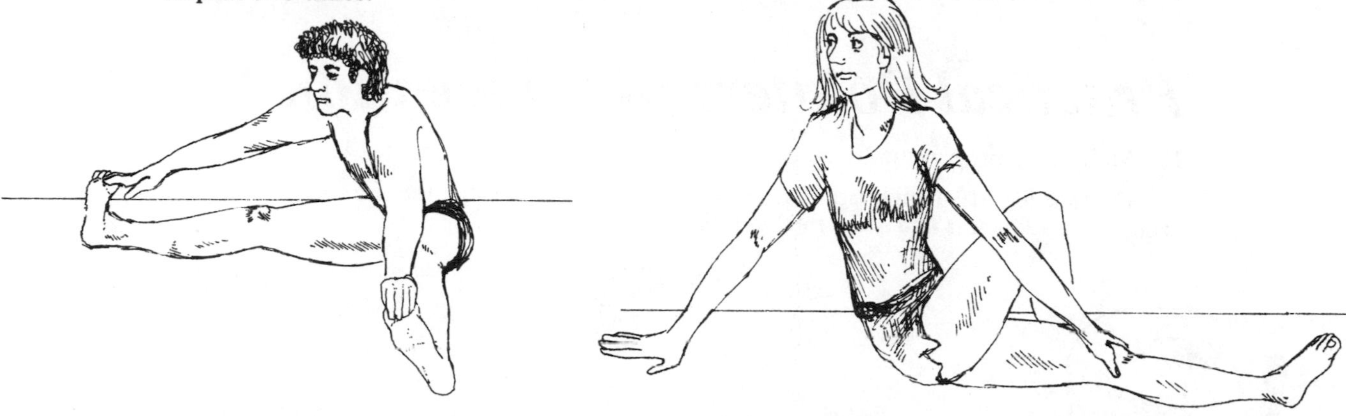

► To stretch the adductor muscles (inside of thigh), sit on the floor, spread your legs apart in front of you as far as you can, and slowly bend forward from the waist trying to touch your head to the floor in front of you.

► To stretch the abductor muscles (outside of the thigh), sit on the floor with your legs straight out in front of you. To stretch the right abductor muscle group, place a bent right leg over a straight left leg (with the left knee locked). Reach your left arm over your right knee toward your left side. Grasp the inside of your left leg with your left hand. Turn your head and body to the right. You should feel the stretch along the outside of your right hip and upper thigh. Hold for 30 seconds. Repeat twice.

5. Before retiring, apply a liberal amount of baby oil to the outside of the affected hip and inner or upper thigh area, and gently massage the area for ten minutes.

6. Hip, groin, and buttocks overuse problems are often associated with excessive pronation (rolling-in of the ankle and flattening of the arch) during running. If you think you are pronating excessively, fit a pair of Spenco inlays to your shoe size. Make a varus wedge out of ¼'' felt (see appendix on Shoe Inserts You Can Make) and attach to the bottoms of the Spenco inlays in the proper position. Place a 1/8'' heel pad cut to the shape of your heel over this varus wedge on the bottom of the Spenco.

7. These problems are often associated with a difference in length between the two legs. If you think you may have one leg longer than the other, see chapter 44.

When ready to resume running...

1. This type of injury can take a long time to heal, and can become chronic if not given enough time to rest. It can take four to eight weeks for some of these problems to completely resolve themselves. Therefore, be careful when returning to running and do not rush or push yourself too soon, lest you become reinjured (see chapter 27).

2. Do not attempt to jog until you have no pain *at all* in walking. Do not run until you have no pain *at all* in jogging.

3. Wear training shoes with good shock absorption in both the heel and the forefoot. Make sure the shoes are kept in good repair (see appendix on Running Shoes).

4. Avoid all hill training, racing, racing shoes and slanted (crowned) road surfaces. When you have been able to sustain painfree running for four to six weeks, you are ready to begin gradually adding hill workouts and speed.

5. Run on soft surfaces initially, using a comfortable stride length and concentrating on landing as gently as possible.

6. In addition to your regular stretching routine (see appendix on stretching), do side stretches if you have pain in the outside of the hip or upper thigh (see appendix on stretching).

7. If possible, heat the area for ten minutes before running and wrap an ace bandage or nylon hose around it to hold the heat in.

8. After running, as long as discomfort is present, lie down for ten to fifteen minutes and repeat the hip exercises with icing later at night. Also, if possible, massage the hip area before retiring (see Treatment #4 and #5).

9. If pain is minimal at the beginning of the run and increases as you go on, stop and stretch the hip (see Treatment #4). Walk 50 yards or so, and start up slowly again. If it is still painful, go home and take two or three days off. If the pain stays low grade or diminishes as you run, you can continue.

Practical Pointers for Prevention

1. Maintain a proper quadricep/hamstring ratio as discussed in chapter 40.

2. Do side leg lifts (thigh isometric exercises) to strengthen the inner and outer muscle groups (the adductors and abductors) as follows:

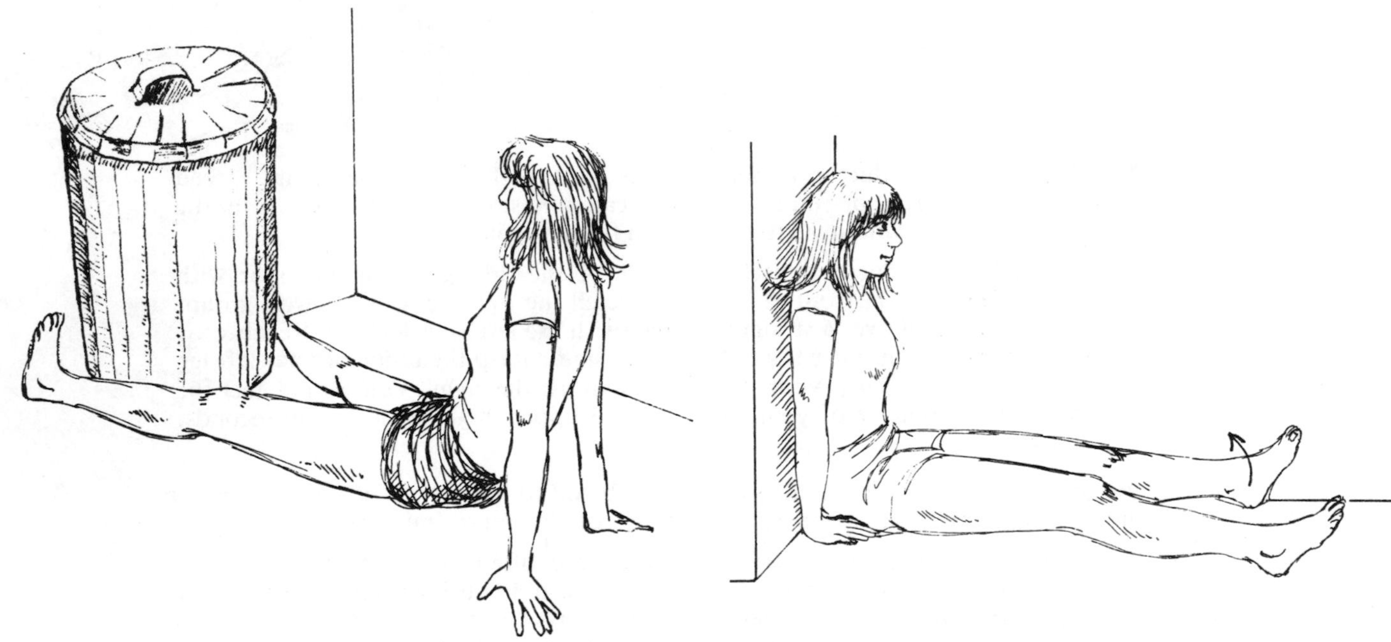

► For the adductors muscle group on the inside of the thigh: Sit erect on the floor with legs apart and a chair or similar object between them. Push the legs together, pressing against the chair. Hold for five to ten seconds, then repeat five times.

► For the abductors muscle group on the outside of the thigh: Sit erect on the floor, legs locked at the knee and straight out in front of you parallel to a wall. For the right side, sit with your right side closest to the wall (about three inches away). Push your right leg hard against the wall (contact usually occurs at the outside of the ankle area. Hold for five to ten seconds, then repeat five times.

When to Call the Doctor

If severe swelling, pain, and/or discoloration persist after up to four days of treatment, see a doctor. If, after a few days of rest, the hip joint gives way, see a doctor. If symptoms return with gradually increasing activity after a long layoff, see a podiatrist. If the injured hip is warmer to the touch than your other one and/or you have a low grade fever, see a podiatrist or sports doctor. Note: If the hip becomes lumpy or severely black and blue, see a sports doctor immediately.

43. Lower Back Pain

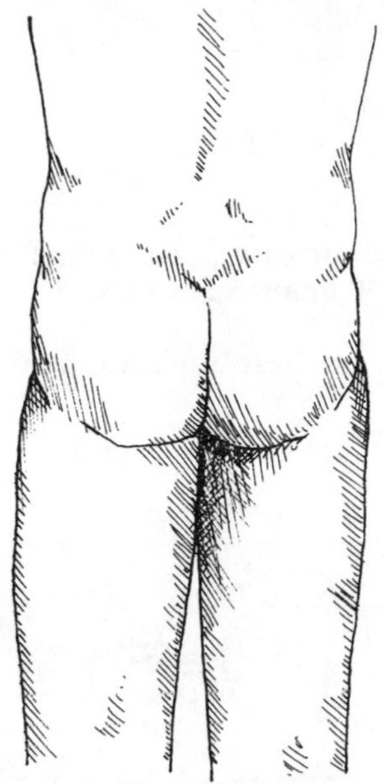

What is it?

Low back pain is often associated with muscle strains or spasms caused by running. If there is "shooting" pain going from the hip down to the thigh and sometimes into the lower leg and foot, then the problem could be sciatica (an irritation to the sciatic nerve).

CAUTION: If you have sustained a direct blow to the back, or if you bend over and find you cannot straighten up or walk without assistance, contact an orthopedist. Also see an orthopedist if you experience numbness going down one or both legs.

> **Special Note:** Pay special attention to back pain and injury. When in doubt, consult a sports physician. Back problems can be serious, and if not dealt with properly can become chronic and disabling.

Things you will need for this treatment

heating pad, rubber backed
heat ointment
terry cloth towel soaked in hot water
baby oil
nitorogen-impregnated foam innersoles
non-adhesive felt ¼"
ice bag
Sacro-Iliac brace
bed board
rubber seat cushion

Caution: *Do not proceed with this treatment until you have read the Guidelines to Treatment in Chapter 2*

Preparation for Treatment

► Make sure all materials and suggested medications are clean and up to date.

► Read through all the instructions which follow, and make sure you understand them before beginning treatment.

Treatment

1. Rest for 24 to 48 hours. In severe cases, bed rest may be necessary. Place an ice pack on the area four times a day, for 30 minutes at a time.

2. After the first 24 hours, apply heat applications three to four times daily for 30 minutes at a time, as follows:

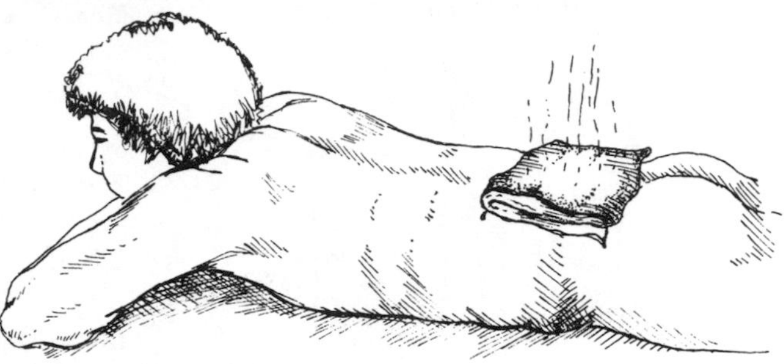

► Lie flat on your stomach
► Place a towel soaked in hot water on your back for three to four minutes. When this cools down, remove the towel.

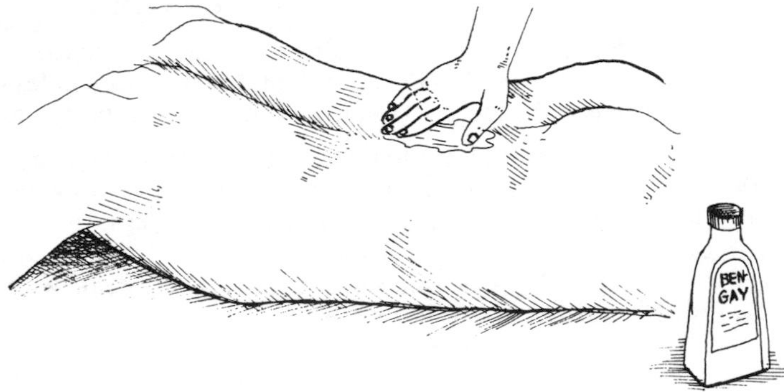

► Take some heating ointment like Ben Gay and apply liberally, directly to the involved area.
► Reapply a newly heated towel for three to four minutes, and when this cools down remove it.

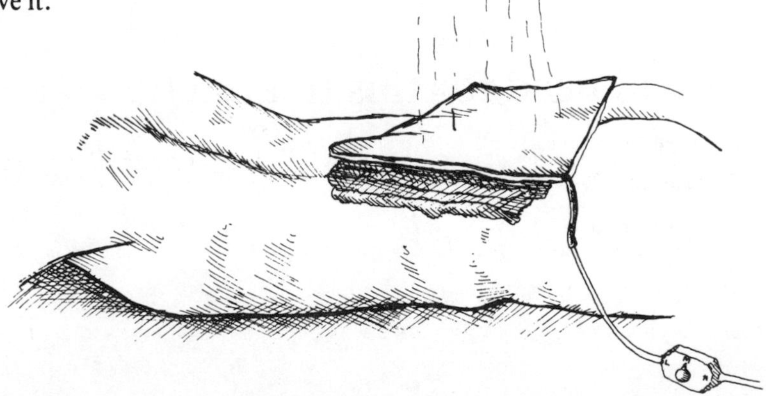

► Cover the area with a rubber-backed heating pad for 20 minutes on medium heat.

3. Take two aspirin every four hours for two days, then two aspirin every six hours for up to one week.

4. Have someone apply baby oil liberally to your back and gently massage the involved area for 10 to 20 minutes twice a day.

5. Some back problems are related to excessive pronation (feet roll inward at the ankles). If you are an excessive pronator, fit a pair of Spenco inlays to your shoe size. Make a varus wedge, extended to the arch, out of ¼" felt. Adhere to the bottom of the Spenco in the proper position (see appendix on Shoe Inserts You Can Make).

6. Low back problems in running sports are often caused or aggravated by a difference in leg length. If you think you have one leg longer than the other, see chapter 44.

7. When you can walk without pain for several days, then you are ready to return to jogging and/or running.

8. Wear training shoes with good shock absorption qualities. Make sure the shoes are in good repair (see appendix on running shoes).

9. Avoid hill training, racing, racing shoes or slanted (crowned) road surfaces.

10. You must be very diligent about giving yourself ample time for proper warmup and warm down. Make sure you do good before-and-after stretch routines (see appendix on stretching).

11. Resume athletic activity gradually, in distance and pace. Try to run erect with a short, comfortable stride, and concentrate on landing gently (see chapters 27 and 28).

12. Apply heat to your back before running by using a heat-producing ointment like Ben Gay and wearing a snug-fitting shirt over it.

13. If you experience minor pain when returning to run, ice down for 10 to 20 minutes afterward.

14. Have someone gently massage your back with baby oil for 10 to 20 minutes nightly.

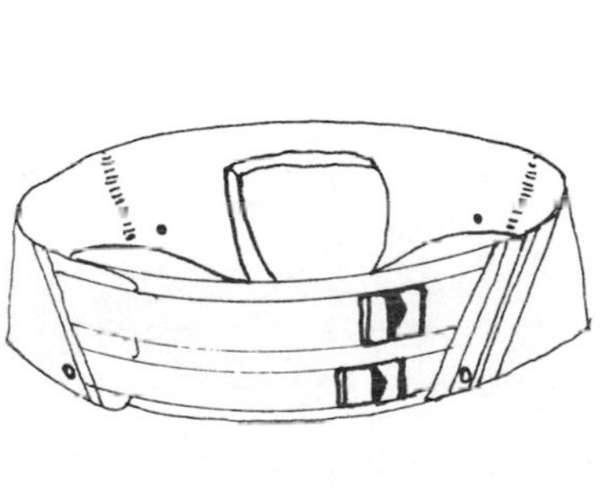

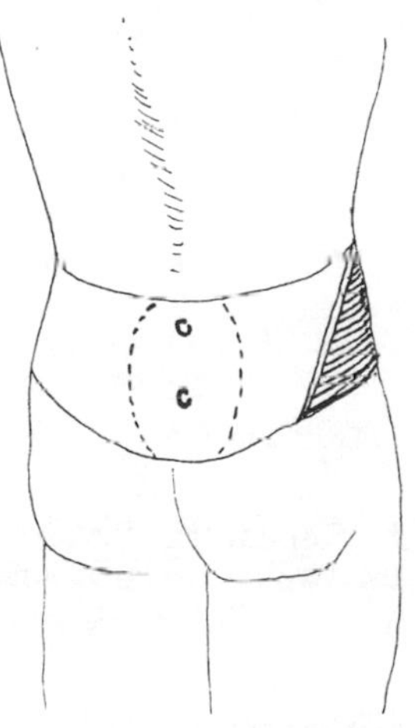

15. Sometimes the use of a Sacro-Iliac belt (available over the counter at most drug stores) is helpful. Be sure to get a proper fit.

Practical Pointers for Prevention

1. Do 25-50 bent-leg situps daily, whether you run or not.
2. Always bend your knees when lifting.
3. If you sit at a desk most of the day, try getting a rubber cushioned seat and a good stiff-backed chair.
4. Change your position in your chair frequently.
5. Try sleeping with a wooden board under your mattress.

6. Do the following stretching exercises daily, in addition to your regular stretch routine.

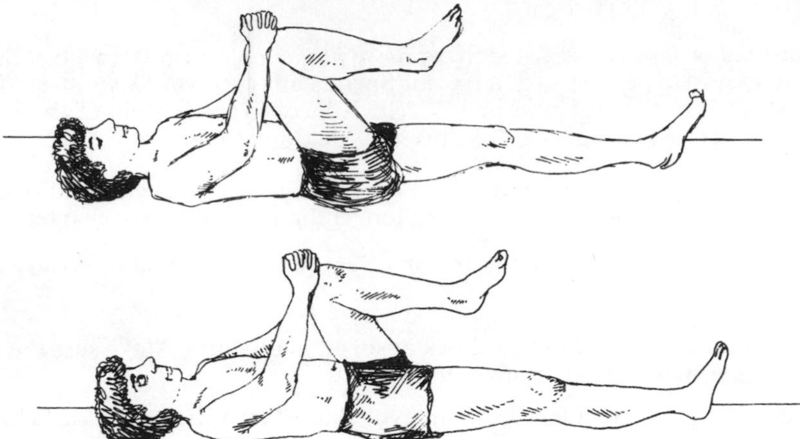

► Lie on your back on a flat surface. Pull one knee up toward your stomach and grasp with the arm on that side of your body. Hold for 15 seconds and lower. Repeat two times.

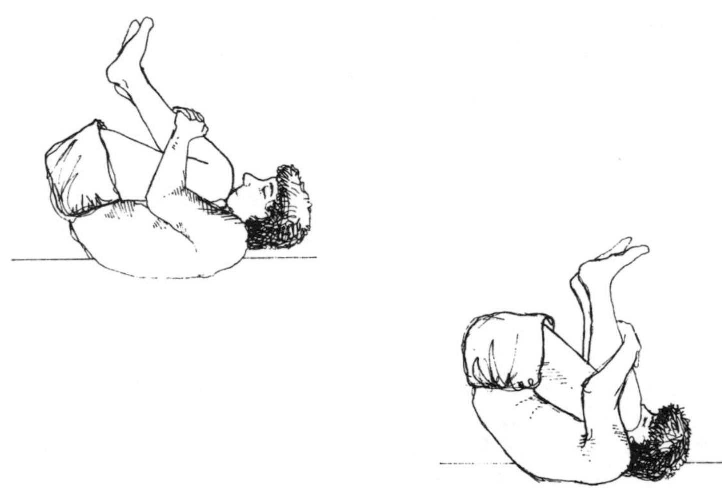

► Repeat the exercise above, with both legs grasped at the same time.
► With both legs grasped at the same time and tucked as close to your chest as possible, roll back and forth four to eight times or until the back feels loose.

DON'TS

1. Don't walk barefoot.
2. Don't lift any heavy objects.
3. Don't wear any shoes which are severely worn in the soles.

When to Call the Doctor

1. If after a day or two of rest, back spasms are severe or you cannot walk without assistance, see a sports physician.

2. If any numbness or tingling sensations are present in your back and/or legs, whether walking or at rest, see a sports physician.

44. Short Limb

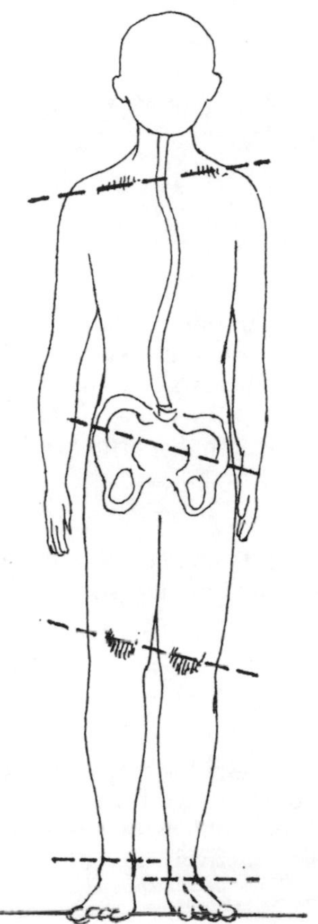

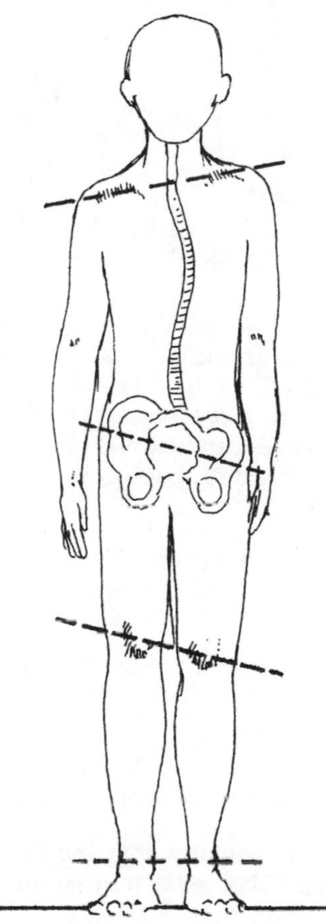

What is it?

It is fairly common for a person to have one leg shorter than the other—or to have one leg which *functions* as though it is shorter than the other. In the first case, there is an actual anatomical difference, and if you were X-rayed from top to bottom, one of the bones on one side of your body would measure shorter than the other. In this situation both feet would look the same. In the second case, called a functional leg length differential, there is probably an asymmetry in the back due to a curvature of the spine. In this case, one foot compensates by flattening out, its arch lowering more than the other.

In either type of case, a difference of five-eighths of an inch or less rarely causes any trouble in walking. But in running and other sports, a small limb length discrepancy can have significant effects.

If you have severe hip pain, back pain, or recurrent injuries on *one side* of your body only, there is a good chance that one of your legs is shorter than the other. Eighty percent of the problems that occur show up on the short side.

How to observe leg length differential:

1. If you get your pants altered and have noticed that the same leg always has to be seamed longer than the other, you may have a limb length discrepancy.

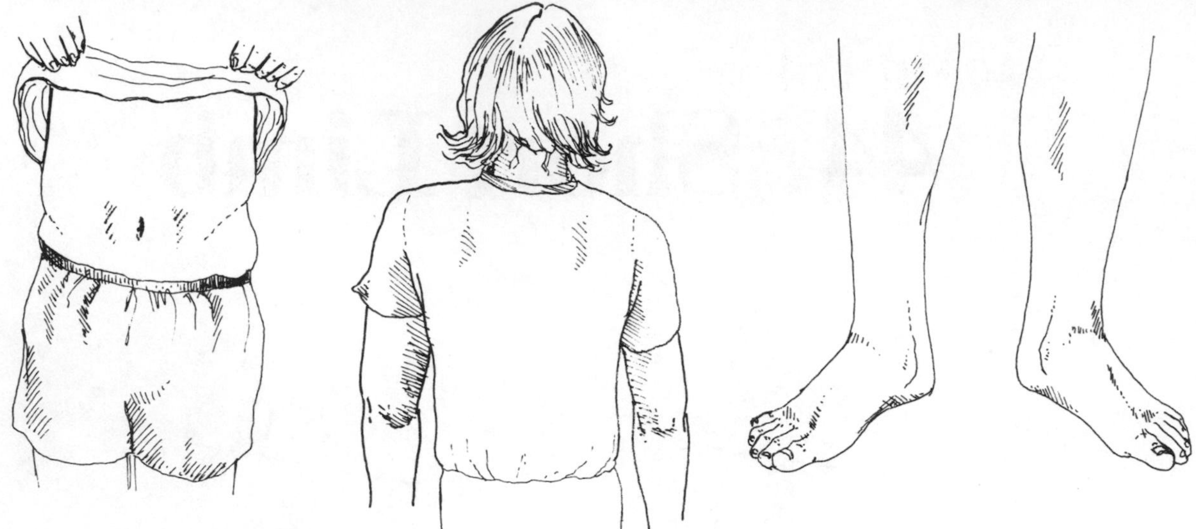

2. To check for a disparity, stand in front of a full length mirror, remove your clothes and observe your body. Stand barefoot with even weight distribution on both feet. Is one hip lower than the other? Is one shoulder lower than the other? Is one knee lower than the other? Do both feet look the same? Is one arch higher than the other? If one or more of these differences can be observed, you may have a limb length disparity (see appendix on foot structure and function).

3. While dressed, have someone watch you walk barefoot. Does one heel seem to come off the ground faster than the other? Do your arms swing differently—one hanging lower than the other?

4. Sit as far back in a straight backed chair as you can and have someone else hold your feet straight out in front of you and let them look at the heel bottoms. If they are uneven, you should suspect a short leg.

5. If you find that you do have a short leg but do not really have any problems or any pain, then do not try to treat it. Your body may have compensated for it already, and you could cause new problems by interfering with the adjustment which has already been made. Only if you feel that the limb length disparity is actively causing you difficulty should you proceed with this treatment.

Things you will need for this treatment

see chapter 2 "Materials List" for brand names and substitutes

non-adhesive felt 1/8" and ¼"
nitrogen impregnated foam innersoles
heel raise
tape measure
pen marker

Preparation for Treatment

► Make sure all materials and suggested medications are clean and up to date.

► Read through all the instructions which follow, and make sure you understand them before beginning treatment.

Caution: *Do not proceed with this treatment until you have read the Guidelines to Treatment in Chapter 2*

Treatment

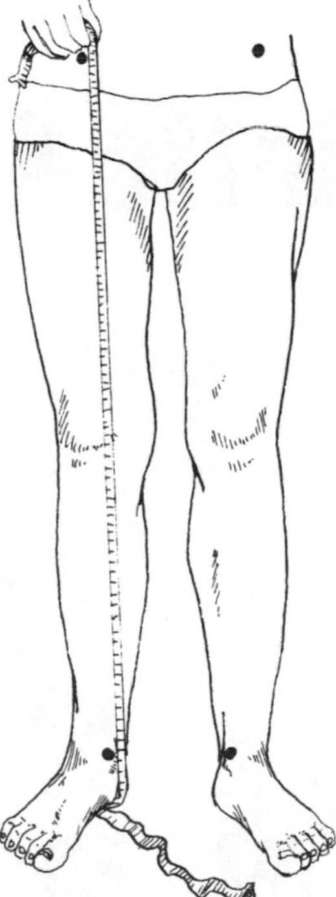

1. If you are going to deal with a short leg, then you first have to determine which leg is shorter. Lie flat on a table or floor and have someone take a tape measure and from a pen mark made at identical points on both of your hip bones, measure to the insides of your ankles (on the bones). Write down the measurements. Then measure from the belly button to the same ankle bones. Write down the measurements. Stand up and do the same two measurements and record. If your measurements show that one leg comes out shorter both lying down and standing, then you have an *actual* shortness. This is important to know for the treatment. If the leg length is equal lying down but different standing up, then you have a *functional* shortness.

2. For an *actual* shortness, the treatment is to compensate with a heel raise. A raise is made out of ¼'' felt or cork, eventually built up to be equal to the heel height differential. The raise should be made so that the front is thinner than the back.

It is important not to add too much compensation too soon. If you have a quarter-inch leg length differential, for example, start with a heel raise of one *eighth* of an inch for a week or two; then go up to one quarter of an inch if necessary. You can either put it directly into the shoe or add it to a Spenco inlay that can be moved from shoe to shoe (see appendix on Shoe Inserts You Can Make).

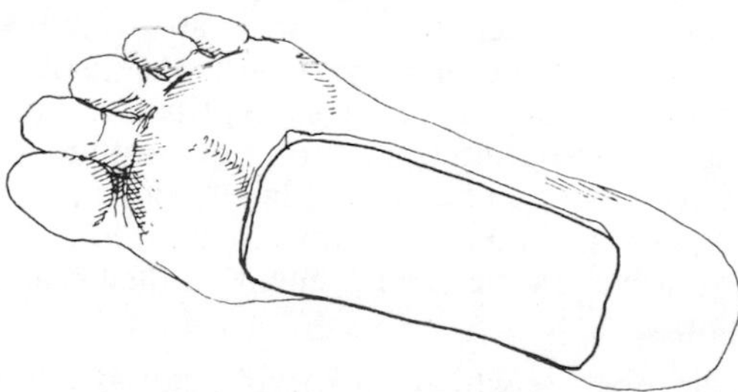

3. If you have a *functional* shortness, the raise should go under the arch. Build up a quarter-inch felt under the arch. Also place a 1/8'' to 1/4'' felt heel pad directly over the heel part of the arch buildup. You can either put it directly into the shoe or add it to a Spenco inlay that can be moved from shoe to shoe (see appendix on Shoe Inserts You Can Make).

4. Repeat all your measurements as described in #1 above with the raise under your bare foot or in your shoe. Make sure you compensated the proper amount. If not, adjust the height of the raise as needed.

45. Athletic Cramps

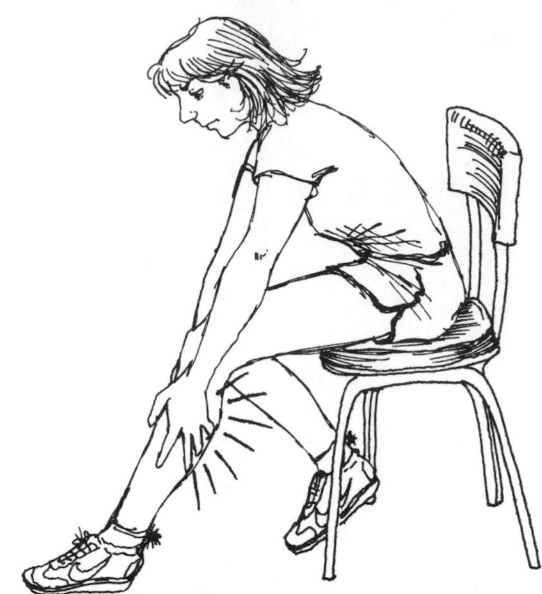

What is it?

A muscle cramp, or spasm, is a sudden, involuntary and abnormal contraction of the muscle. It commonly occurs in athletes, and can have many causes, including: (1) a blow to the muscle causing slight internal bleeding, (2) overstretching of the muscle causing ruptures of some of the fibers, and (3) strain of the muscle against resistance. Muscle fiber tears and contusions often occur in healthy, active children, but usually they heal up rapidly.

A "charley horse" is a tear which involves bleeding into the muscle belly. The muscle is painful to use, and becomes swollen and sensitive to touch.

Occasionally a severe muscle cramp or spasm will occur for no apparent reason in the calf of a seemingly normal athlete. While running at full speed, he experiences a sudden, violent contraction of the calf muscle which pulls the foot down and causes severe cramping pain. This may even happen when actual exertion is at a minimum. There are several causes of this condition, some curable and some not. The depletion of minerals in the body by excessive perspiration may increase susceptibility. Sudden changes in temperature, local impairment of circulation (pants too tight around the calf, or calf muscles strapped too tightly) and even diet can be factors in cramping. Most of these factors can be controlled by an adequate training program. In addition, foot and leg structural weaknesses can lead to excessive muscle use fatigue, and then cramping (see appendix on foot structure and function).

There still remain some cramps for which no specific causes have been pin-pointed. In most instances the athlete has exhibited no preliminary symptoms; the muscle suddenly jumps into severe spasm and the athlete is rendered helpless by both pain and lack of mobility. The muscle is not particularly tender and there is no swelling.

Muscle spasms or cramps are particularly prevalent in the neck, back, hamstrings and calf muscles. They are common in weight-bearing portions of the body, but relatively infrequent in the arms.

In most cases, treatment of cramps is simple and can be self-administered.

Caution: *Do not proceed with this treatment until you have read the Guidelines to Treatment in Chapter 2*

Things you will need for this treatment

see chapter 2 "Materials List" for brand names and substitutes

heating pad
heat ointment
wet heat
aspirin
nitrogen-impregnated foam innersoles
non-adhesive felt ¼"
adhesive felt 1/8"
weights, 5 pounds
ace bandage
ice bag

Treatment (Immediate)

1. Apply local pressure to the spastic muscle and try to guide it firmly through a normal range of motion.

2. For a calf cramp, sit on the ground and grab the calf firmly with one hand while pulling the top of the foot toward you with the other. Hold this position until the muscle knot is released.

3. The cramp may also be released by contraction of the opposing muscle group, so that for example, if there is a cramp on one side, stretching the muscle by leaning to the opposite side will frequently relieve the spasm.

4. For arch or toe cramping, hold the arch with one hand and the toes with the other, and slowly pull the toes and the foot toward your face. Hold this position until the cramping disappears (see chapter 24, #1).

5. For a thigh cramp, grab the thigh with one hand and the lower leg with the other. Slowly, straighten the leg and massage the thigh until the cramp relaxes.

► If you need help in relaxing the spasm have someone else apply steady, even, firm, local pressure. The results will often be dramatic. So will simple stretching of the muscle. A combination of the two appears to be even more effective.

6. Using a back-and-forth motion, massage the calf, arch, and toes with baby oil for five to ten minutes. As the muscle spasm relaxes, a relatively gentle massage toward the direction of your head may be useful. The muscle may be tapped gently from side to side by the two hands by rolling the muscle between the two palms. Once this cramp is gone, you may continue to compete, although the condition is quite prone to reoccur. If the cramping is more persistent it will require further treatment. This consists of local heat applications by whirlpool baths, warm packs, or in fact any heat modality. Wet heat appears to be more effective than heating pads. Massage is valuable in restoring circulation to the muscle.

7. Take two aspirin immediately and two more after four hours.

Treatment (Long-term)

1. Fit a pair of Spenco inlays into your shoes. Make a varus wedge long enough to extend from the back of the heel to the arch (see appendix on Shoe Inserts You Can Make). Attach to the bottom of the Spenco inlays in the proper position.

► For calf or thigh cramps, add a heel pad made of 1/8" felt, and attach to a varus wedge on the bottom of the Spenco inlay. This heel pad is made by cutting 1/8" felt into the shape of the heel, and attaching it to the bottom of the varus wedge at the heel. If you do not pronate (roll in at the ankles) excessively, just use the heel raises.

2. Apply moist heat applications to the affected muscle each day until there is no trace of cramping (see chapter 2). Do the following exercises four to seven days a week. For each exercise, each leg should be stretched 30 seconds, twice (see appendix on stretching).

► Wall pushes with the back leg straight
► Wall pushes with the back leg knee bent inward
► Hamstring stretches
► Toe touches

3. *For Arch and/or Toe Cramps Only:*

► With your weight off your feet (sitting or lying on your back), move your toes up and down as far as possible in each direction. Hold for ten seconds each time and repeat five to ten times (see illustration in chapter 24).

► From a flat footed standing position, move up and down on your toes 10 to 20 times.

4. *For Calf Cramps Only:*
► Sit on a table with legs hanging down. Hang five pounds of weight from the top of your feet (use an old pocketbook with a strap or a paint can with a padded handle, and fill with rocks or other objects to the desired weight). (See appendix on stretching.)
► Pull your toes toward your face, without moving your leg. Repeat five times, holding for five seconds each time.
► Repeat the same exercise with the foot turned inward.
► Do these exercises twice a day, four days a week.

5. For thigh cramps, quadriceps and hamstring muscle balance must be checked and corrected if necessary with strength exercises as explained in chapter 40.

6. If you suspect excessive perspiration as a possible cause, drink more water before and during your training and actual competition.

7. Make sure none of your clothes, elastic bandages, or tapings are too tight. If they are, loosen them.

Treatment for Trauma-Related Cramping

1. See Immediate Treatment Section #1 through 6.

2. Rest the injured area and partially immobilize it with an ace bandage (also used here for compression), for 24 to 48 hours depending upon the severity of the swelling and/or discoloration.

3. Apply ice packs along with the compression bandaging, for 30 minutes on and 30 minutes off, for up to 48 hours (see chapter 2).

4. Take two aspirin every four hours for two to three days and then every six hours for up to one week.

5. For calf injury, use the treatment described in chapter 38, from #3 on.

6. For thigh muscle cramp injuries, refer to chapter 41.

DON'TS

1. Don't overstretch the muscle, as you are only trying to restore a normal range of motion. In hamstring spasm, the knee should be extended but straight leg raising should not be carried out. In calf spasm, the foot should be pushed up to ninety degrees but not forced further. In passive exercise, force should be applied steadily and smoothly with no jerk or swing.

2. Don't apply massive force with leverage against the muscle spasm, as this may result in a rupture of the muscle fibers or even tearing of the tendon away from the bone. In this case a relatively simple condition can easily be replaced by one much more serious.

3. Don't walk barefoot.

4. Don't use negative-heel shoes for every day wear.

When to Call the Doctor

If after following all the above instructions, including taking several days of rest, the cramps continue to occur and worsen in either frequency or intensity, see a podiatrist or sports physician. If swelling or black-and-blue discoloration persists after four days of treatment, see a podiatrist or sports doctor. If the involved muscle group is warmer to the touch than the other leg and/or you have a low grade temperature, or you cannot move your foot downward at the ankle joint off of weight bearing, or you have extreme pain when you move your knee and/or hip joint, see a sports doctor.

46. Apophysitis of the Heels

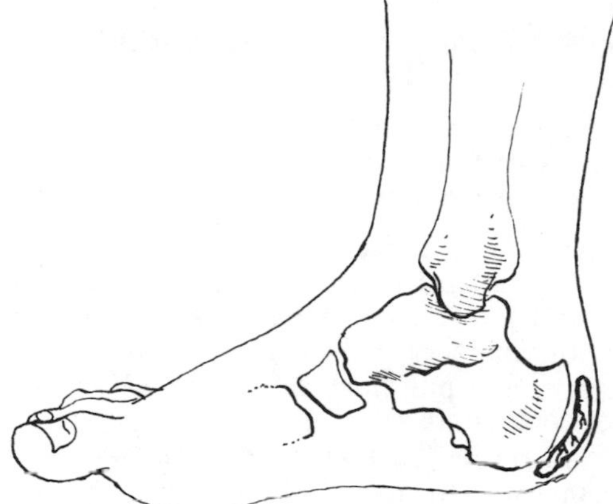

What is it?

Apophysitis of the Heels is an irritation or irregularity of the growth plate (cartilage) in back of the heel bone. It usually occurs in young people between the ages of eight and fifteen (most often in males). This is a period of rapid growth and the bones are growing so fast that the muscles, tendons and other soft tissues cannot keep up the pace. Therefore the soft tissue is literally stripped off the heel bone.

Things you will need for this treatment

see chapter 2 "Materials List" for brand names and substitutes

ice bag
slant board
adhesive felt ¼"
soap & water
adhesive spray and skin protectant
adhesive tape 1½" to 2"
nitrogen-impregnated foam innersoles
aspirin

Preparation for Treatment

► Make sure all materials and suggested medications are clean and up to date.

► Thoroughly scrub the entire foot with warm soapy water and a terry wash cloth. Pat dry with a soft clean towel.

► Read through all the instructions which follow, and make sure you understand them before beginning treatment.

Caution: Do not proceed with this treatment until you have read the Guidelines to Treatment in Chapter 2

Treatment

1. If the pain is so noticeable that the child limps, all athletic activity should be discontinued. It will probably take from one to two weeks for the problem to abate enough to permit a resumption of activity. In isolated cases the condition could last for up to three months.

2. Initially, apply ice to the bottom or back of the heels (wherever the pain usually occurs) for 10-20 minutes once or twice a day.

3. Use aspirin to reduce the initial inflammation.
► Take two aspirin every six hours for two to seven days.
► If you are allergic to aspirin or any of its contents, don't touch it (see chapter 2).

4. Do the following stretching exercises daily. If they irritate the problem (they shouldn't), do them with less intensity. Do each exercise slowly; avoid bouncing or making jerking motions; and if you feel a burning sensation with the stretch, let up a little.
► Sit on the floor with your legs stretched out straight; grab your toes with your hands or a piece of rope, and pull back slowly for 30 seconds. Release slowly and repeat (see chapter 35, treatment #4).
► Do 10 seconds of wall pushes (back knee straight), twice (see appendix on stretching).
► Repeat the wall pushes with the back knee bent.
► Alternatively, use a slant board or purchase a pair of Flex-Wedges

► For best results, do these exercises three times a day. If you can, do your ice treatments after you finish the stretching.

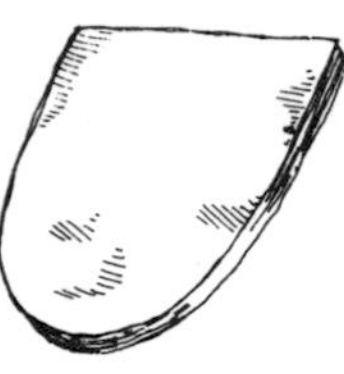

adhesive felt pad

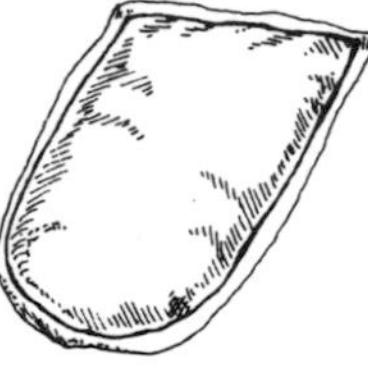

sponge rubber pad

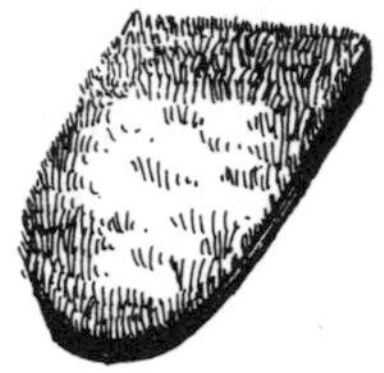

indoor-outdoor carpet pad

5. Fit heel pads into the shoes (see appendix on shoe inserts you can make). You can either cut a piece of ¼" adhesive felt to the shape of the heel, or purchase a ready-made heel cushion or sponge rubber pad. It is also possible to make your own pad from a scrap of indoor-outdoor carpeting.

6. Unless you have a disparity in leg length, add the same thickness of pad to both feet even if you are only treating one.

7. Tape the foot with an "equinus taping" as follows (see chapter 35):
► After cleaning the area well with soap and water and rinsing down with alcohol, spray tincture of Benzoin on the bottom of the foot and back of the legs to allow the tape to stick better and protect the skin from irritation.
► If you are using a heel pad, you can attach it directly to the heel and then incorporate the tape afterwards.
► Cut three strips of 1½-2" tape, about 8-12 inches long depending on the size of the foot and leg.
► Center the first strip on the front of the heel pad (or heel) and pull the tape up over the foot.
► Make sure the foot is relaxed, with the toes in a downward direction (equinus position).
► Repeat with strips 2 and 3, covering the entire heel or heel pad. Anchor down on foot and leg with two 4-inch strips of 1½-2 inch tape.

8. An alternative is to use the tape separately and place the heel raises directly in the shoes.

9. If the child is a runner and is bow-legged or has excessive wear along the outside of the heel of his shoes, place a varus tilt of up to ¼" on the inside of the heel of his running shoe or shoes. This can be done by using a piece of ¼" felt thinned down so that the outside portion is thinner than the inside (i.e., the left-hand side of a left shoe insert is thinner than the right side). This wedge can also be added to the bottom of a Spenco inlay, so they can be moved from shoe to shoe (see appendix on making your own shoe inserts).

10. If pain is present in walking, the foot should be either taped all day or protected by using the varus wedge and heel raise. Also, if walking is painful, the child should not be allowed to participate in sports.

When Returning to Action...

1. When athletic activities are resumed, make sure the running shoes or athletic shoes have a rigid heel counter and a very flexible sole (see appendix on shoes).

2. When athletic activities are resumed stretching exercises should be done both before and after each practice or competition.

3. If there has been a layoff from athletic activity of a week or more, resumption should be gradual (see chapter 27).

When to Call the Doctor

If pain is still present after a week of treatment, see a podiatrist. If swelling and/or black and blue discoloration occurs and is still present after four days, see a podiatrist. If the child cannot move the foot downward, see a podiatrist.

DON'TS

- Don't go barefoot.
- Don't wear negative-heel shoes, loafers, or exercise sandals
- Don't let your heels get run down.

Appendix A
All About Podiatrists

1. Definition:

"Podiatry is that profession of the health sciences which deals with the examination, diagnosis, treatment, and prevention of diseases, conditions, and malfunctions affecting the human foot and its related or governing structures, by employment of medical, surgical or other means." —*Adopted by American Podiatry Association House of Delegates.*

2. Education:

The pre-requisites for admission and criteria used in the admissions process by schools of podiatric medicine are identical to those of the traditional medical schools. A minimum of three years of pre-medical study at an accredited college or university, and a satisfactory score on the New-Medical College Admissions Test (New-MCAT). Better than 90% of those students entering a school of podiatry have Baccalaureate Degrees or higher, prior to the admission to the four year course in a college of podiatric medicine.

3. Colleges:

There are five colleges of podiatric medicine in the United States. They are located in New York City, Philadelphia, Cleveland, Chicago and San Francisco.

4. Curriculum:

The curriculum at the colleges of podiatric medicine is, in effect, a "single tract" medical education with special emphasis on the lower extremity, but provides a general medical curriculum parallel to that of traditional medical schools. Curricula offered by the individual colleges consist of more than 4,000 hours of instruction distributed throughout four academic years. Curricula in the first two years are predominantly in the basic sciences, and the final two years concentrate on clinical training and practice. Required courses include anatomy, physiology, biochemistry, pharmacology, microbiology, pathology, general and podiatric surgery and general and podiatric medicine, in addition to specific courses which relate to clinical practice. All the colleges confer the degree Doctor of Podiatric Medicine (DPM). During the last two years of the educational program, the student spends a major portion of his time in the study of podiatric medicine and surgery and its relation to the general health, well being and emergency care of patients. This study is accomplished in the clinics of the colleges, their allied clinical programs, affiliated teaching hospitals, long term care facilities, and private offices.

5. Podiatric Residency:

Over 50% of the graduates from the colleges of podiatric medicine enter post-graduate residency training programs of one, two or three years' duration. Such programs are carried out in teaching hospitals. The resident receives additional training in podiatric medicine and surgery and serves in rotation and emergency services, anesthesiology, radiology, general medicine, pathology, general surgery, and podiatric surgery. Programs also include experience in other services such as pediatrics, dermatology, neurology, orthopedics, and physical medicine and rehabilitation. Both the professional and post-graduate education programs stress an awareness of the vital need to promote cooperative relationships between podiatry and the other primary health professions in the appropriate delivery of quality health care services.

6. Licensing

Podiatrists are licensed in all 50 states to treat the foot medically, mechanically and surgically. Foot and leg problems seen on an everyday basis by podiatrists include:

A. Infants and children
   1. Foot deformities requiring correction through bracing, casting or surgery.
   2. Flat feet
   3. Pidgeon toeing
   4. Outtoeing
   5. Leg cramps
   6. Skin conditions

B. Injury
   1. Fractures and dislocations
   2. Sprains and strains
   3. Lacerations, cuts and bruises
   4. Foreign bodies; splinters, glass, stings
   5. Burns

C. Skin conditions
   1. Fungus infection (athletes foot)
   2. Allergies
   3. Nail disease
   4. Corns and callouses
   5. Plantar warts
   6. Skin tumors
   7. Foot odor and excessive sweating
   8. Blisters

D. Sports medicine
   1. Prevention of athletic injuries
   2. Treatment of athletic injuries

E. Bone and joint problems
   1. Bunions
   2. Arthritis
   3. Heel spurs
   4. Hammertoes
   5. Arch problems

F. Aged
   1. Diabetic foot problems
   2. Circulatory problems

Appendix B
Foot Structure and Function

The foot has two basic functions. One is to adapt to the surfaces on which we walk or run, and absorb the shock of impact; and the other is to accept the body weight from above and move it forward.

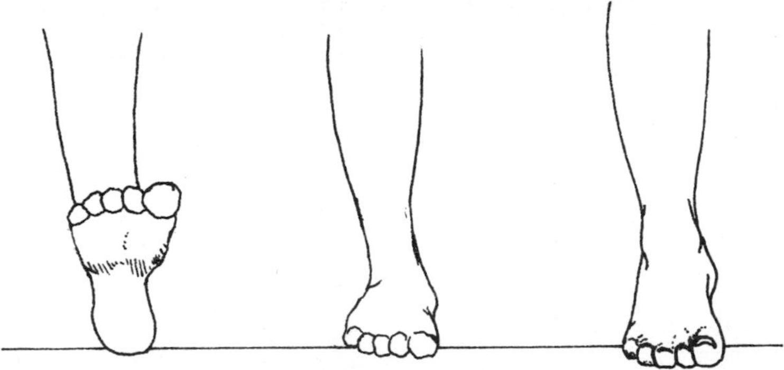

When the "normal" foot strikes the ground, it contacts on the outside of the heel and then rolls inward and downward and the arch lowers a little. This series of motions is called *pronation*. It allows the foot to become loose and mobile in order to be an effective adapter and shock absorber. After the foot has landed firmly, and is bearing the full weight of the body, the directions of the foot movements reverse. The arch starts to rise, and the foot starts to roll upwards and outwards, becoming very rigid and stable in order to lift the weight of the body and move it forward. This series of movements is called *supination*.

In order to accomplish these movements, the joints and muscles of the entire lower extremity, from the ankle to the hip, go through a special sequence of motions. The timing is extremely important. If the foot goes from pronation to supination smoothly and on time, no strain or loss of efficient motion occurs. However, if it pronates excessively, the weight of the body falls on the foot at the wrong time. Instead of being a rigid, stable structure, the foot is a "loose bag of bones" and cannot possibly propel the body forward efficiently. Instead of being in a strong supinated position, it is in a pronated or weakened state. This is the cause of many overuse injuries in athletics. It also explains why people who pronate excessively may have their performance adversely affected. Muscles which are designed for stabilization are called upon to help propel, and propeller muscles are forced to help with the stabilization. When the various muscle groups of the lower extremities are called upon to do work that they were not intended to do, they become strained and performance levels are diminished. Another problem with excessive pronation is that body weight is thrust on the foot at a time when it is unstable. The bones are subjected to abnormal stresses, which can lead to stress fractures, bone spur formations, enlargements of bones called exostoses, joint injuries, bursitis, and arthritis. And, with the muscles forced to do the wrong work, as described above, stresses are created which can lead to muscle and tendon injuries. In some cases, excessive stresses are transmitted through the legs to the skeletal structure above, producing many of the knee, hip, and lower back injuries seen in runners. Because of evolutionary failures, most of us—something like 80 to 90 percent of us—have feet which are sufficiently imperfect in structure to cause them to function defectively to some extent.

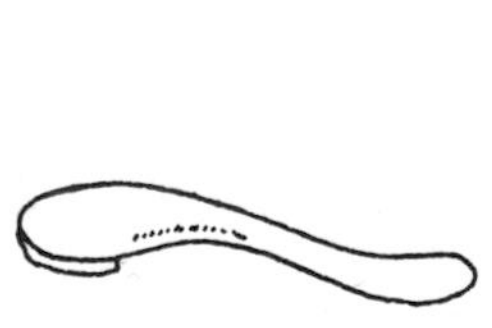

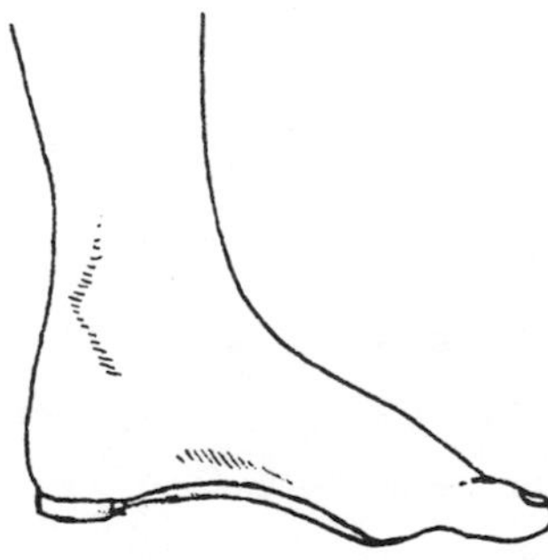

Each one of us is born with a particular structural relationship between the front of the foot, back of the foot, leg, and supporting surface. This is known as the neutral position. This position is neither "normal" or "abnormal," but is the one an individual must function with. If a person's neutral position is such that he or she strikes the ground at heel contact excessively to the outside of the heel or front of the foot (forefoot), then it is obvious that this foot must pronate excessively or abnormally in order to get the inside of the foot to contact the ground. To alleviate this problem, an orthotic device can be made which eliminates abnormal pronation and allows the foot and leg to function with maximum efficiency. An orthotic is a scientifically fabricated device which is contoured to fit each individual foot and may have rearfoot and forefoot posts which represent specific degrees of biomechanical correction in order to retain a proper relationship between the forefoot, rearfoot, and leg, and the supporting surface. To have such a device made, see a podiatrist.

Self Examination

Stand in front of a mirror nude, or have someone directly observe your structure.

1. *From the front:*

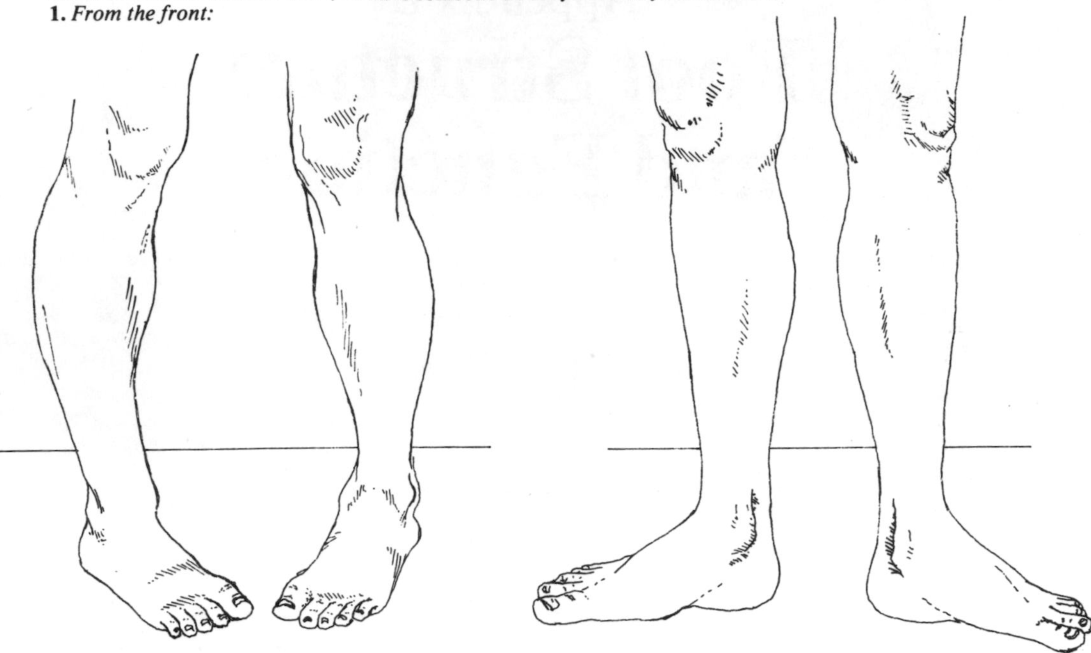

► Do your toes turn in, toward each other (toe in; pigeon-toed)?
► Do your toes turn out, away from each other (toe-out; duck-walk)?

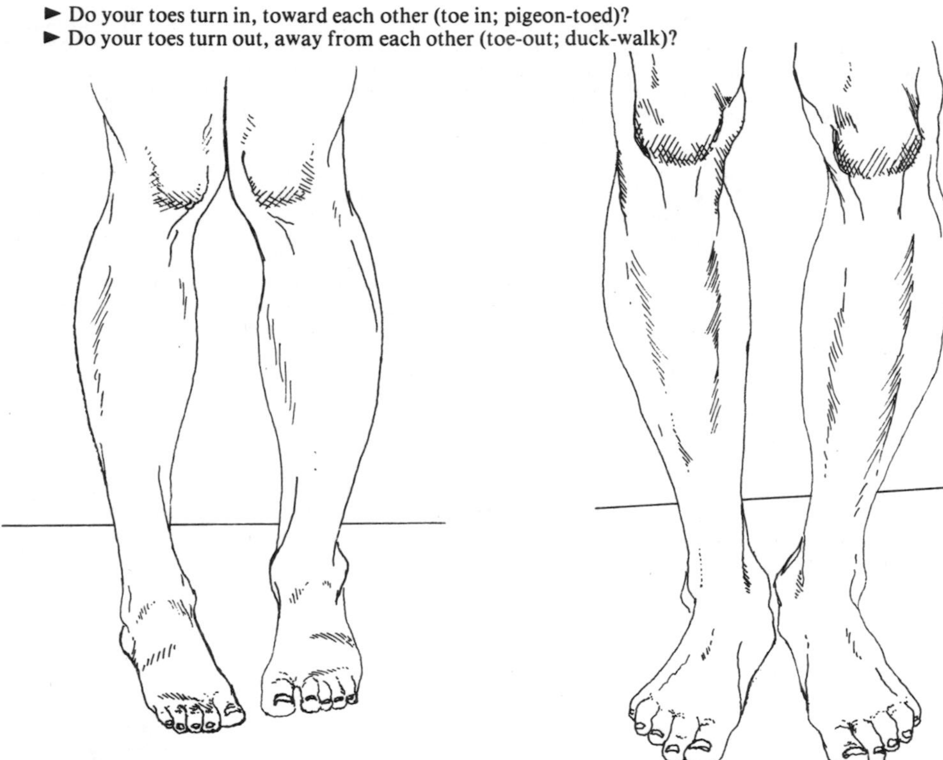

► When your legs are together, do your knees touch, and is there a space between your ankles (knock-knees)?
► When your legs are together, do your ankles touch, and is there a space between your knees (bow-legs)?

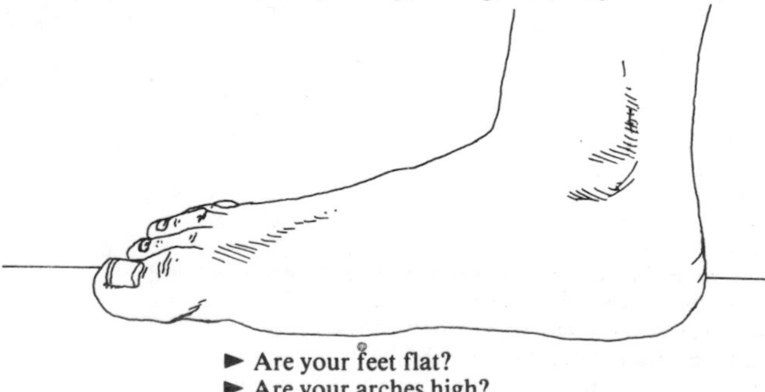

► Are your feet flat?
► Are your arches high?

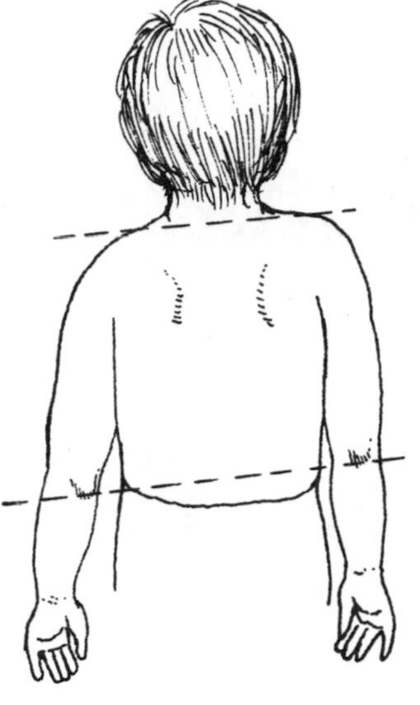

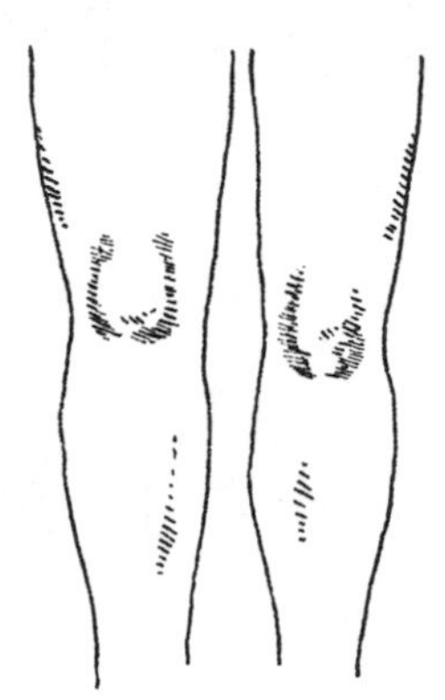

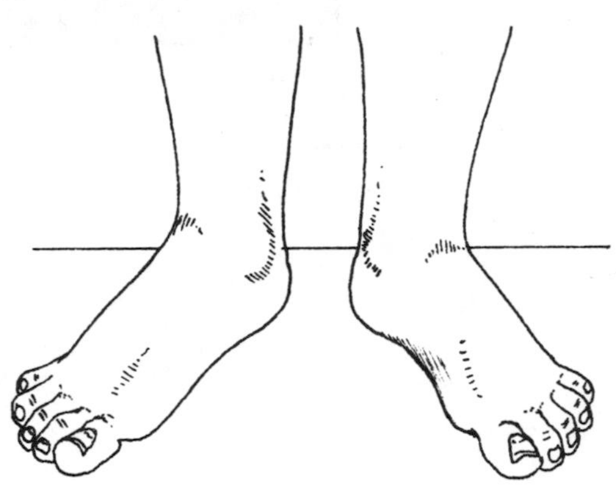

► Is one shoulder lower?

► Is one arm longer?

► Is one hip higher?

► Is one knee cap higher?

► Is one foot flat while the other has a high arch?

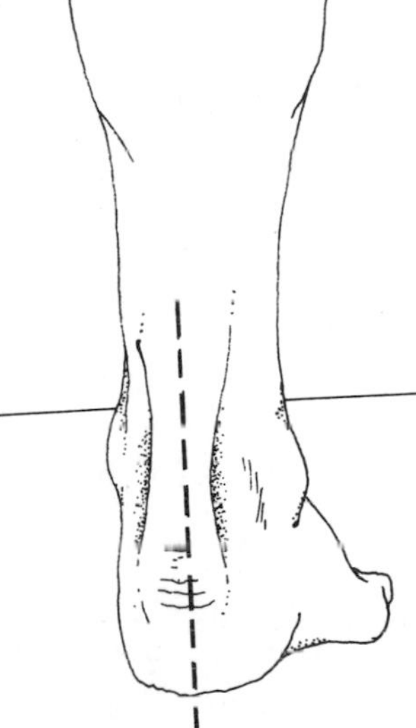

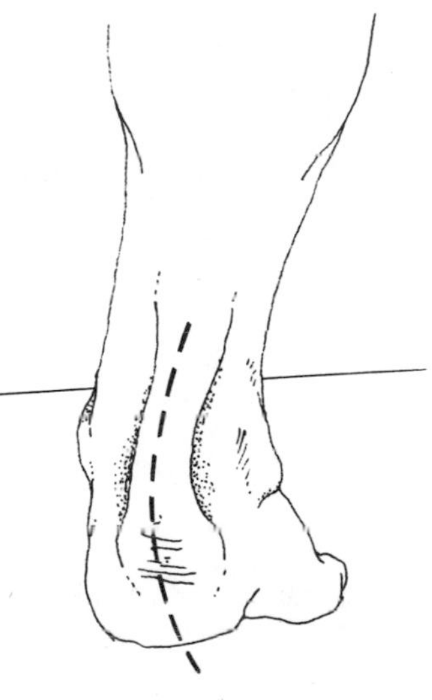

3. *From the back:*
► Does the achilles tendon look straight up and down at the back of the leg . . . or does it curve outward when it gets to the heel level? If it curves, you probably pronate excessively.

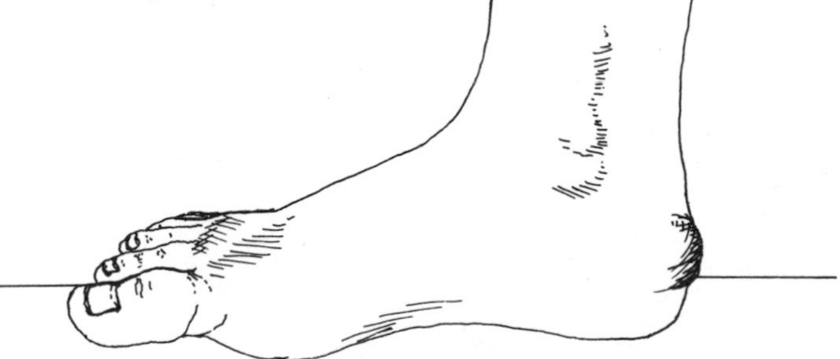

4. *From the side:*
► Does your head project in front of your shoulders?
► Are your shoulders rounded forward?
► Do you have a small pot belly that exercise and diet won't take away?
► Do your buttocks protrude excessively?
► Do your lower legs curve from front to back?
► Do you have bumps in back of your heels?

If in your self-examination you have found one or many of the faulty alignments listed, your improper alignment can make you susceptible to various mechanical problems, or lead to injury.

NOTE: If your answer to any of the questions in #2 is "yes," turn to chapter 44.

To realign your body, see the appendix on Shoe Inserts You Can Make.

If these measures do not improve the alignment (recheck alignment with proper insert in place in shoe and shoes on the feet), see a sports medicine podiatrist.

Appendix C
Children's Problems

1. Babies

► Babies do not need shoes or socks until they can stand and/or begin to walk.

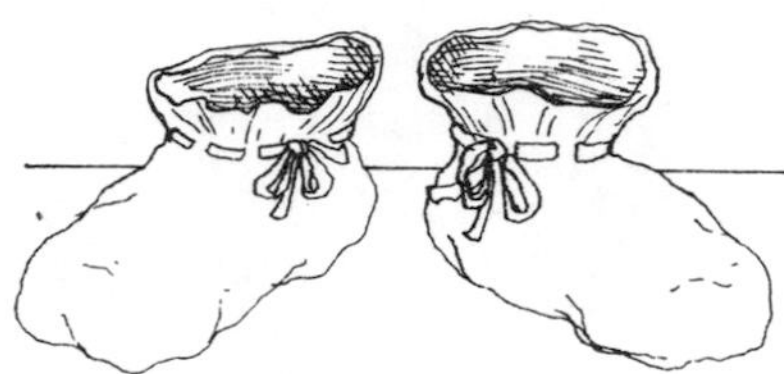

► Any foot coverings at this time should be loose and provide warmth. The soles should be flexible. If using booties, check the length and fit every time you put them on the baby.

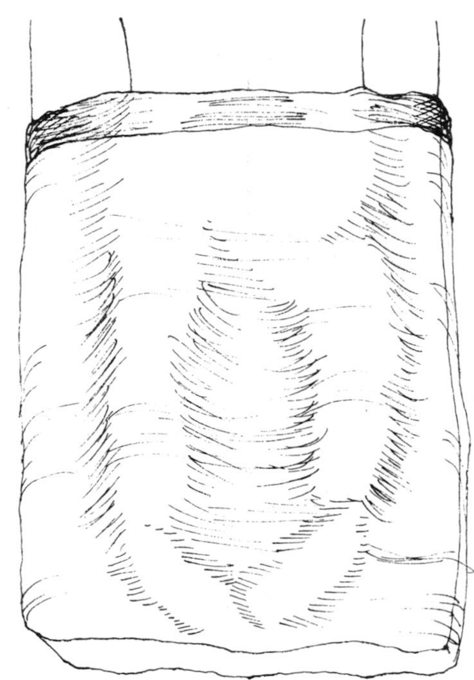

► No binding bed covers should be placed over children's feet, as they can retard development by not allowing the child to exercise the feet and legs as they prepare for walking.

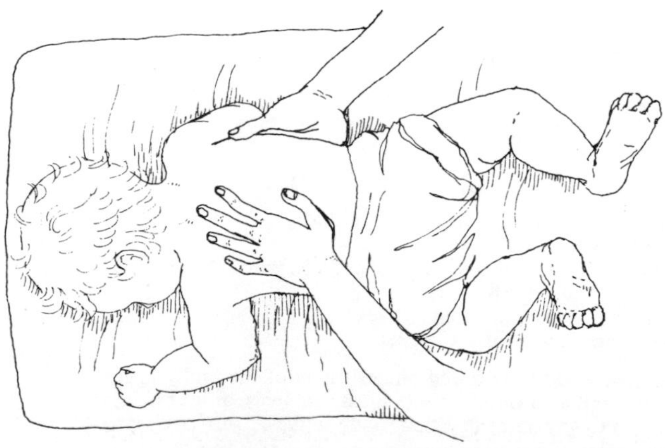

► Change the baby's lying position several times each day. Prolonged lying in one position, especially on the stomach, can put excessive strain on the foot or leg.

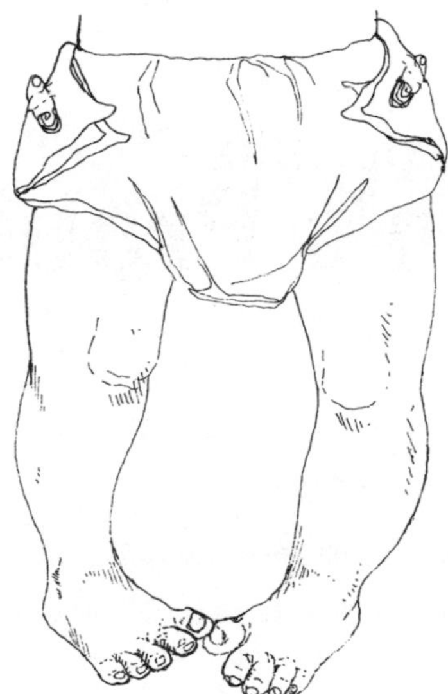

► Too many layers of diapers can sometimes cause the child to assume a bowlegged-type position. More than a double layer is unnecessary unless there is a specific reason. Have your podiatrist check the legs carefully, if more than a double layer of diapers is needed.

► Do not rush a child to walk. Do not compare him to other children. The average walking age is between ten and eighteen months, but there are large differences among individuals.

2. Children

Here is an examination you can perform with your own child, to determine whether there are any structural weaknesses present. Many problems with children's feet, legs, hips and back may be avoided by early recognition and proper attention.

► Watch your baby or child walk and run.

a. Does he like it or dislike it or complain about it?
b. Does the walk seem peculiar?
c. Does the child stumble or fall down excessively?
d. Does he always take his shoes off?

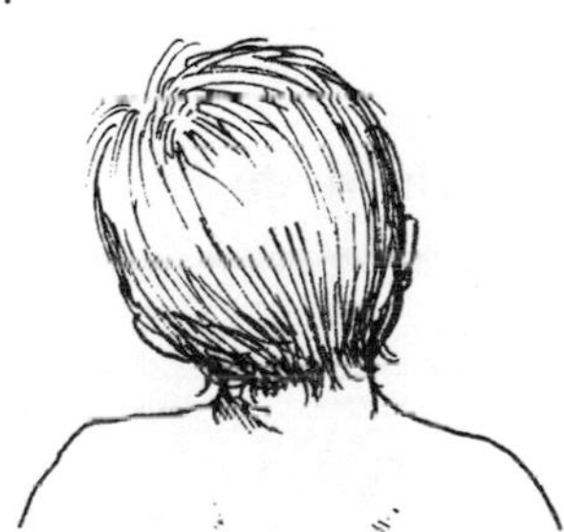

e. Does his head usually tilt to one side or another?
f. Is one shoulder lower than the other? (See appendix on foot and leg structure.)
g. Do the hips seem to be level? (See appendix on foot and leg structure).
h. Does one arm swing lower than the other?

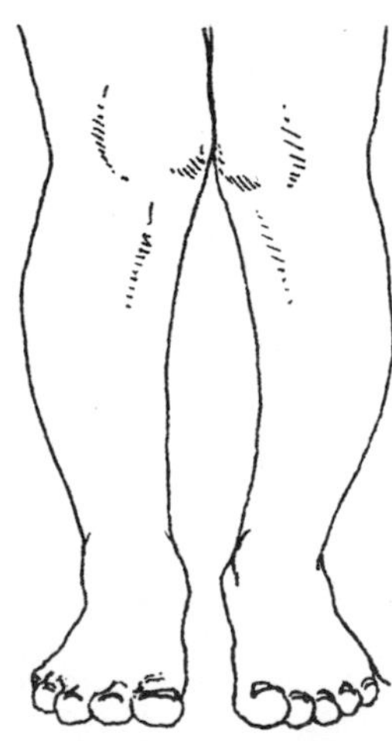

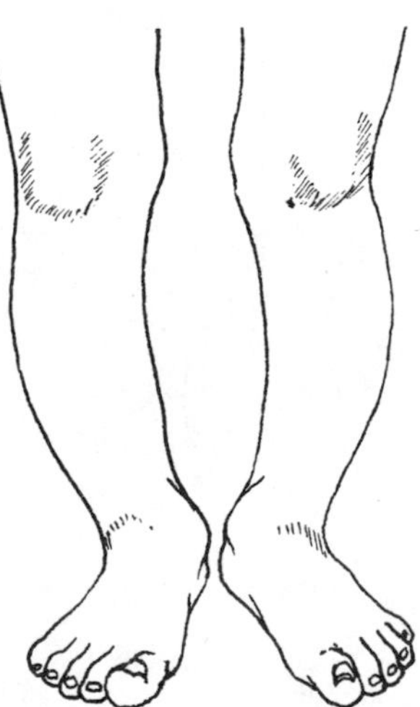

i. Do the knees seem to be pointed inward or outward (rather than straight ahead)?
j. Do the feet turn in or out?
k. Does the child toe-walk?

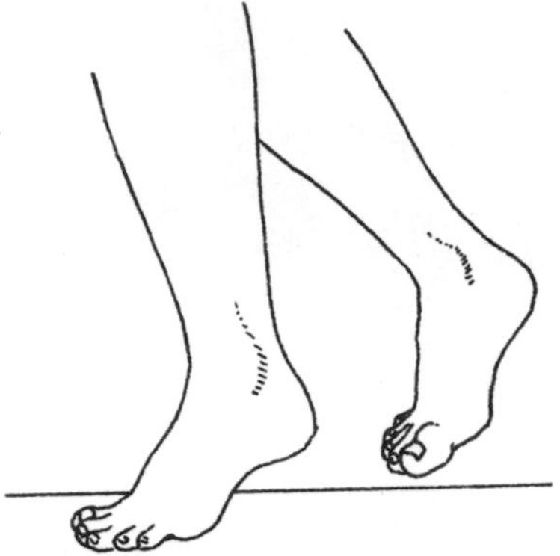

l. Is there a premature heel lift? (Does the child lift his heels off the ground too quickly?)

► Does the child complain of night cramps or wake up in the middle of the night with cramping or muscle spasms in the legs?

► Have your child stand.
a. When you put the ankles together, do the knees touch first? Is there space between the ankles (are the legs knock-kneed)? (See appendix on foot and leg structure.)
b. When the ankles are together, is there a wide space between the knees (bow-leg)? (See appendix on foot and leg structure).
c. Do the arches appear very flat or very high? (see appendix on foot and leg structure)
d. Ask the child to turn around with his back to you. Do the tendons in the back of the lower leg bow outward? (See appendix on foot and leg structure).

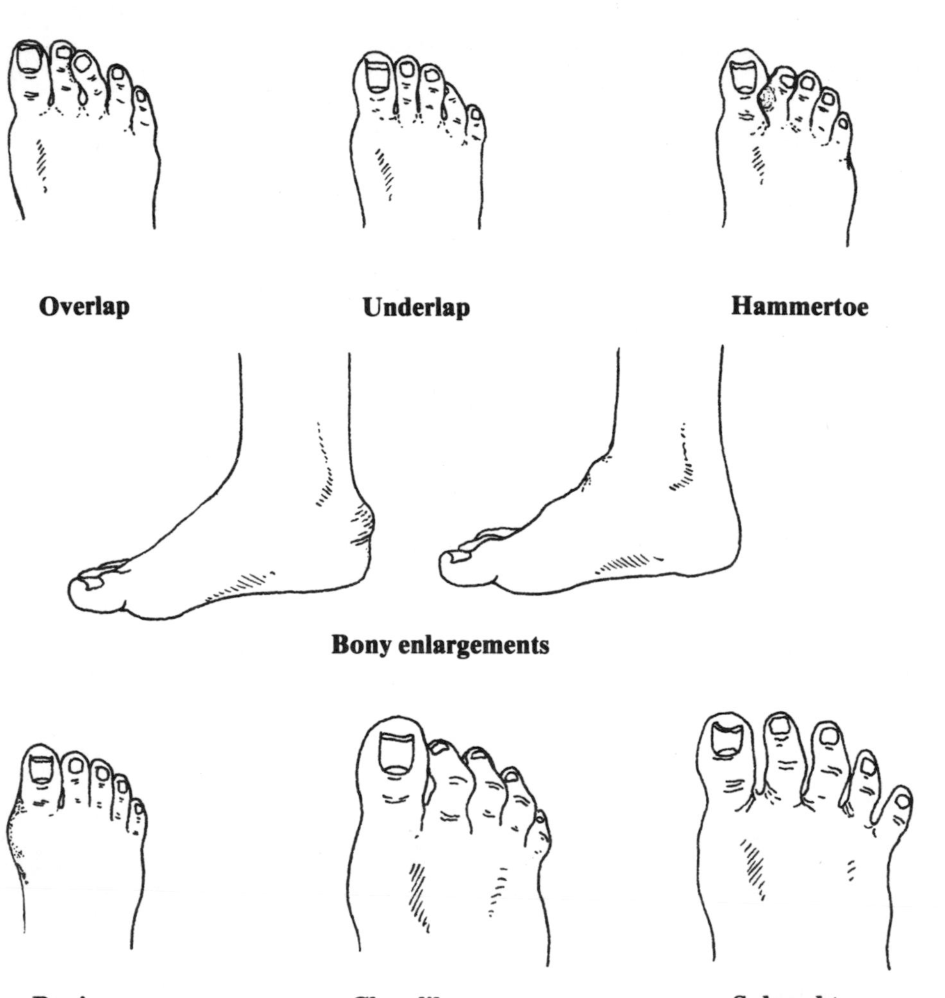

e. Have the child sit down and take his shoes off. Does one toe overlap another? Does one toe underlap another? Are there any hammertoes, bunions, or bony enlargements in back of the heel and on top of the foot? Are the toes claw-like when the child stands? Do the feet splay out with the toes wide apart and looking very loose?

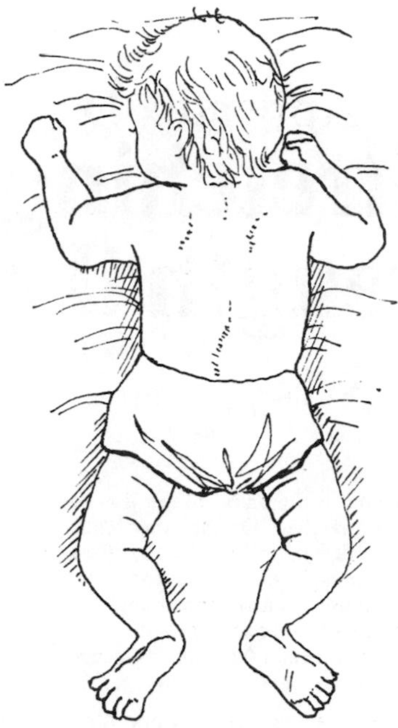

f. If the child is very young, have him lie down and put the legs together. Do they appear different in length? Do the heels seem to touch at different points? Do creases in the thigh look more pronounced on one side than the other? Are there more creases on one thigh than the other?

Children may not complain much about their feet, but check the following:
1. Do the feet perspire too much?
2. Are there any infections, blisters, spots, or areas of redness?
3. Are there any rashes?
4. Are there any unusual growths?
5. Is there any redness or pain around the toe nails?
6. Does the child complain of pain anywhere in the feet?
7. Is there bad posture?

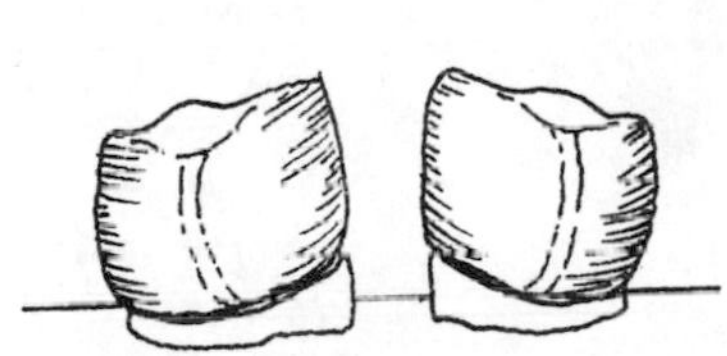

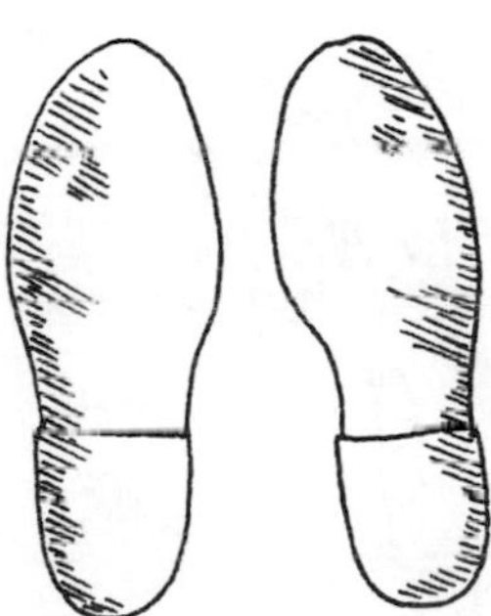

8. Do the heels or soles wear out and run down peculiarly on one side?
9. Does the child usually get tired and cranky easily? Does he complain of pains in other parts of his body (back, neck or hip) after play or after standing for long periods of time? Does he like to play?

► Does the child always seem to want to sit down a lot?

If the answers to any of these questions are "yes," see a podiatrist or have your pediatrician refer you to a podiatrist.

Appendix D
Stretching and Strength Training

Running tends to tighten the muscle groups at the backs of the legs and the lower back. To compensate for the effects of running, these muscles must be stretched. On the other hand, certain muscle groups at the front of the leg and body are used relatively little in running, and need to be strengthened. Stretching before and after running is essential to prevent injuries due to muscle imbalances and lack of flexibility. Each stretch should be done for at least 30 to 60 seconds. If you are not used to any of the stretches, then add them to your routine gradually, just as you gradually increase your running distance and the time spent running. Add one new stretch every few days, and gradually increase the time spent on each from 30 to 60 seconds. Pay close attention to how the exercises feel. Remember that when a stretch is beneficial, the tissues generally feel good.

All stretching should be done in a relaxed frame of mind. Concentrating on deep and rhythmic breathing will help you to relax. Move slowly into the stretch with no bouncing or jerking motion. There should be no burning or actual pain caused by the stretch. If you feel pain, you may be stretching too far, too soon, causing muscle tissue damage (and increasing muscle tightness rather than alleviating it). If you reach the threshold of pain, let up a little and then hold the stretch in a motionless position.

Do not compare yourself to anyone else with your stretching, because some of us are naturally tighter or looser than others. Just keep working at it gradually, and you will eventually increase your own muscle range of motion. For example, many of us have congenitally tight calf (back of the leg) or hamstring (back of the thigh) muscles, and no matter how much we try, we may never be able to touch our fingers to the ground when doing the toe touch stretch. Most of us also have one side tighter than the other. For right-handed people it usually is the right side. If you are like many runners, you will have a tendency to slack off and hurry your stretching once you get started, so it is a good idea to stretch your tight side first.

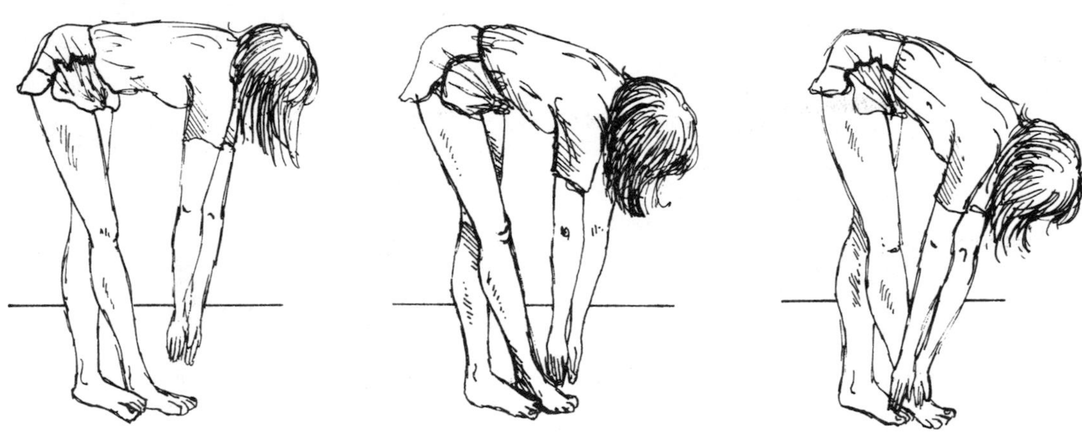

With each exercise, stretch as far as you can (but stop if you feel pain or strain), then let up a little and hold still for a few seconds (say ten to twenty seconds), as you feel the fibers loosening up. Then stretch for another ten to twenty seconds. For example, in the toe touch, bend forward with the front of the leg bent at the knee to take the strain off the lower back. The right leg can be crossed over in front of the left, so you are stretching the left hamstring. Bend forward as far as you can comfortably, and hold for ten or twenty seconds. Go a little further for ten to twenty more seconds, and if you feel like you can, go a little further and hold for still another twenty seconds more. Then switch legs. Each time you straighten up, remember to bend both knees so the effort is placed on the upper leg muscles rather than the lower back muscles, which are easily strained.

Here is a good ten minute exercise routine for use both before and after athletic activity.

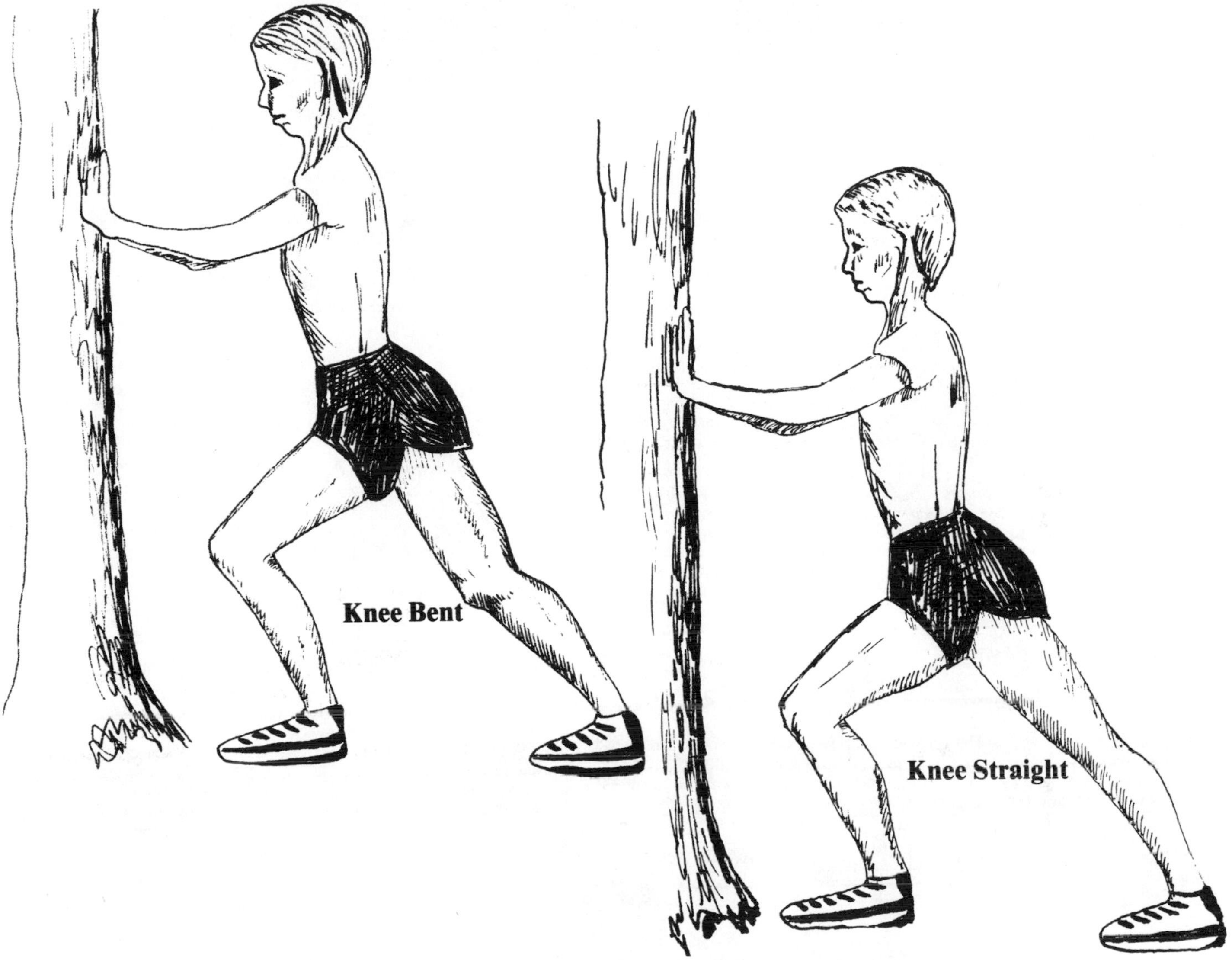

Knee Bent

Knee Straight

► Wall pushes with the knees bent, 30 seconds for each leg, twice. In this exercise, keep your feet flat on the ground (*don't* lift the heel), with your weight on both legs. Repeat with the knees straight.

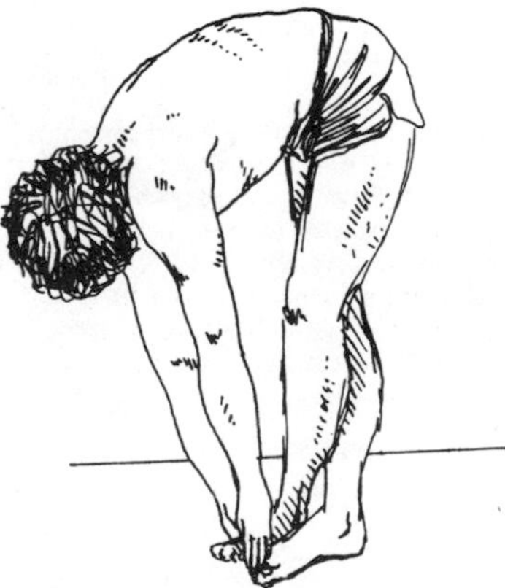

► Toe touches, 30 to 60 seconds each side (left leg crossed over right knee, then vice versa), twice. Go down *slowly* and do not bounce. Do not twist yourself that last inch in order to "touch" your toes momentarily; it will only make you tighter—and could cause injury. The only good stretch is one you can hold comfortably for 30 seconds.

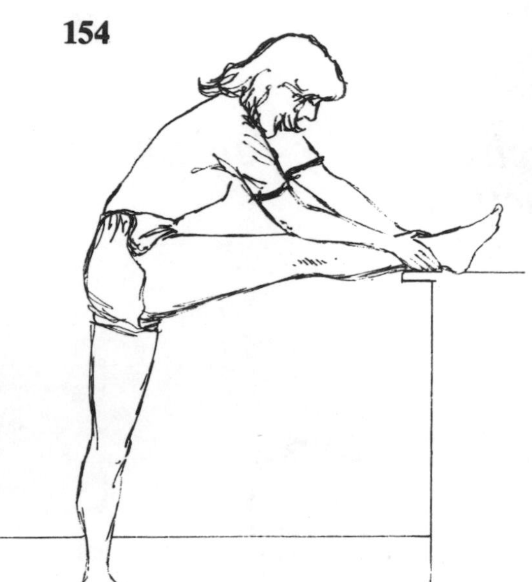

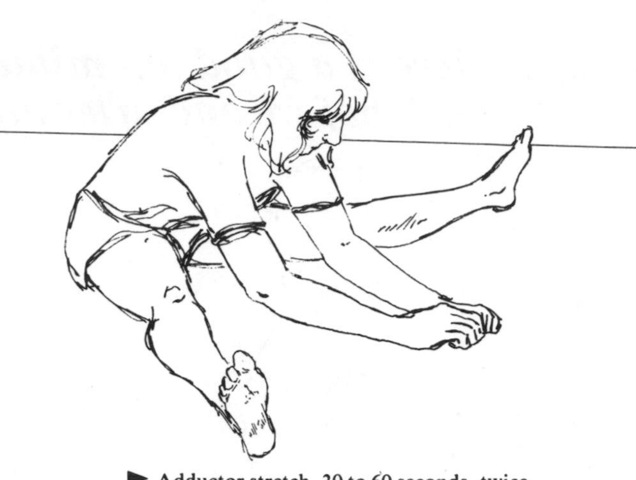

► Adductor stretch, 30 to 60 seconds, twice.
Try to lower head slowly to floor.

► **Hamstring** stretch, 30 to 60 seconds, twice.
Try to move head slowly down to knee of outstretched leg.

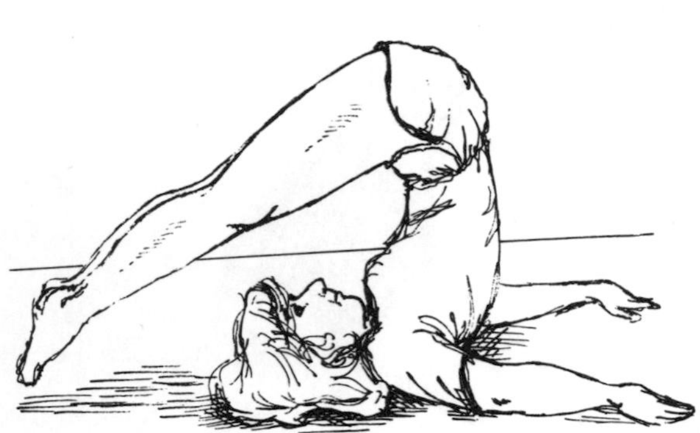

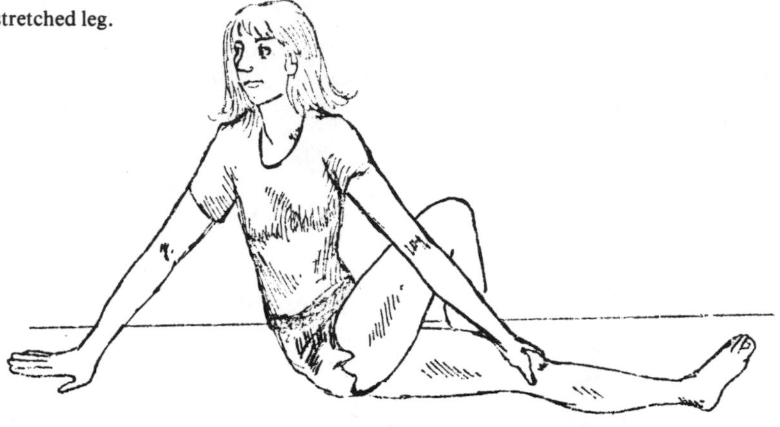

► To do the "plow", lie **flat on your** back with arms at your sides. Bend your knees up toward **your chest. Then** raise your legs straight up and lower slowly over your **head as shown. If you** feel pain in the back or neck, retreat slowly to a more comfortable **position.**

► To stretch the abductor muscles (outside of the thigh), sit on the floor with your legs straight out in front of you. To stretch the right abductor muscle group, place a bent right leg over a straight left leg. Reach your left arm over your right knee and grasp the inside of your left leg with the left hand. Extend the right arm to the right side of the body, twisting slowly toward the back. You should feel the stretch along the outside of your right hip and upper thigh. Hold for 30 seconds and repeat twice.

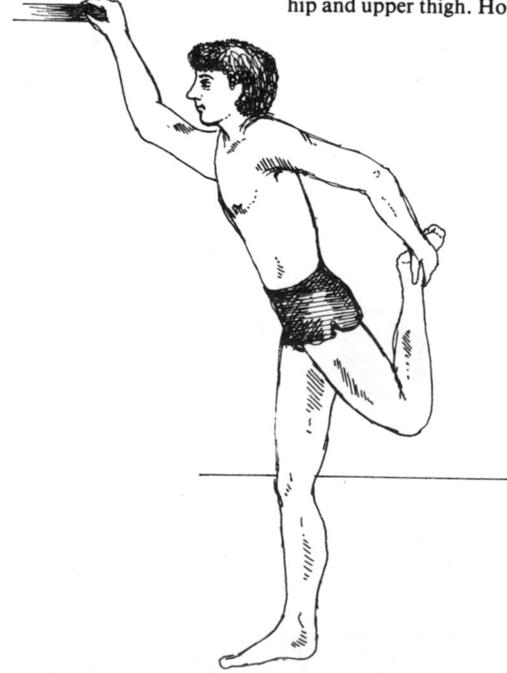

► **The quad stretch, 30 seconds**, twice. Slowly try to pull your foot up to your buttocks.

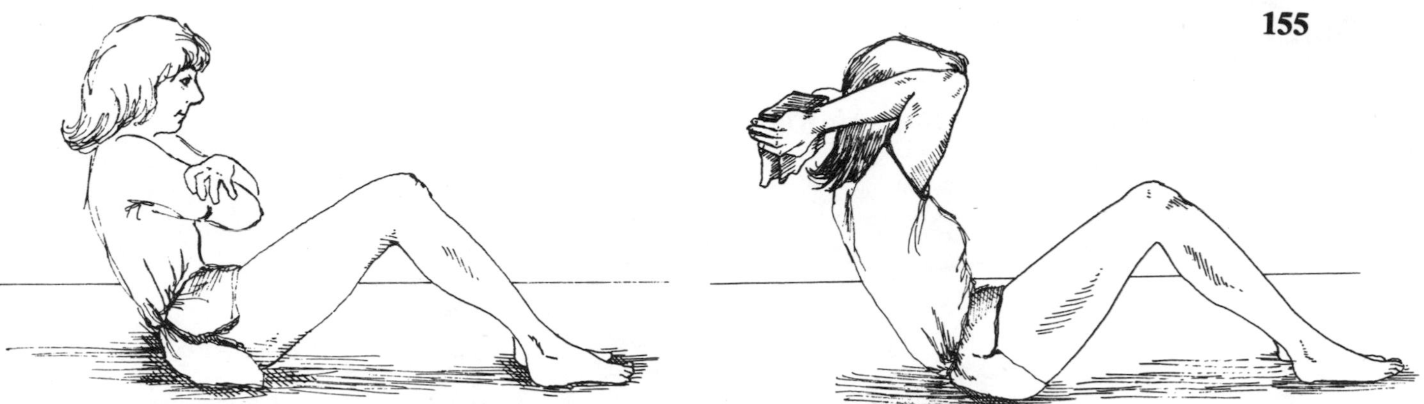

To balance up the muscles in the lower back with those in the stomach, do 25-50 bent-leg situps every day.

► With your knees bent in front of you, do 25 to 50 bent-leg sit-ups. You need not have your feet held by anyone.

► With your arms folded in front of you at your chest or clasped behind your head; come to a sitting position; then lie flat down and repeat.

To increase the difficulty of the situp, hold weight behind your head (wrapped in a towel to prevent head from injury).

Testing Your Flexibility

Here are three tests to determine whether the key muscle groups in the back of your body are too tight. If you fail one or more of these tests, either you are not stretching enough (or not using the right techniques), or you have congenitally tight muscle groups, in which case you should simply continue to do the best you can, and not worry. In either case, make sure you have read this section carefully.

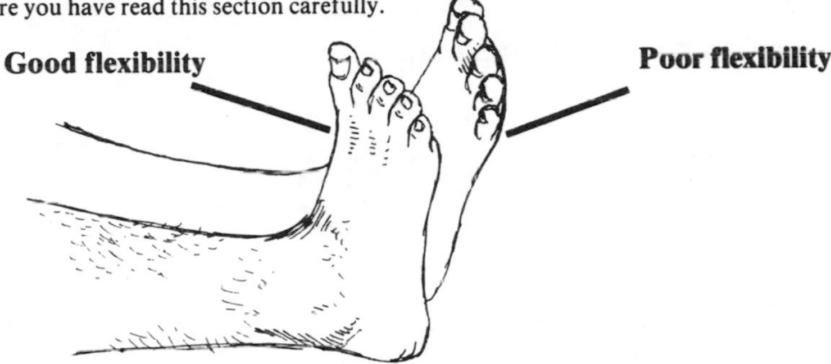

To Test for Tight Calf Muscles

► Lie on your back on a flat surface. Without moving your leg, pull your foot back as far as you can at the ankle-joint. You should have about 10° of motion from a perpendicular starting position. If you don't, your calf is too tight.

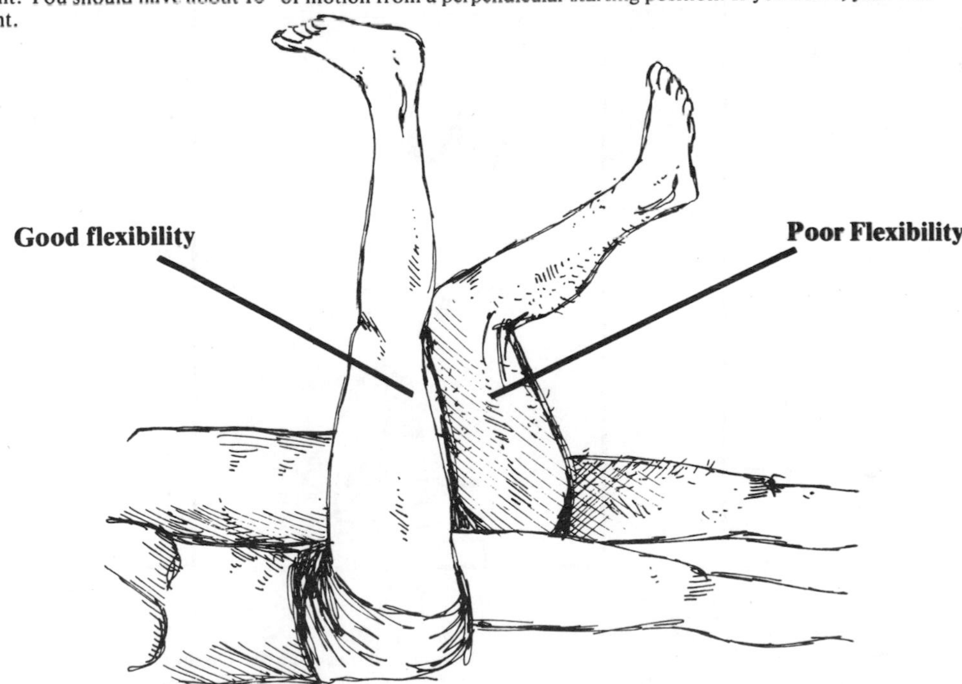

To Test for Tight Hamstring Muscles

► Lie flat on your back on a flat surface. Keeping your entire leg straight (knee locked), raise the leg straight up in the air. You should be able to raise the leg up to a 75° position to your hip. If you can't, you have a tight hamstring muscle.

To Test the Lower Back Muscles

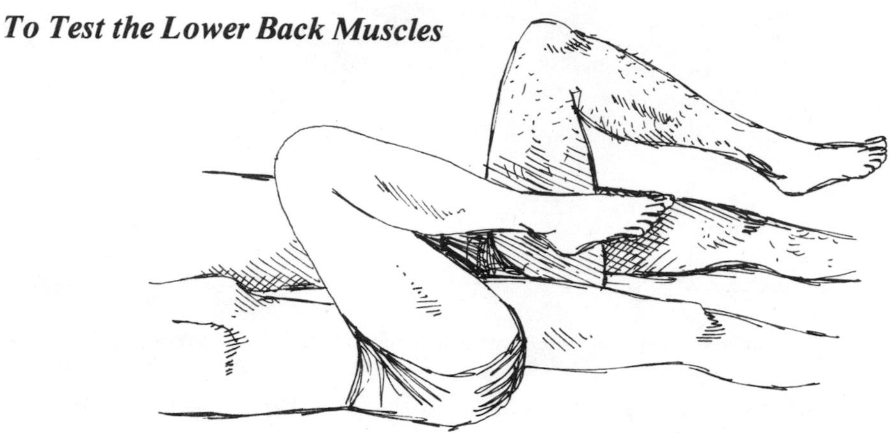

► Lie flat on your back on a flat surface. Bend your leg at the knee joint and bring it back toward your chest (trying to have top of thigh touch your chest). Your other leg (the one not being moved), should not be allowed to come off the surface at the hip. You should be able to bring your bent leg back 45° toward your chest. If you can't, your back muscles are too tight.

Exercises for the Slant Board

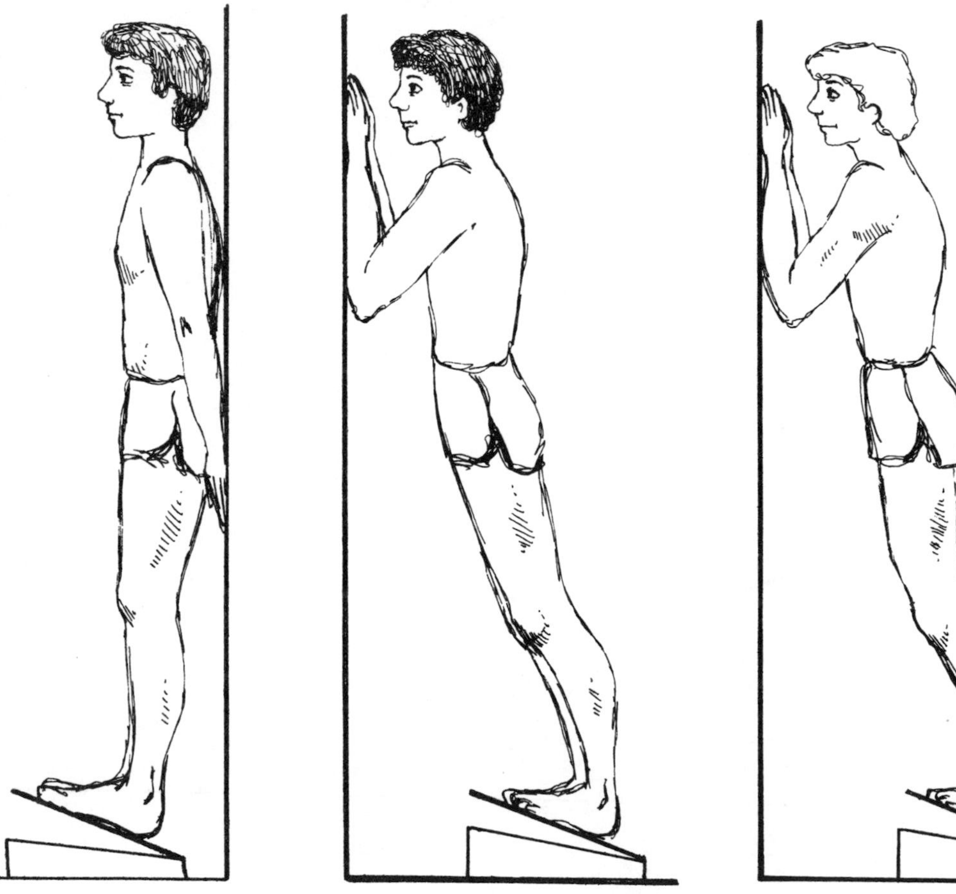

1. Place the boards so the downhill ends are 2-3" from the wall.
   ► Stand on the boards with your heels at the bottom and toes pointed "Uphill."
   ► Lean back to the wall, allowing your knees to bend slightly. Hold for ten seconds and repeat.

2. With the boards 8" to 12" from the wall and the uphill edges facing the wall, stand with heels at the bottom and toes pointed "uphill." Lean toward the wall, keeping your knees straight.
   Concentrate on keeping your buttocks forward and heels down. Repeat with the knees bent.

To Make a Slant Board . . .

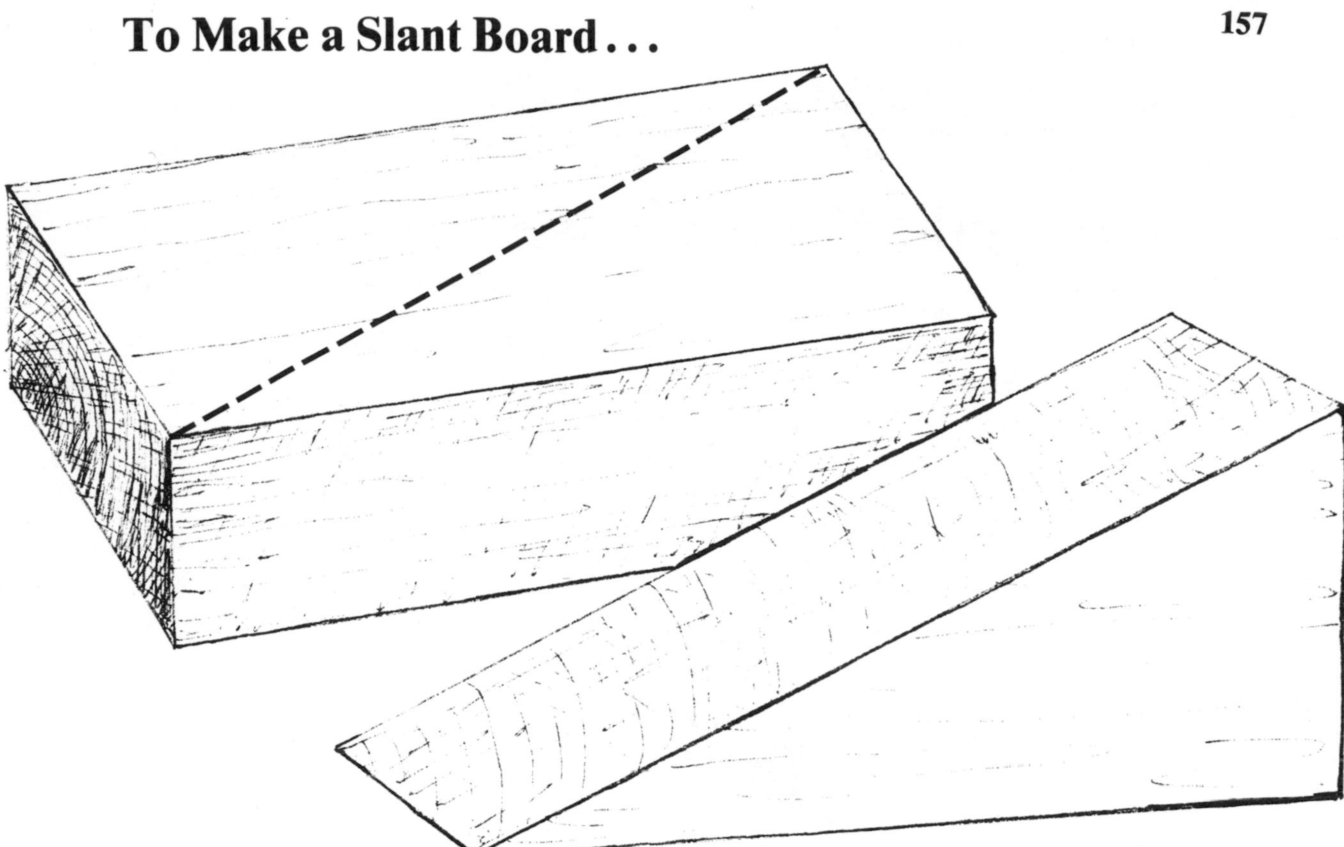

► Take a one foot section of 2x4 lumber and cut it diagonally the long way.

► Sand it smooth, apply wood sealer, and allow to dry. Coat with shellac to provide a smooth surface for barefoot stretching.

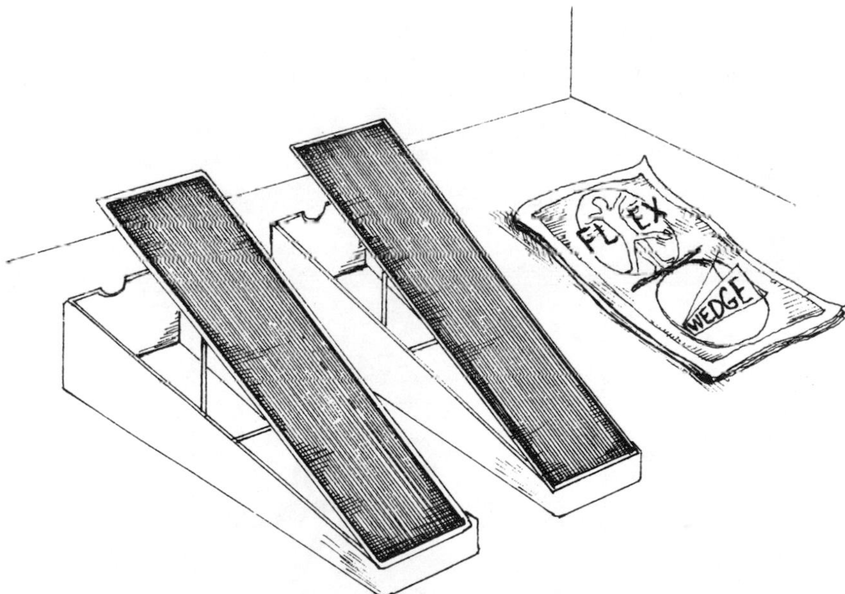

► As an alternative, you may wish to purchase a pair of Flex-Wedges

Guide to Stretching Time

If you are a runner, the amount of time spent stretching should increase as your distance does. If you run:

- ► 20-40 miles a week, stretch 10 minutes before and after;
- ► 40-60 miles a week, stretch 10 minutes before and after and another 10 minutes at night;
- ► 60-90 miles a week, stretch 15 minutes before and after and another 10-25 minutes at night; and
- ► 90 or more miles a week, stretch 15 minutes before and after and another 30 minutes at night.

Stretching vs. Warmup

Remember that stretching and warming up are *not* the same thing. Stretching makes the muscles more flexible, while warming up increases the flow of blood to prepare them for hard work. After you have finished a pre-run stretching routine, allow a few minutes of additional time for warming up. One way is to start your run at a slower pace, then gradually pick up speed. On cold days, it may be better to do some warming up *before* you stretch.

Strengthening Exercises

Since running naturally tightens the muscles in the back of the body, the muscles in the front of the body generally do not get enough activity.

1. A good way to avoid shin splints and help maintain muscle balance is to strengthen the muscles in the lower leg.

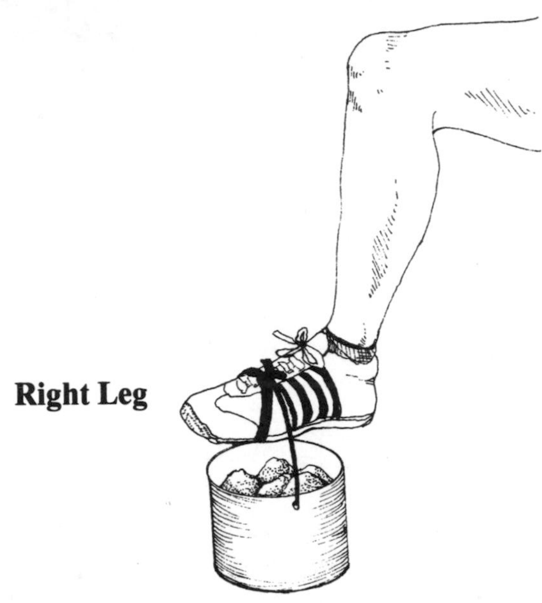

► Take a paint can or an old pocket book and fill it with five to ten pounds of weight.
► Sit on a table so that your leg is hanging down at a right angle (90 degrees) and suspend the weight from the top of your foot. It is helpful to tie the handle of the paint can or the strap of the pocket book onto your foot so that it doesn't roll off.

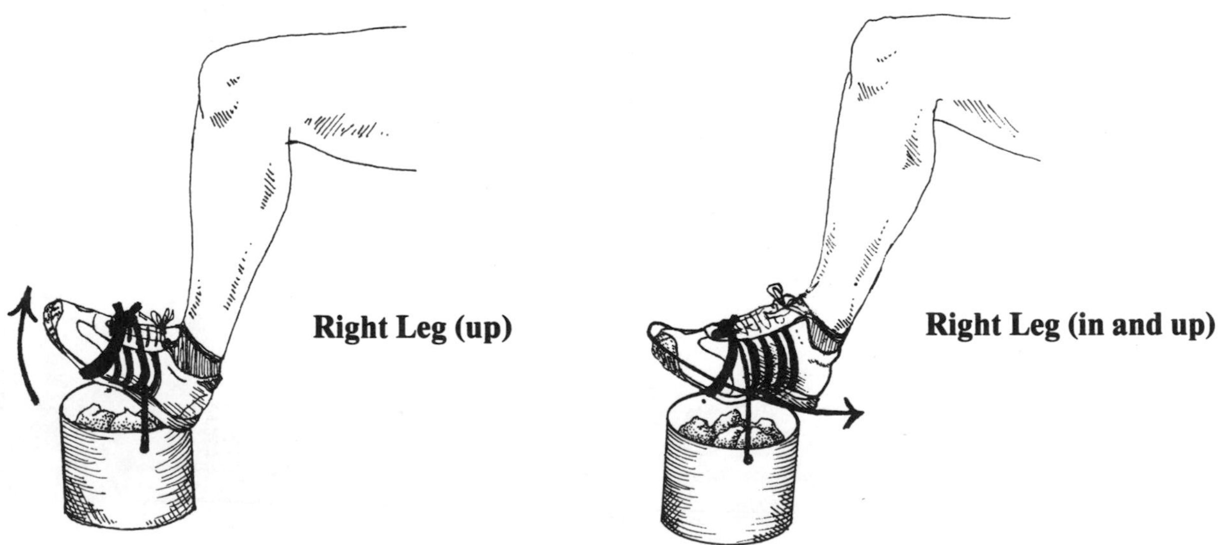

► Move your foot straight up (without lifting the leg) for a count of five, and relax. Repeat five times.
► The same exercise should be repeated with the foot turned inwards. The first exercise strengthens the muscles in the front of the leg, while the second strengthens the muscles on the inside of the leg.

2. For the knee, the following basic exercises are recommended:
► Tie a weighted paint can or pocket book (as described above) to the foot and raise the leg up from a 90° angle to a 180° angle, ten times for ten seconds each time.

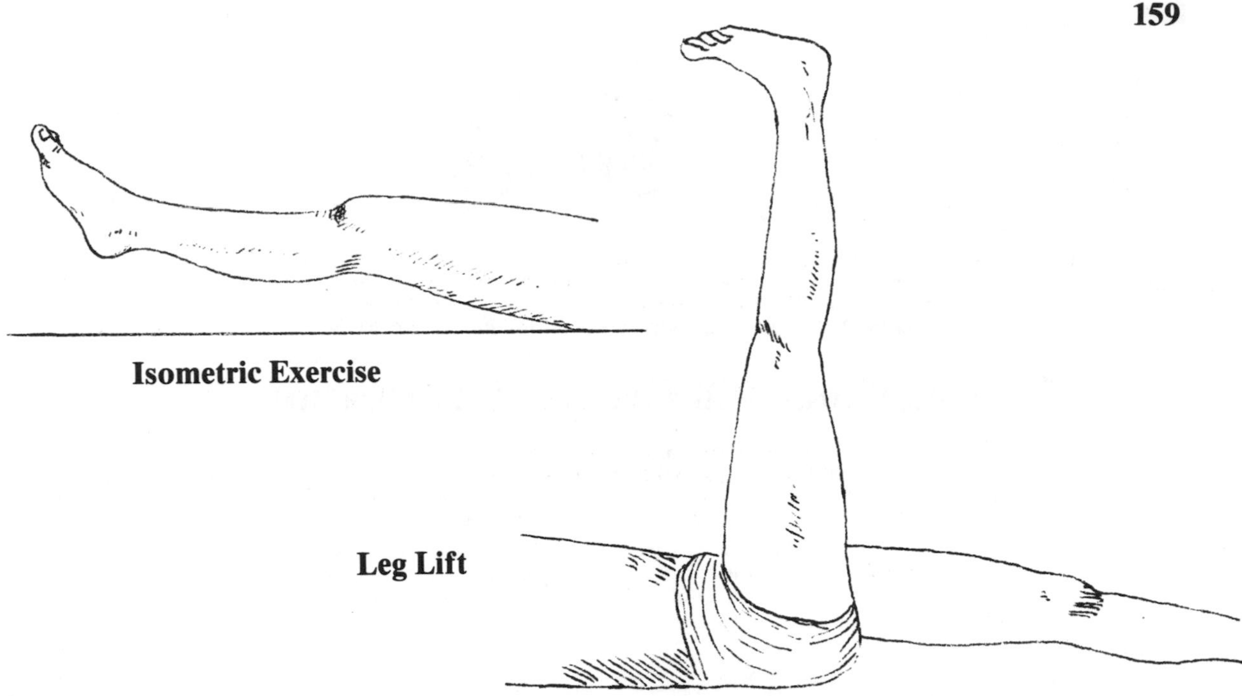

Isometric Exercise

Leg Lift

► Use isometric exercises. Sit on the floor with legs straight out in front of you. Lift one leg about two inches off the floor and lock your knee as hard as you can 15 times, holding for 15 seconds each time. The foot should be held straight. Repeat this exercise with the foot curved in.

► Use leg lifts. Lie completely flat on the floor and very slowly raise your leg straight up, coming as close to 90° as possible. Repeat 20 to 40 times and hold each time for approximately two seconds when you have gotten the leg up as high as you can go.

3. When doing strengthening exercises for the muscles which act on the front of the knee as above, it is often important to do strength work for the back of the upper leg muscles.

   ► Lie flat on your stomach on a counter or table top with your legs hanging down over the edge; attach the weight system to the ankle; lift your leg slowly to the perpendicular and then slowly lower it to the beginning position ten to fifteen times. Take a minute rest in between and do three sets of ten repetitions all together.

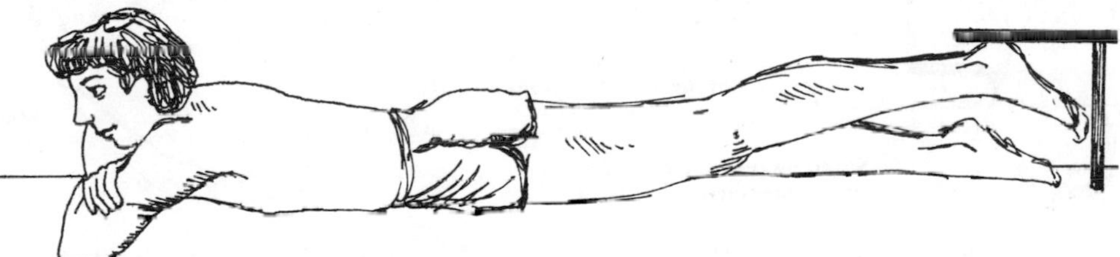

► To use isometric exercises, lie flat on your stomach on the floor and have the back of your heels about two inches or so below a counter or dresser. Keeping your lower extremity straight (locked at the knee), try to raise your leg up through the immovable counter or dresser. Contact should be made between the back of your heel and the immovable object. Push up as hard as you can 10 times, holding for 10 seconds each time. See illustration in chapter 40.

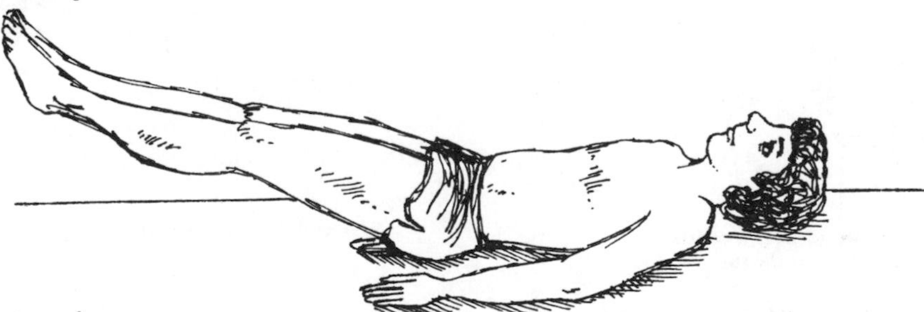

4. For the lower stomach group:

   ► Lie flat on your back with your legs straight and locked at the knees.

   ► Lift your strengthened lower extremities together about ten inches off the ground and hold for 10 seconds.

   ► Repeat 10 times.

Appendix E
Shoes

Shoes should be made to accommodate not only the shape of the foot, but the function of the foot as it helps the body to move. Since the feet function quite differently with different kinds of activity, this appendix is divided into four sections—the first dealing with walking shoes and questions of a general nature; the second with shoes for babies; the third with shoes for older children; and the fourth with running shoes.

Walking shoes and General Information

1. What is the best material for shoes to be made of?

Leather has important features that make it superior to so-called man-made materials. It has some of the same properties as human skin. It is moldable and readily adapts to the shape of the foot. Since the foot may change size and shape during the day, the leather will accommodate it by stretching or contracting.

When shoe leather "breathes," an exchange of moisture and absorption takes place. Leather is a superior absorber of moisture and has the ability to vaporize this moisture into the air. This capability plays a key role in hygiene and comfort within the shoe. If this vaporization does not occur, the feet get hot and perspire profusely.

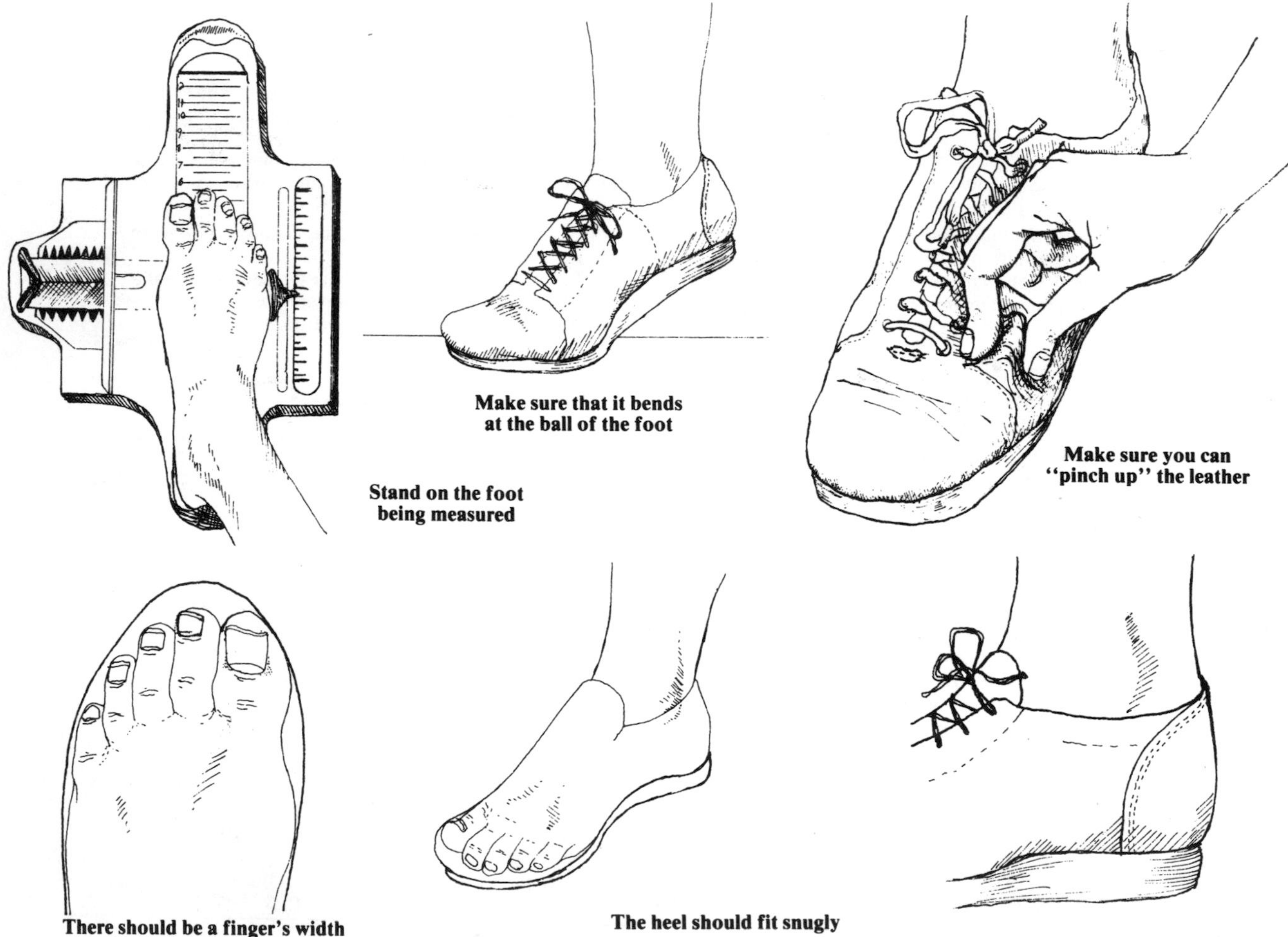

Stand on the foot being measured

Make sure that it bends at the ball of the foot

Make sure you can "pinch up" the leather

There should be a finger's width of extra space at the toe

The heel should fit snugly

2. What should you look for in trying on a new pair?

Consumers are often advised to buy shoes at the end of the day, when the feet are more likely to be tired and swollen. But there are also more part-time salespeople manning the shoe stores during the peak selling hours in the evenings, so beware. If the salesperson asks you your shoe size instead of measuring you, you may be in the wrong store. When you are being measured, stand on the foot being measured. When you examine the shoe, make sure that it is leather, that it bends easily at the ball of the foot, that it is not concave between the arch and heel, and that the shoe slips easily over the instep without "cutting" (you should be able to "pinch up" the leather across the ball). There should be about a finger's width of extra space at the toe, but the heel should fit snugly. The shoe should not slip or rub anywhere, and it should feel good when you put it on. It should not have to be "broken in." For a good fit, your best bet is the smaller family or independent shoe store.

3. Do shoes cause foot problems?

Most people blame shoes for their foot problems, but there is evidence that in many cases the causes lie elsewhere. If you have a deformity such as a bunion or a hammertoe, you probably would have developed it whether you had worn shoes or not. Shoes, however, can certainly aggravate foot problems that already exist. And shoes—particularly athletic shoes—can protect the feet from shock, friction and stress that might otherwise be intolerable. The best answer to the question of what causes foot problems is that shoe design and materials play a role, but so do heredity, hard surfaces, and other factors. A prominent podiatrist once said "a pair of shoes will not make the feet well, any more than a new hat cures a headache."

4. Do "orthopedic" or "corrective" shoes really help?

Unfortunately, there is no ready-made or even custom-made shoe that has a sound mechanism built into it to control the way we walk. Most authorities agree that "corrective" shoes do not correct. Rather, abnormal stresses put on the feet by unhealthy motion patterns will be directly transferred to the shoe itself and the shoe will then conform and break down.

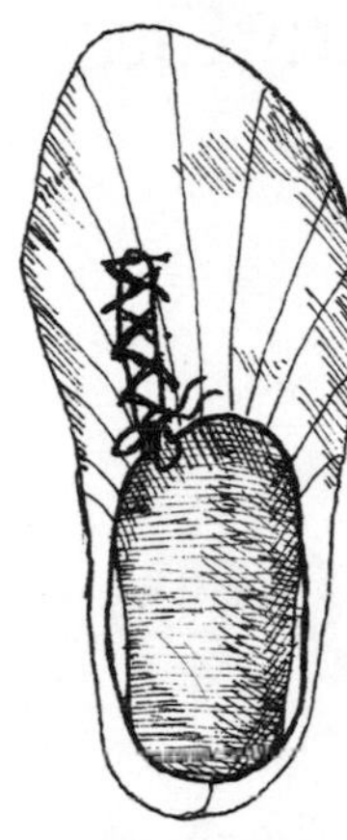

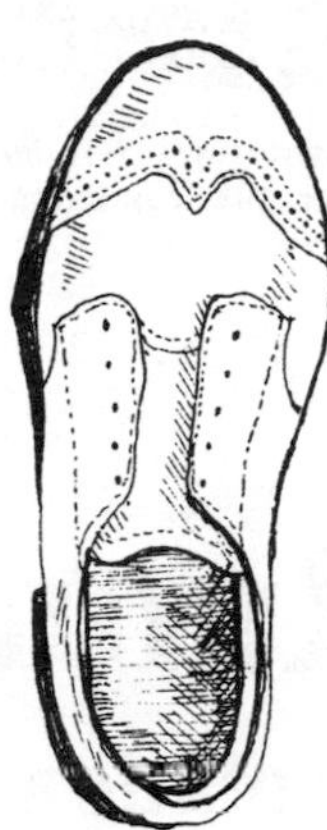

A word about children's orthopedic shoes. We have seen too many cases of children who have had a deformity at birth and were put into "corrective" shoes. Orthopedic shoes for children should be used *only* temporarily to retain a correction made by something else (casting or surgery) or in the mildest of foot deformities. Even in these cases, the shoe will only work until the abnormal forces and stresses placed upon it break it down. These shoes are so stiff that the amount of force it takes to bend the sole may actually be more than the child weighs. Therefore, due to the lack of flexibility, such shoes actually cause more foot problems than they prevent.

5. What about repairs?

When shoes are repaired, the uppers tend to diminish in size, so you are better off getting new shoes than trying to repair the old.

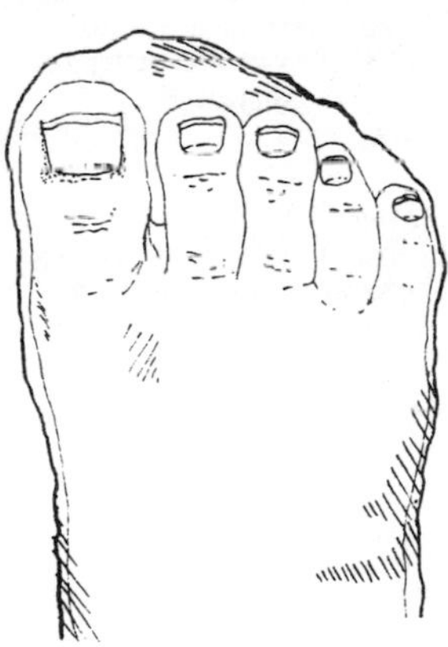

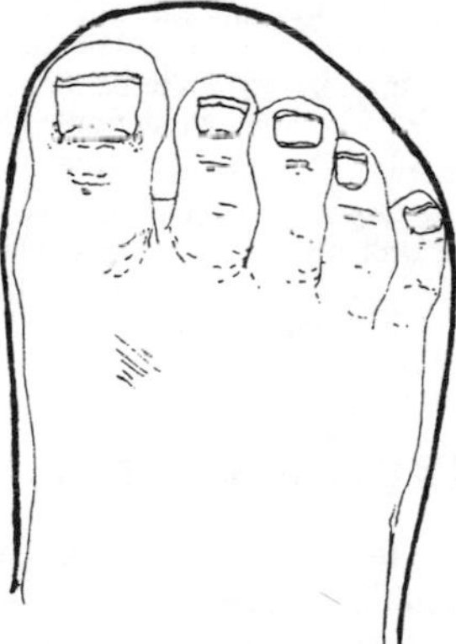

6. What about socks?

Select socks about half an inch longer than the longest toe—lest they cause blisters. Avoid tube socks, which generally do not fit well.

Shoes for Babies

When a baby takes his first steps, he is ready for shoes.

1. The shoes should be high with laces over the ankle to make it harder for the baby to kick the shoes off and pull his foot and heel out of them. The shoe should be hard enough to protect the soft, pliable bony structure at the front where it must be able to bend. The shoe should be made of leather.
2. Shoes and socks should be about one half inch longer than the baby's foot and slightly wider. The size must be changed as soon as the child has outgrown them. The size may have to be changed every month or so for the first year.

3. A child may appear to have no arch when he stands. This is not necessarily a problem. Children have fat pads in the arch area, which may create the appearance of flat feet to the untrained eye.
4. If the child walks with his ankles either rolled out or rolled in with his feet flattened out, he should be checked by a podiatrist. Early treatment can prevent a lifetime of discomfort.

Shoes for Older Children

1. Children's shoes should be purchased in stores that specialize in children's foot wear. Avoid part-time sales people, and seek out an individual who is experienced in fitting children's shoes. Make sure the store has a system to check the date and size of the shoe bought each visit. If you find such a store and you are satisfied, keep going there (children's feet and shoe sizes should be checked every three months).
2. Between the ages of one and six, the shoe size changes every four to eight weeks; between ages six and ten, the shoe size changes every 12-16 weeks; and between ages 12 and 15, the sizes change every 16 to 20 weeks. Do not get fitted solely by number. Get *both* feet measured.
3. Never accept special shoe pads or inserts from salespersons without the advice of a podiatrist.
4. Never use hand-me-down shoes. Besides probably being worn down too much, the shoes will be forcing a child's foot into another child's mold and this will lead to trouble.

Running Shoes

General Information

Buying a running shoe is like buying a car. In a car, there are a number of criteria—gas mileage, performance, frequency of repair, and comfort, to name a few—by which the value of a particular model can be measured. What can make the choice of a car difficult is the fact that a car which rates high on one criterion (such as performance) will usually rank lower on another (such as fuel efficiency).

In the selection of running shoes, the first question to be answered is whether the shoes are to be used for serious training, for casual jogging, for racing, or for facilitating the rehabilitation of an injured limb.

There are also a number of *personal* variables to be considered. How much do you weigh? How fast do you run? Are you a heel-runner or a toe-runner? How much do you pronate? The answers can make an enormous difference!

Finally, there are some questions of personal preference. Not just questions of style, but of function. For example, at some point in your deliberations over which shoes to purchase, you may have to choose between having more *shock absorption* and more *flexibility*. Not that we can't recommend shoes which are strong in both—we can. But if you want the shoe with the very *best* shock absorption, you'll have to settle for a little less than the best in flexibility—and vice versa. The are a number of tradeoffs like this, where you are better off making intelligent choices than letting some panel of experts (who don't know your needs) dictate the choice for you. In fact, some of these tradeoffs are so unescapable that many runners make no attempt to find one all-purpose shoe that will satisfy all of their requirements.

Consider the difference between training and racing. For most runners, the first job of a training shoe is to provide protection from injury, whereas the job of a racing shoe is to perform. As it happens, the features which characterize the most protective shoe (such as thick heel wedge) are not the same as those which characterize the fastest shoes (such as high flexibility and light weight). For this reason, comparing shoes for racing with shoes for training is like comparing apples and oranges.

Characteristics to Look For

— A full, rigid **heel counter** to fit snugly around and cup the heel to give it good support.

— **Heel Elevation:** The heel should be elevated about one-half inch higher than the front of the shoe in order to reduce the strain on the calf muscle and achilles tendon.

— **Heel Width:** Should measure about three inches across to allow enough stability and surface area to absorb heel impact.

— **Outer Sole:** Should be durable, should compress and should be approximately one-half inch thick.

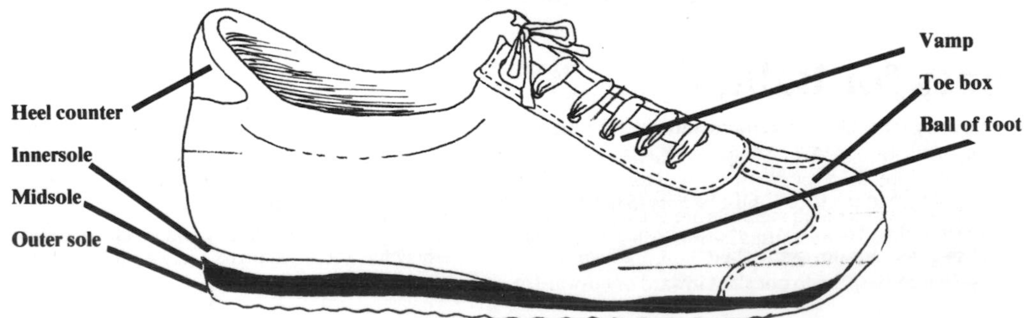

— **Sole Flexibility:** Soles should bend easily at the ball of the foot. If they are rigid, excessive stress is placed on the back of the leg and the bottom of the foot.

— **Midsoles:** The material between the outer and inner sole adds cushioning, but should end where the foot bends.

— **Inner Sole:** The material next to the foot should be smooth, soft and non-irritating. All shoes should have innersoles. If your choice doesn't, buy some insoles, preferably Spenco or Scholl's insoles, at your shoe or drug store and place them in your shoes.

— **Flat Bottom:** The sole should be flat on the ground from heel to toe, especially under the middle of the foot.

— **Arch Supports:** These are usually made of sponge rubber, and actually offer little or no support. However, make sure they feel comfortable and are placed in both shoes so they don't cause blistering and/or irritation.

— **Uppers:** Should be soft and smooth and not have rough seams that cause irritation. Preferably they should be made of nylon or a nylon/suede combination.

— **Toe Box:** Should be rounded and approximately one inch in depth, providing enough space for your toes to wiggle

— **Weight of Shoe:** A lighter shoe may allow you to run a few seconds faster, but you are more likely to get hurt.

Checking for Fit

Note that these considerations apply to ordinary walking shoes as well as to athletic shoes.

— Have shoes fitted after a run or at the end of the day, because your feet will have a tendency to swell. Try to get service from an experienced salesperson, not a part-timer.

— Have shoes fitted while you are standing, and try walking or even jogging on a hard surface, away from the store carpeting.

— If one foot is larger than the other, fit the larger foot.

— Be sure to wear your regular foot attire (i.e. double socks, peds, etc., including any pads, orthotics or supports).

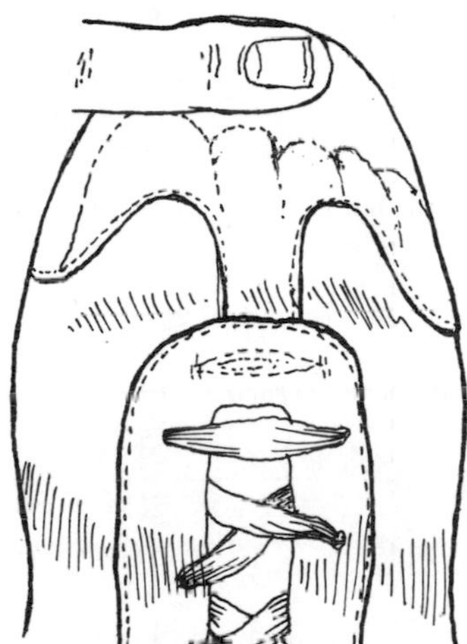

— Be sure that there is a thumb's width between the end of the shoe and the end of the longest toe.

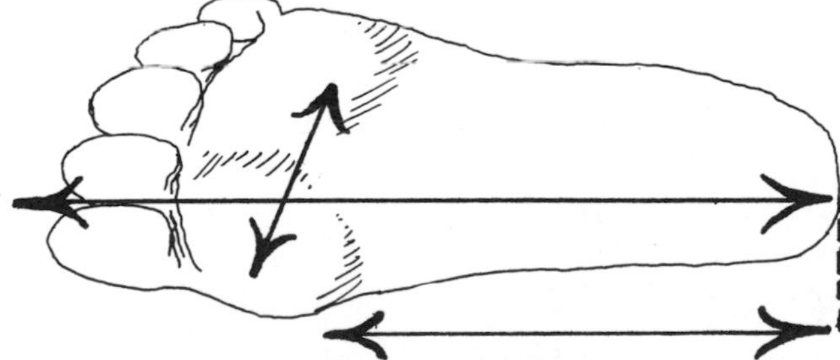

— Width should be measured at the widest part of the foot (the ball).

— Make sure that when shoes are laced, no part of the foot bulges out.

— Uppers should hold the foot securely and be shaped so as not to cause irritation.

— The heel counter should fit snugly and securely.

— Occasionally a pair of running shoes will be defective. Therefore, be sure to examine the shoes closely, and if any of the following items are not right, return the shoes to the store.
—That they are symmetrical
—That the heel counters are equal in height and width
—That the inner arch supports are equal in size and in the proper place.
—That there are no unusual seams or tears.
—That heel heights are equal
—That the uppers do not slant inward or outward.

Breaking in New Shoes

— Wear the shoes around for several days, a few hours each day before running in them.
— Wear the same number and kind of socks and arch supports, inlays or orthotics that you will be regularly wearing with the shoe.
— At first use new shoes only for shorter runs.
— Never race in a brand new pair of shoes. Run 25-50 miles before racing in them.
— After one or two runs, make sure that the uppers have not caved in and that the shoes retain their basic shape.
— If you insert any inlays or arch supports, make sure that you first remove the inner arch cookies that were put into the shoes by the manufacturer.

Interpreting Wear Patterns

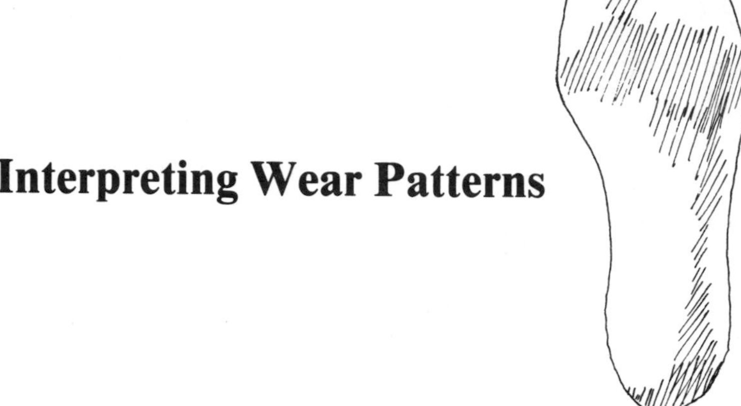

— Normal wear patterns are from the outside of the heel to the middle of the sole toward the middle of the forefoot and onto the big toe.

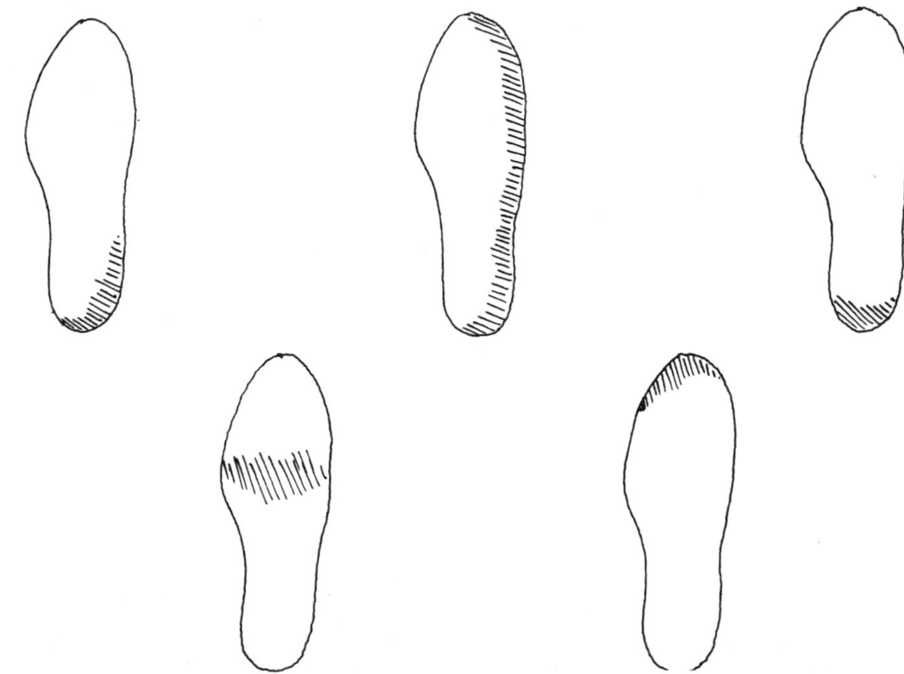

— Other patterns are indications of imbalances.
— Excessive outside heel wear occurs in people who are bowlegged or have a rearfoot varus imbalance. This must be built up with Shoe Goo or Shoe Patch.
— Wear along the entire border, inner or outer, indicates severe imbalance.
— Excessive wear throughout the center of the heel indicates overstriding, which is a common source of knee problems.
— Excessive forefoot sole wear (with very little heel wear) could indicate a tight achilles calf complex. Whether this is a problem or not depends on your training and racing pace and your preference for this running form.
— Excessive tip of the sole wear indicates the shoes are the wrong size. It can be the cause of toe blistering, toe irritation or toe jamming.

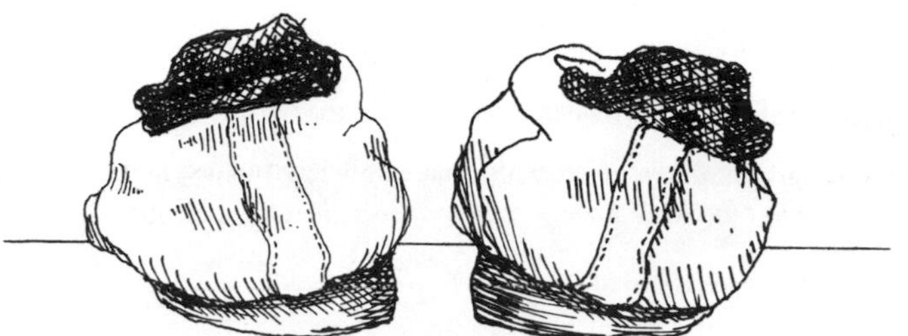

— Uppers caving inward or outward indicate that the shoes do not fit properly or that you have a foot imbalance problem. The uppers should be perpendicular to a flat surface.

— Inward tilting of the entire shoe indicates a pronation problem, and usually leads to injuries.

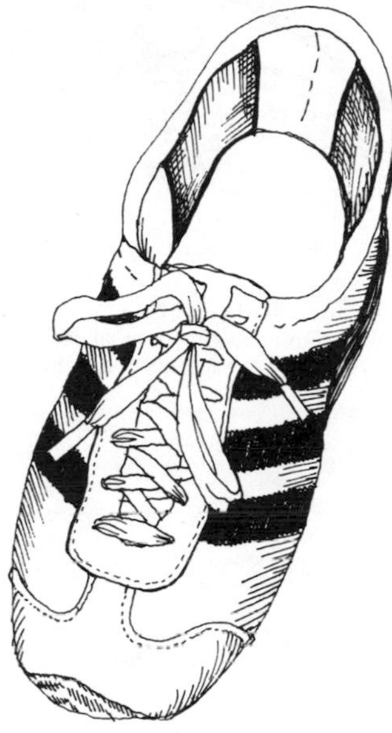

— A loose fitting heel counter will lead to poor motion control and will increase the chance of injury.

— If the shoe is too wide and the foot slips out or moves around, try moleskin around the inside of the heel counter, not in the back. If not thick enough, use 1/8 inch foam. Also try putting 1/8 - 1/4 inch foam in back of the tongue.

— To make shoes narrower, add an extra innersole, preferably a Spenco inlay. This will equal approximately one letter in width (c to b, d to c, etc.).

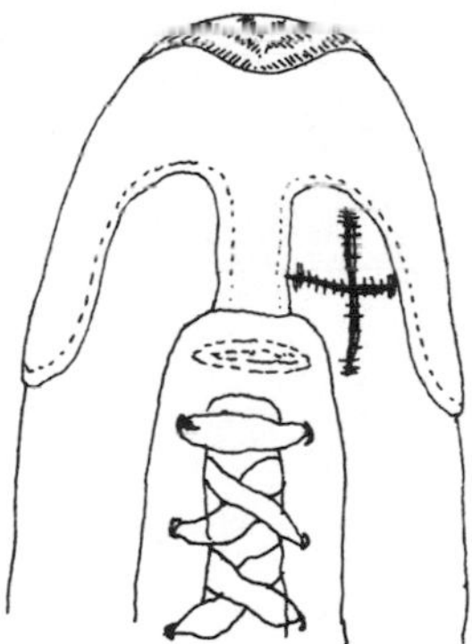

— If you want to increase space in the toe box depth, slit a hole in the nylon upper (above the toes) to relieve pressure.

— If a nylon shoe gets smelly or especially dirty it can be washed in the washing machine. A leather shoe cannot. In either case:
—Air shoes out between runs
—Use more than one pair of running shoes
—Apply foot powder to the inside of shoes before runs (Desenex spray)

Maintenance and Repair

— If shoes get wet, dry slowly
—If the shoes are leather, dry them with shoe trees in them.
—Never use heat to dry shoes.
—Never start a run with wet shoes on.

— Excessive sole wear should be corrected, especially in the outside heel area.
—One way is to take inner tube material, cut to proper shape, skive down with a knife, glue with Barge cement or contact cement (available in a hobby shop).

—You can cut portions of soles of older shoes where the sole is not worn too badly, and place the piece on as directed above.
—An alternative to the above is to buy rubber sheets from a shoe repair store and use this material for your repair work.
—You can get rubber taps in various sizes from a shoe repair or sports store, glue the taps on as above.

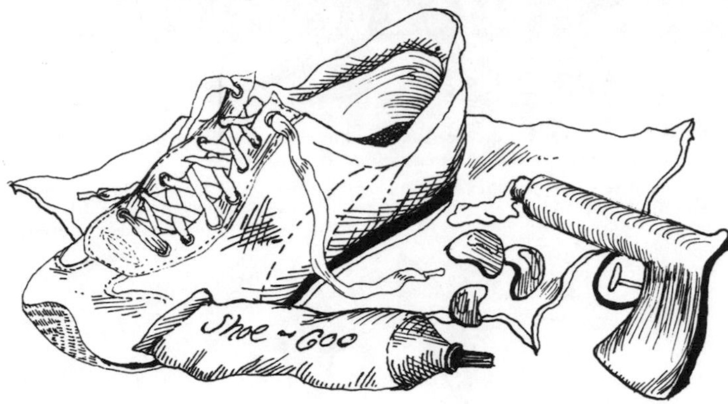

—You can use the various goos: "Shoo Goo," "Shoe Mend," and "Shoe Patch," or hot glue from a glue gun.
—Shoes can be resoled . Some running shoe stores will do this for you.
—To repair spaces between the uppers and the sole, use a piece of leather. Take the smooth side of the leather and glue it to the inside of the upper. Separate the leather from the upper with tweasers and allow 15-20 minutes for the drying of the glue.

Socks

— Use clean, dry socks daily

— 100% cotton or wool blends are the best socks.

— Avoid tube socks and stretch socks.

— During cold weather use double socks—cotton socks underneath and wool socks on top.

Appendix F
Shoe Inserts You Can Make

This section contains instructions for making inserts (1) to balance your foot to relieve corns and callouses; (2) to provide a temporary orthotic-type device or varus wedge; or (3) to compensate for a difference in length between your two legs. The conditions under which each of these adjustments may be called for are described in the chapters on specific types of foot conditions.

Materials:

1. A pair of your shoes
2. Graph paper (10'' x 12'')
3. Lipstick
4. Two 4'' x 8'' squares of adhesive foam
5. 1/8'' adhesive foam
6. Piece of calf or kidskin leather
7. Spenco inlay or other store bought inlay as an alternative

Caution: Minor muscle aches in the legs, hips, feet or back are normal during the break-in phase for these inserts. Wear them for one hour the first day, adding on an hour each day until you can wear them comfortably all day long. Once you can wear them comfortably walking for six to eight hours straight or more, you can use them for athletic activity. If unusual discomfort develops, see a podiatrist.

Note: Unless you have one leg longer than another, whatever you make to put under one foot or in one shoe, you should do for the other.

1. To balance your foot . . .

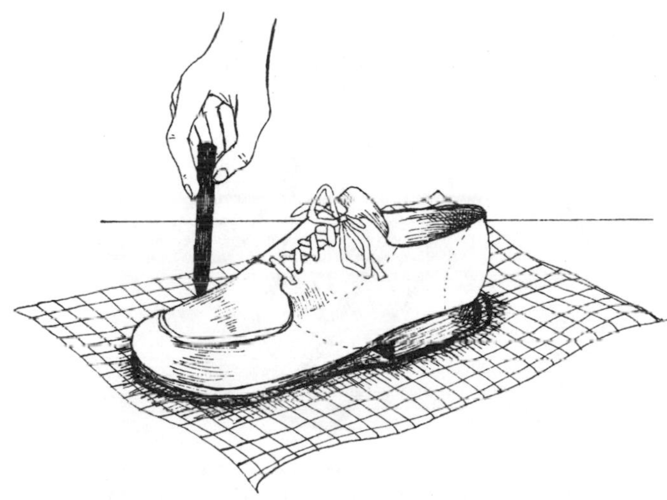

1. Place your shoe on a sheet of paper (preferably graph paper) and trace its outline.

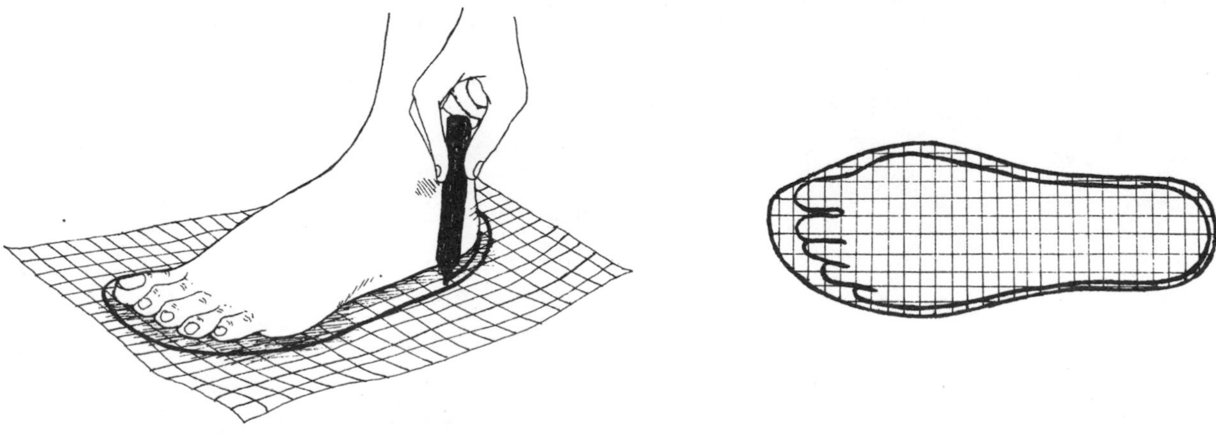

2. Step onto the shoe outline (center your bare foot in it) and trace the foot.

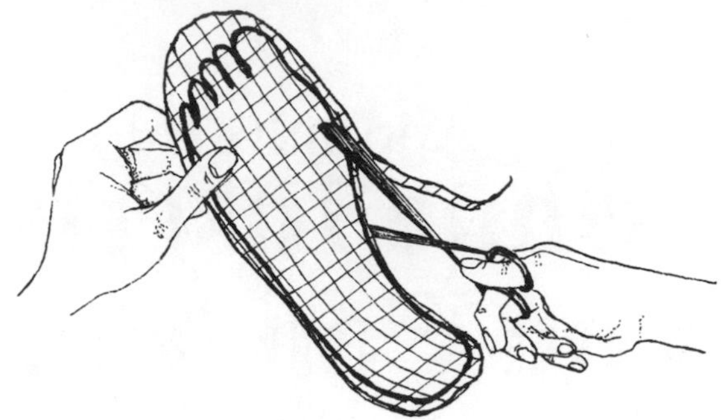

3. Cut out the foot pattern (it should end up about ¼" smaller all around than the shoe diagram). The pattern should fit inside the shoe.

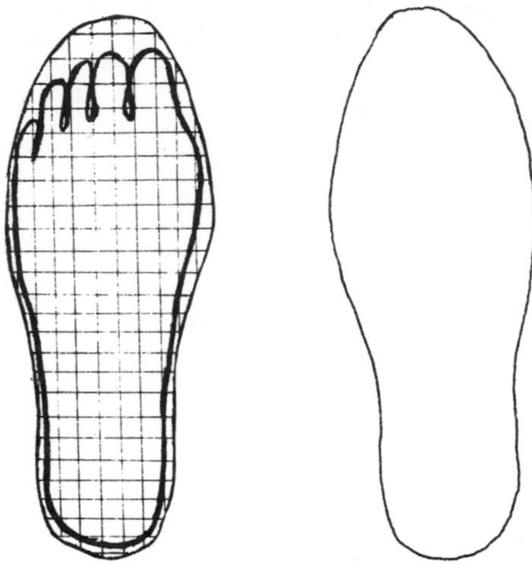

4. Cut a second pattern identical to the first, then turn it over for the other foot.

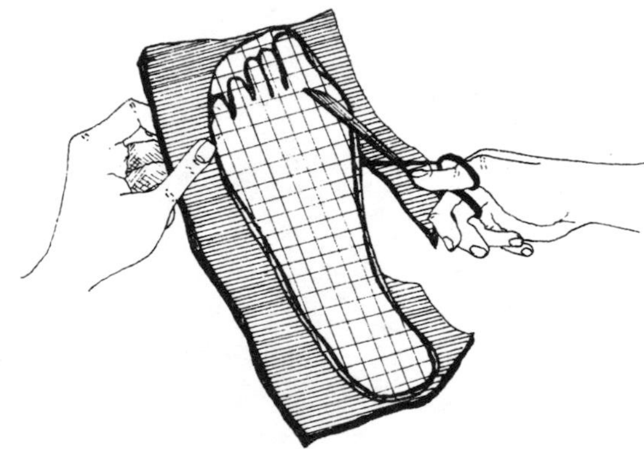

5. Tape each pattern onto kidskin leather and foam (leather on top) and cut out. (A full length, commercially available, innersole sized according to shoe size or a Spenco type insole may be substituted for the leather and foam that you are making from scratch. If you decide on this substitution then skip step six; and where it specifies kidskin and adhesive, use the store bought insert instead.
6. Attach the adhesive side of the foam to the underside of the piece of kidskin leather. If you don't have *adhesive* foam, you may glue the foam to the leather using rubber cement, barge cement or one of the new instant-stick glues.
7. Color the callouses on the bottom of the foot with lipstick.

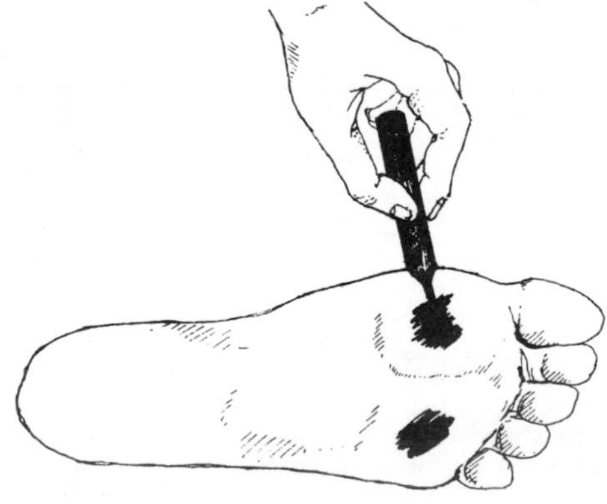

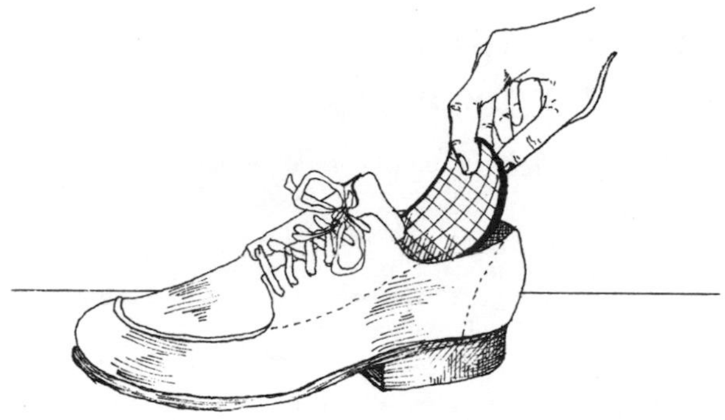

8. Put patterns into the shoes, then walk around for five minutes (do both feet at the same time).

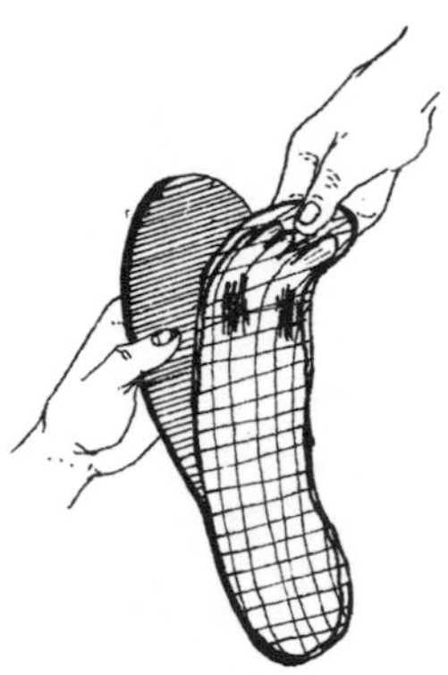

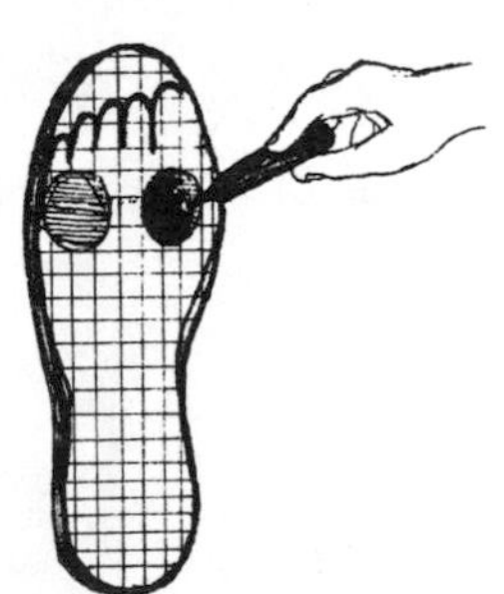

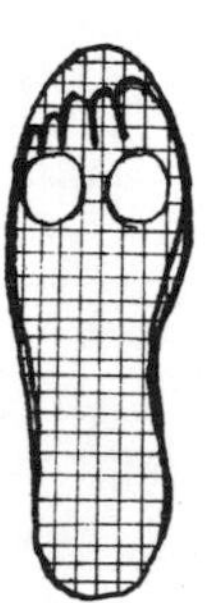

9. Remove the shoes and take the patterns out. Put circles around the lipstick marks on the pattern and cut out circles. Then tape the pattern onto the bottom (foam) side of the insole and color in the circles. Make sure you use the proper pattern for each foot.

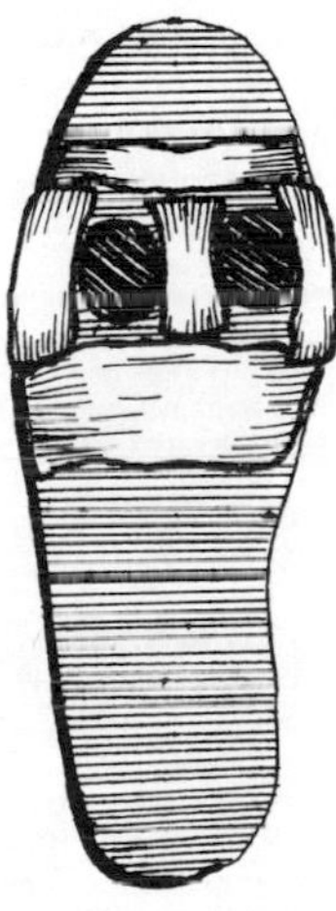

10. Place 1/8'' foam strips around the circles as shown, and you've balanced your foot.
11. Wear this inlay in all your shoes, and you will walk in comfort; in fact your corns or callouses in many cases may disappear altogether.
12. If you need more support, or if the insert wears down, just add more foam.
13. For additional support, add double padding in the arch or heel, depending on the pain.

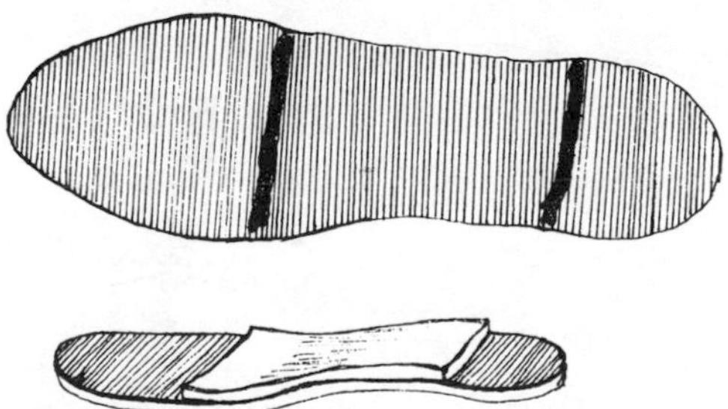

14. For heel pain or arch pain put a line of lipstick across the front of your heel, and another behind the ball of your foot. Step on the pattern in shoe as above. Fill the area between the two lines with a double thickness of 1/8'' foam.

2. To Make a Temporary Orthotic-type insert (varus wedge . . .)

1. Purchase a pair of Spenco inlays or make a full length leather and foam insert as described in steps one through six.
2. On the bottom of the inlay, mark the center of the heel (bisect lengthwise) with a pen.
3. Mark the widest portion (across the ball joint), bisecting the ball widthwise (extend from behind big toe to just behind little toe). Mark another line parallel and one inch behind the ball joint line (both of these lines will course slightly diagonally across the bottom of the inlay).

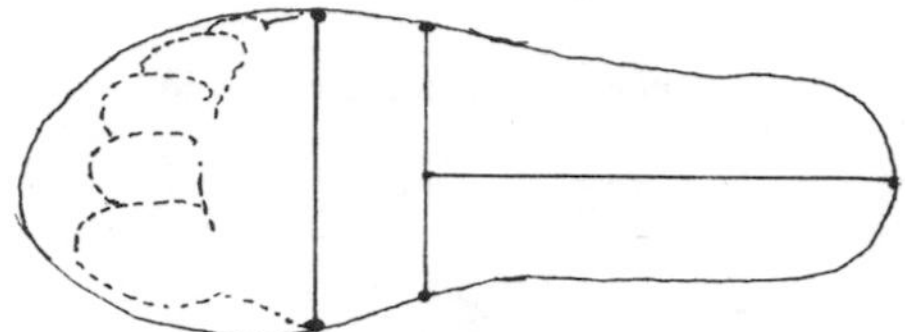

4. Bisect the second line, extend the heel bisection line until the two lines intersect.

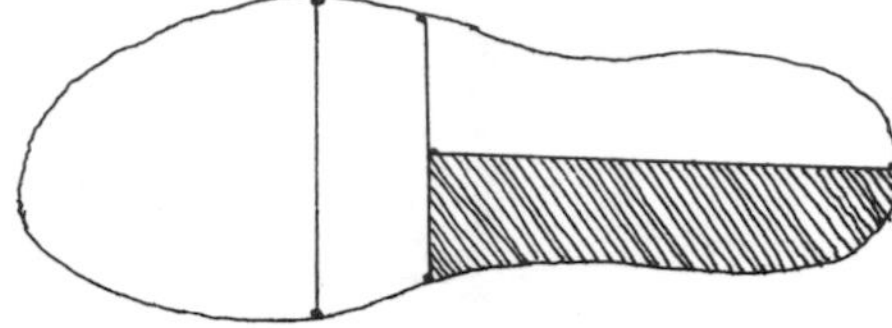

5. Fill the entire *inside* portion of the inlay between the lines with 1/8" to 1/4" adhesive foam or felt (if you don't have access to the adhesive, use glues previously discussed).
6. Bevel the edges of the foam or felt with scissors or file.
7. When this insert is placed into your shoe it will hold your foot in a varus position.

3. Heel Pads—Heel Lifts

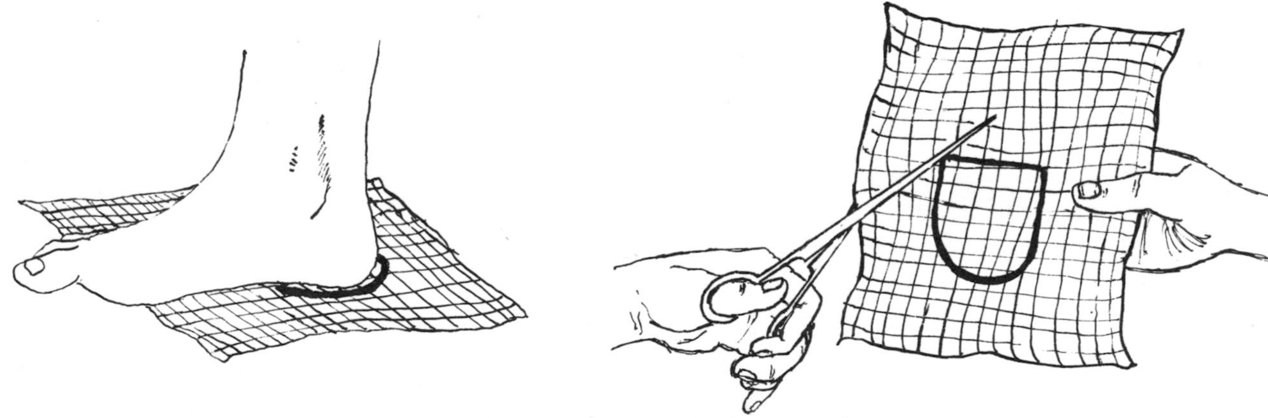

Trace the outer perimeter of the heel onto a piece of paper and cut out.

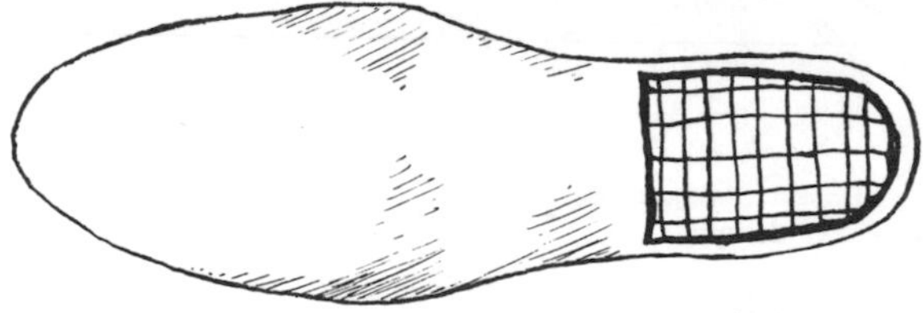

Trim the patterned shape of the heel all around so that your pattern now is ¼" smaller than the heel of your shoe.

Take a piece of 1/8" or 1/4" felt (you may want to increase thickness later as needed) and tape the pattern onto it. Cut out the pattern and you will wind up with a heel lift that will fit into all of your shoes.

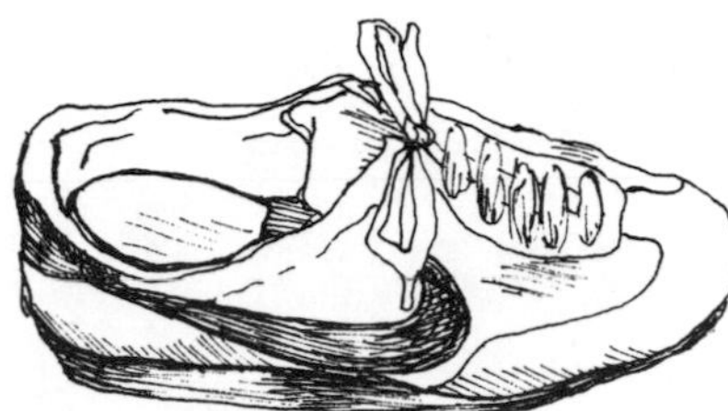

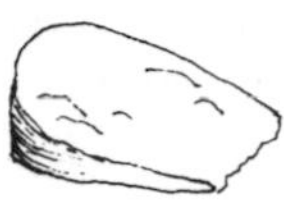

Thin down the lift toward the front if indicated.

For those conditions that require two lifts, place the pattern on the second piece of felt, cut out, and thin down the front as described.

4. Varus Heel Wedge

1. Repeat steps one through four in the heel pad section.
2. Place the completed heel pad on a flat surface right side up (sticky side down if adhesive).

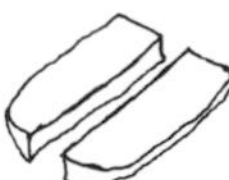

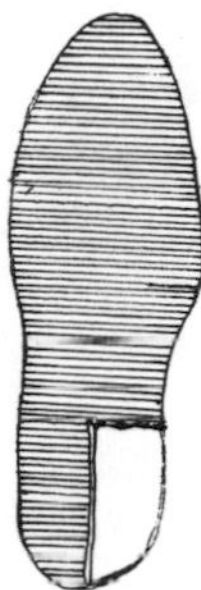

3. Cut the heel pad in half lengthwise, and you now have two varus heel wedges.

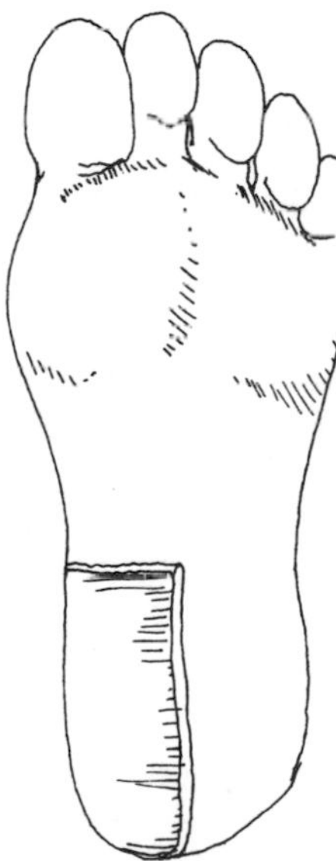

4. For placing the wedge directly onto your heel, or onto the bottom of an inlay, take the left half of the pad thin down the inner (straight) edge. Turn the pad upside down (sticky side up, if adhesive) and adhere to the inside of the bottom of the left heel.
5. Use the left half for the left heel.
6. For placing the wedge directly into your *right* shoe, take the *left* half of the pad and thin down the inner straight border. Place right side up (sticky side down if adhesive) into the inside of the shoe on the left side over the heel.
7. For placing the wedge directly into your left shoe, take the right half of the heel pad and follow step six above.